BEING A CAREGIVER IN A HOME SETTING

Elana Zucker

PEARSON

Boston   Columbus   Indianapolis   New York   San Francisco   Upper Saddle River
Amsterdam   Cape Town   Dubai   London   Madrid   Milan   Munich   Paris   Montreal   Toronto
Delhi   Mexico City   São Paulo   Sydney   Hong Kong   Seoul   Singapore   Taipei   Tokyo

Publisher: Julie Levin Alexander
Publisher's Assistant: Regina Bruno
Executive Editor: Joan Gill
Associate Editor: Bronwen Glowacki
Editorial Assistant: Mary Ellen Ruitenberg
Editorial Assistant: Stephanie Kiel
Director of Marketing: David Gesell
Marketing Manager: Katrin Beacom
Senior Marketing Coordinator:
  Alicia Wozniak
Production Manager: Susan Hannahs

Senior Art Director: Christopher Weigand
Cover Designer: Kevin Kall
Cover Art: Fotolia
Full-Service Project Management:
  Nitin Agarwal/Aptara®, Inc.
Composition: Aptara®, Inc.
Printer/Bindery: R.R. Donnelley/
  Crawfordsville
Cover Printer: Lehigh-Phoenix Color
Text Font: 10/12 Palatino

Credits and acknowledgments for content borrowed from other sources and reproduced, with permission, in this textbook appear on the appropriate page within the text.

Library of Congress Cataloging-in-Publication Data

Zucker, Elana D.,
Being a caregiver in a home setting / Elana Zucker.—1st ed.
  p. ; cm.
  ISBN-13: 978-0-13-274189-7
  ISBN-10: 0-13-274189-X
  I. Title.
  [DNLM: 1. Home Care Services. 2. Caregivers. 3. Home Health Aides.
4. Home Nursing—methods. WY 115.1]
  LC Classification not assigned
  362.2'4—dc23

                                                          2011047158

10 9 8 7 6 5 4 3 2 1

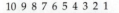
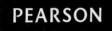

ISBN 10:   0-13-274189-X
ISBN 13: 978-0-13-274189-7

PREFACE

With today's growing population of individuals over the age of seventy, younger people may be placed in the role of caring for a loved one at home. In addition to issues related to aging, some individuals may be asked to provide care in the home of a friend or family member who is struggling with a physical and/or mental challenge. If you find yourself in the position of accepting responsibility of caring for someone in her or his home, it is important to be equipped with the necessary skills to care for this person successfully. Through simple explanations and examples, *Being a Caregiver in a Home Setting* provides important information on how to care for someone properly in the home. As a member of the home health care team, the caregiver plays a critical role in the successful care of a patient in his or her home. The materials in this book focus not only on how to accomplish the various daily tasks required when caring for an individual, but also on the importance of being efficient in these tasks while demonstrating a sensitive and caring attitude toward both the person who is receiving care and the patient's family members.

All the material in *Being a Caregiver in a Home Setting* is designed to assist you, the home health aide, in developing your role within the home health care system and alerting you to your responsibility to observe, report, and act responsibly in many situations and cultural settings. All activities are geared toward encouraging and creating an atmosphere of patient safety and independence and toward helping you build your confidence in the role of caregiver.

TOPICAL HIGHLIGHTS OF BEING A CAREGIVER

Here are some examples of the various topics discussed throughout *Being a Caregiver in a Home Setting:*

- *Children under stress:* Children under stress are discussed as patients and as family members affected by the illness of others. The caregiver's role in observing and reporting is emphasized.
- *Elderly patients:* Elderly patients are discussed in both the home and the community, with elders' special needs of socialization, sex, and fulfillment. The role of culture is highlighted throughout.
- *Terminally ill individuals:* The text discusses not only the individuals' physical and emotional needs but also those of family members and friends. The role of palliative care and advanced directives are highlighted.
- *Patients with physical and mental disabilities:* The text reviews these patients as both patients and family members. Also reviewed are the effects on the family members and the caregiver's role in relating to both the patient and the family members.

- *Rehabilitation in the home:* The text stresses the relearning process and helping a person learn ways to function with a disability.
- *Diseases common in patients:* The text reviews the diseases commonly found in patients receiving care in their homes and the role of the caregiver in assisting these patients with living with the respective diseases.
- *Nutritional information:* The text includes instruction on food allergies and aspects the caregiver should consider when caring for individuals with food allergies.
- *Emergency and first aid procedures:* The text's discussion meets current standards of delivery and content.
- *Communication:* Principles to enhance the communication among health care team members, the patient, and the caregiver are examined.
- *Infection control:* The text examines the role of infection control in everyday activities to create a safe environment. It also emphasizes the importance of the chain of infection and daily activities to protect all members of the home.
- *Patient satisfaction:* The role of patient satisfaction is incorporated throughout the text. The patient's role in his or care, is also emphasized.
- *Patient independence:* Patient independence is a major focus throughout the text. All chapters emphasize the role of the caregiver in assisting both family members and the patient in setting and maintaining realistic activities when the aide is no longer in the home.
- *Identifying abuse:* The text discusses the role of a caregiver in abuse cases. It gives specific guidelines to follow and stresses the importance of the aide examining her or his feelings on this subject.
- *Standard precautions:* The latest guidelines for infection control are addressed throughout the text.

BUILT-IN STUDY AIDS

This manual provides a simple, clear, and concise framework for learning. It can be used both as a primary learning tool and as a vehicle for future review of procedures, theoretical information, and ideas for teaching families how to cope when the caregiver leaves the house.

Step-by-Step Procedures

Each procedure gives a logical, step-by-step approach to tasks performed in the work setting and includes detailed illustrations. A rationale introduces each procedure. A task is an assigned duty, something you are expected to do. In this text, each task has been divided into a logical, orderly series of actions or steps. The full set of steps is a procedure.

Guidelines

Guidelines are important basic principles, ideas, and methods that must be remembered for overall patient care. In some situations, the order in which the tasks are done doesn't matter, and such pieces of information are often presented as guidelines.

Clinical Alerts

Clinical alerts highlight important facts and concepts relating to the discussions in the text.

Illustrations and Photographs

Visuals are integrated throughout the text to enhance discussions, make critical visual connections, and to show readers how a particular action is performed.

TO THE READER: TIPS FOR SUCCESS

Welcome to *Being a Caregiver in a Home Setting*. You are or will be working as part of the home health care team. This team cares for people who require care in the home for a period of time.

You will work with nurses, doctors, and technicians; speech, physical, and occupational therapists; and nutritionists. You can take pride in your work. The most important person in the health care system is the individual you are caring for (i.e., the patient). Everyone strives to meet the needs of the patient and his or her family. You will play a pivotal role in helping the patient and the patient's family members learn new skills for meeting and coping with the illness of one of its members. You will learn new skills, too. You will become familiar with different cultures and a variety of coping skills.

This book has been written to help you do well in the tasks required of you when taking care of an individual at home.

TIPS TO REMEMBER

When caring for someone in the home, you will most likely work with team members of the health care profession. Typically the nurse, team leader, or therapist is considered the supervisor of all the activities that are performed for the patient. Keep the following points in mind:

- If you don't know how to do a procedure or are unsure of your role or abilities, ask the appropriate team member for assistance. Communicate any doubts that you may have to the supervisor who is in charge or to the appropriate health care team member. It is better to get help than to do something wrong.
- Use this book. Read the procedures until you remember every step.

CONTENTS

PROCEDURES

The number shown for each procedure gives the page where the procedure begins.

GUIDELINES

The number shown for each guideline gives the page where the guideline begins.

ACKNOWLEDGMENTS

We would like to express our thanks to the following individuals.

REVIEWERS

Chris Cosgrove, MSW, LCSW, CACIII, NHA,
Nursing Home Administrator,
Camellia Healthcare Center,
Aurora, CO

Theresa Pavnica, RN, BSN, HHA
Instructor, Inservice Educator,
Home Care Nurse,
South Bend, IN

Beth Schoenfeld, RN, MSN,
Indiana Home and Hospice Care Foundation,
Indianapolis, IN

CONTRIBUTOR

Lori Tyler, MS
Innova Inc.
President/Owner
Denver, CO

Chapter *1*

Providing Care in the Home

SCENARIO

Andrea, a forty-year-old single woman, cares for her mother in her mother's home. Andrea's father passed away several years ago from lung cancer. Until recently, Andrea's mother has been independent in caring for herself and her home. A year ago, Andrea's mother was diagnosed with diabetes and has since had several toes removed, which causes her difficulty in walking and managing her home. Andrea has moved in with her mother to care for her while Andrea returns to school to start a new career (see Figure 1.1)

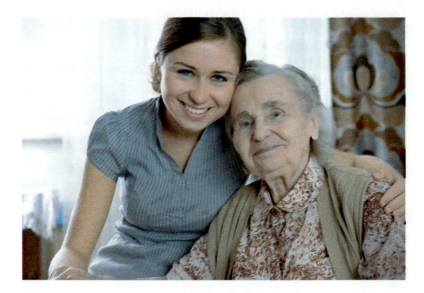

FIGURE 1.1

INTRODUCTION: CARING FOR SOMEONE AT HOME

The concept of caring for someone at home is not new, but it is becoming a more popular form of care as the population continues to age and health care costs continue to soar in the United States. In addition to caring for the elderly person, home care can involve the care of a disabled person, new mother, or individual suffering from a terminal illness.

Providing care to a person at home requires a team of health care members. Some of these members are trained professionals such as physicians, nurses, medical assistants, nutritionists, and home health aides. Sometimes individuals are asked to take on the role of home health aide without any training. These caregivers are often family members and/or friends who have agreed to take on the role of helping to care for the homebound patient. The purpose of this book is to provide a comprehensive guide to individuals who find themselves in the home health aide/caregiver role and need basic training to be able to perform the tasks of caring for an individual at home.

Whether you are in a similar situation to Andrea, caring for a parent at home or for a disabled spouse or child, this handbook provides easy, step-by-step instructions for common tasks performed when caring for someone at home.

Common Tasks Performed by the Home Health Aide/Caregiver

When caring for an individual that is ill, disabled, injured, or dying, the role of the caregiver can involve any or all of the following:

1. Assisting the individual in walking or ambulating
2. Maintaining the individual's personal hygiene (feeding, bathing, grooming, dressing, toileting)
3. Ensuring the individual is properly taking his or her medication
4. Performing minor health care tasks such as taking vital signs, ensuring oxygen is at the prescribed level, changing a dressing, assisting a patient with hanging the patient's feeding tube, adjusting an oxygen tank
5. Conducting housekeeping chores as required
6. Shopping for groceries, meal planning, and cooking
7. Providing companionship for community events, leisure activities, or at-home activities
8. Acting as a liaison with health care providers, supply companies, and other participants that provide care for the individual

Common Health Care Needs

When providing care to an individual in her or his home, there may be some health care–related duties that require a home health care agency to be involved. When home health is prescribed by a physician, most insurance plans will cover procedures that must be performed by a licensed professional (i.e., a licensed nurse). These procedures may include:

- Inserting an IV
- Drawing blood for a lab test
- Measuring the progress of a wound
- Changing a catheter, tracheostomy or g-tube (feeding tube)
- Providing physical, occupational, speech, or mental health therapies
- Prescribing, distributing, and administering medications

Depending on the insurance, home health care is often prescribed as an alternative to remaining in the hospital, going to a rehabilitation center, or making frequent trips to a medical clinic.

Insurance Coverage

At times the home health aide may be asked to assist in submitting insurance claims or obtaining information for submission of claims. Each insurance company has clear and strict rules for obtaining reimbursement. It is important to follow the rules related to the individual's insurance coverage. The home health aide may need to call the insurance company to determine the types of equipment and/or supplies that may or may not be covered under the patient's insurance plan. If you assist the individual in calling his or her insurance company, it is important to be prepared. The insurance company will want to know, at minimum, the individual's name, date of birth, and insurance information. The insurance company may be looking for specific information about the progress of an individual. If health care providers are involved, the home health care aide should have the provider report the progress of the individual. This will help to ensure that no incorrect information is given, which could affect coverage. Documenting a communication with an insurance company is critical. It would be wise to keep a file that contains any communication that does occur with the individual's insurance provider. The date, the name of the person with whom you spoke, and the information given should be documented. If any issues arise having to do with coverage, the information contained in this file may be very useful. Table 1.1 is a list of common insurance plans and coverage. However, it is important to verify individual insurance coverage.

In 2011, new insurance rules were implemented by the passage of the 2011 Affordable Care Act. This act mandates that insurance providers can no longer do the following:

Deny coverage to children with preexisting conditions. Health plans cannot limit or deny benefits or deny coverage for a child younger than age 19 simply because the child has a preexisting condition like asthma.

Put lifetime limits on benefits. Health plans can no longer put a lifetime dollar limit on the benefits of people with costly conditions such as cancer.

TABLE 1.1   Sources of Payment

Source of Payment	Eligibility	Services Covered
Medicare: federally financed health care plan. Often clients choose to use a different health care provider in lieu of Medicare (the benefits are usually fairly similar).	Over 65 years old or disabled more than two years, or on dialysis.	Nursing, physical therapy (PT), occupational therapy (OT), speech therapy (ST), social worker (SW), home health aide (HHA), some supplies, formulary medications, and equipment.
Medicare hospice: federally financed program providing care to terminally ill patients.	Eligible for Medicare with prognosis of six months or less to live, uses certified hospice.	All necessary services (possibly with copayment).
Medicaid: state health care for persons without financial means to obtain health care.	Financial eligibility differs from state to state; services must be provided under medical doctor (MD) supervision.	Nursing; HHA; medical supplies/equipment; possible coverage for PT, OT, ST, audiology, personal care, day care, transportation, and medication.
Health insurance: private.	Individually purchased coverage.	As per policy.
Special.	Workers' compensation, auto insurance.	As per situation.

Cancel an individual's insurance policy without proving fraud. Health plans can't retroactively cancel insurance coverage solely because an honest mistake was made on an individual's insurance application.

Deny claims without a chance for appeal. With the passage of the Affordable Care Act, individuals can demand that a decision to deny payment for a test or treatment be reconsidered, including an external appeal to an independent reviewer.

In addition to these restrictions placed on insurance companies, the act also gives customers in new health plans and renewed policies after 2011 the rights to:

Receive cost-free preventive services. New health plans must provide access to recommended preventive services such as screenings, vaccinations, and counseling without any out-of-pocket costs to the insured.

Keep young adults on a parent's plan until age 26. Unless a child is employed and has her or his own health insurance, a parent can keep a child on the parent's health care plan until the child turns twenty-six years old.

Choose a primary care doctor, obstetrician/gynecologist (OB/GYN), and pediatrician. New health plans must allow the individual to choose the primary care doctor or pediatrician from the health plan's provider network and let the individual see an OB-GYN doctor without a referral from another physician.

Use the nearest emergency department without penalty. New health plans can't require one to get prior approval before seeking emergency department services from a provider or hospital outside the individual's insurance plan network. The individual must also not be subjected to higher copayments or co-insurance for out-of-network emergency department services

Individual Rights

Every individual has certain rights and expectations of the people who provide care (see Figure 1.2). It is important to know the rights of those for whom you are caring. These rights include the right to:

1. Exercise civil and religious liberties
2. Voice complaints without fear of retribution
3. Refuse care, medical care, and/or medications
4. Have an active part in establishing an individualized, appropriate care plan
5. Be treated with respect and dignity
6. Be free of physical and mental abuse
7. Be free of chemical or physical restraints
8. Privacy and confidentiality
9. Private communication with family, friends, and medical care providers
10. Have competent personnel caring for them in a dignified manner

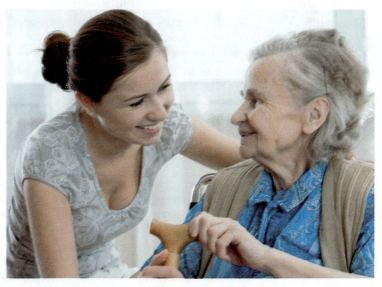

FIGURE 1.2 Honoring patient's rights.

TASKS, RESPONSIBLITIES, AND DELEGATION

As a home health aide, you will work with a health care team comprised of health care providers such as a physician, social worker, and nurse. Some health care must be performed by a specified licensed person, whereas other tasks can be delegated to others. Although the actual task completion may be taught to the home health aide, the licensed person cannot delegate responsibility for the task and is always accountable to be sure that the task is completed correctly. Table 1.2 provides a list of health care

TABLE 1.2 Health Care Professionals	
Physician (MD) or doctor of osteopathy (DO)	Graduate of an accredited medial program licensed by the state to practice medicine.
Registered nurse (RN)	Has graduated from a two- to four-year RN program and is licensed by the state to practice nursing.
Physician's assistant (PA)	Has graduated from a physician's assistant graduate program and is licensed by the state to work under a physician's license as a practitioner. Usually has prescriptive rights.
Nurse practitioner (NP)	Has graduated from a nurse practitioner graduate program and is licensed by the state to work under a physician's license or sometimes in private practice. May have prescriptive rights, depending on the state regulations.
Licensed practical nurse (LPN) or licensed vocational nurse (LVN)	Has completed a one- to two-year program in nursing and has a license from the state to work under the direction of a registered nurse, physician, or dentist.
Physical therapist (PT)	Licensed by the state to practice physical therapy. Concerned with restoring function and preventing disability following disease, injury, or loss of a body part.
Occupational therapist (OT)	Graduate of an approved occupational therapy curriculum and granted a certificate and/or license from the state. Concerned with patient's ability to perform essential daily living tasks.
Occupational therapy assistant	Has specialized training to carry out the treatment plan of an occupational therapist. Certification is required in some states as a certified occupational therapy assistant (COTA).
Speech therapist (ST)	Graduate of an approved speech pathology program and granted a certificate of clinical competence. Treats persons with speech, swallowing, and cognitive disorders caused by physical or mental illnesses
Respiratory therapist (RT)	Graduate of an approved respiratory therapy program and granted a certificate and/or license from the state. Concerned with evaluating breathing, assisting with prescribed breathing treatments and/or regimes, and equipment.

TABLE 1.2 *(Continued)*	
Registered dietician (RD)	Graduate of an approved RD program and registered by the state to practice as a dietician. Applies the science of food consumption and utilization to the growth, maintenance, and repair of the human body.
Social services worker	Has special training in resource and referral management for patients in need.
Social worker with a bachelor of social work (BSW), licensed social worker (LSW), certified social worker (CSW)	Has a four-year degree in social work. Concentrates on intake, treatment planning, assessment, resource management, and discharge planning.
Social worker with a master of social work (MSW), licensed clinical social worker (LCSW), licensed independent social worker (LISW)	Has a master's degree in social work. This is required to provide assessment and treatment planning for the psychosocial needs of individuals, families, groups, and/or communities. An LCSW (in some states called an LISW) is an MSW with a license to practice clinical work with patients. Examples of clinical work include diagnosis, treatment planning, and counseling for psychosocial issues.

professionals who may be involved with providing care to an individual at home. See also Figure 1.3.

Responsibilities are duties expected of you. The medical provider (physician or licensed nurse) will discuss with the caregiver which activities the caregiver is responsible for performing. Usually this information is provided

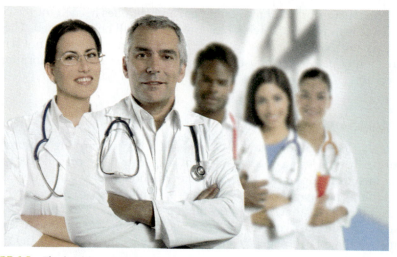

FIGURE 1.3 The health care team.

both verbally and in writing. If the home health aide does not understand or is unsure about what is being conveyed, it is important to discuss this with the medical provider.

Each member of the health care team will have expectations of each other, including you as the home health aide. In addition to the expectations of the other members of the team, the individual you are caring for will have her or his own expectations of the type of care that you will be providing. Knowing your responsibilities and the expectations of others will help to ensure success in your position as home health aide.

Responsibilities of the caregiver include completing assigned procedures correctly, documenting the completion of the procedure, and noting how the individual tolerated the activity. If you cannot complete a task or the individual's condition has changed during or as a result of the activity, communicate this to the medical provider. Documentation of conversations with doctors, supply companies, and observations of changes in physical or mental condition is important to ensure continuity of care among all caregivers.

Equipment and Supplies

As a caregiver in the home, it is necessary to have the proper supplies, medications, and equipment to perform your tasks. When you know what procedures are needed, make a list of the equipment and supplies you require. Try to purchase or order enough supplies to ensure that there are enough supplies available until the next health care professional examines the individual. The health care provider will often make changes in the type of wound dressing, medication, or tube feeding formula, and once distributed, most supplies are not returnable. You want to have enough on hand but not too much that you end up not using the supplies.

Next, plan storage of the equipment and supplies needed for the procedure in a clean place near where the procedure will be performed. The goal is to stay with the individual during the entire procedure and not have to go to another part of the house for supplies in the middle of performing the procedure.

Personal Safety

Personal safety should always be addressed when performing a procedure. Ensuring that the home is safe while providing care is important. This preparation includes keeping walkways clear in the home so that the safety of the individual is maintained and so that there is enough space for caregivers to perform their tasks. In addition, posting emergency (police, ambulance, poison control) and key contact (doctor, medical supply company, insurance company, home health agency, and family) phone numbers near the phone

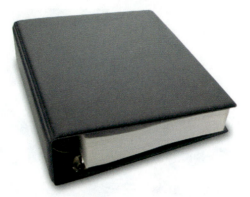

FIGURE 1.4   Communication notebook.

allows you or other involved parties to make phone calls quickly. Keep a communication notebook that has insurance policy numbers, names and dosages of current medications, medical conditions, and so on, close at hand to give accurate information to callers and health care providers (see Figure 1.4). For safety purposes, adaptive equipment may be recommended by the health care professional. This equipment can include a gait belt, step stool, commode, or shower chair. The prescribed equipment will depend upon the abilities of the individual for whom care is being provided.

Finally, it is wise to arrange for backup caregivers to assist you when you are sick, fatigued, or just need an extra pair of hands to complete a task. Ideally, backup caregivers would be volunteer neighbors, friends, or family members; however, respite programs are available through a home health agency (if involved), the insurance company, or local human service agencies (adult, children, and disabled departments exist in all state or county human service agencies). Once you have established a working relationship with people from one of these agencies, keep their contact information near the telephone with instructions for who and when to contact the agency communication notebook.

Establishing and Maintaining a Positive Relationship

Establishing a relationship is vital to a successful experience for you and the individual for whom you provide care. To establish a positive caregiving relationship, establish an agreed-upon list of duties you will be performing. Discuss with the individual and any other interested parties (i.e., other family members or friends invested in the care of the individual) your responsibilities, tasks, and hours of work.

It is your responsibility to perform the duties agreed to and to do them to the best of your ability. You are expected to provide care with thought, consideration, and respect. You are also expected to provide care as is appropriate for the individual's age and cognitive functioning. This is covered in depth in Chapters 4 and 19 (see Figure 1.5).

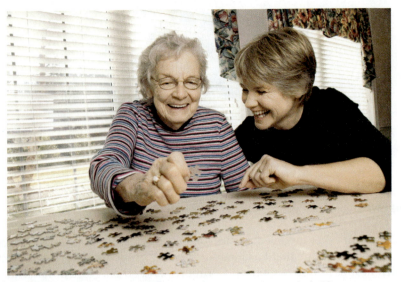

FIGURE 1.5 Caring for someone at home can add dimension to their life.

Summary

The role of the caregiver or home health aide is important to those who need or want to receive care at home. The caregiver is a vital part of the health care team. To be a successful member of the caregiving team, the caregiver must not only understand how to correctly perform the various tasks required of him or her, but also recognize the importance of documenting and reporting any issues related to the patient's care to other members of the team. In addition to establishing a good working relationship with the other health care professionals, the caregiver provides companionship to the individual for whom she or he is providing care. The caregiver can help create a strong supportive environment for the individual who is receiving care at home.

Chapter 2

Communication Skills

SCENARIO

Mrs. Garcia has been suffering from leg ulcers and decreasing vision. She has always enjoyed her hobbies of crocheting and going to bingo once a week. Recently, poor vision and pain in her legs have forced her to remain indoors. She spends the days in her chair with the curtains drawn and the radio on. Her daughter-in-law has assumed responsibility for staying with Mrs. Garcia during the daytime to assist her with activities of daily living and in hopes of getting her back into the community. Mrs. Garcia speaks primarily Spanish and her daughter-in-law speaks little Spanish (see Figure 2.1).

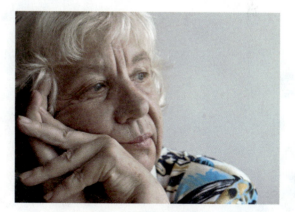

FIGURE 2.1 Depression in the elderly is not uncommon due to the physical and mental changes that can occur with aging.

COMMUNICATION

Communication means exchanging information with others. We exchange information about feelings, opinions, or facts. People let others know how they feel or what they want all day and even during the night. You can tell if your friend, family member, or patient is happy, in pain, sad, or bored. They can tell the same about you. You can tell if someone sleeping is in pain or resting comfortably. Communication takes place in several ways: through verbal exchange, written words, body language or nonverbal methods. Communication is necessary so that people can function together—in other words, so they can "get along" (see Figure 2.2). Developing the ability to get along with people is an important part of taking care of someone. Being a good communicator is essential.

Verbal Communication

Verbal communication is the exchange of ideas or information through the spoken word. When you say, "Good morning" to someone, that is verbal communication. The tone of your voice, the speed at which you speak, your inflection, and your actual choice of words are all part of the verbal picture you paint. Many cultures communicate different pieces of information to different family members. For example, in some cultures, finances are only discussed with the eldest male, and intimate health-related information is only discussed with the eldest female. Determining whom to talk to about specific information will save time and avoid misunderstandings later.

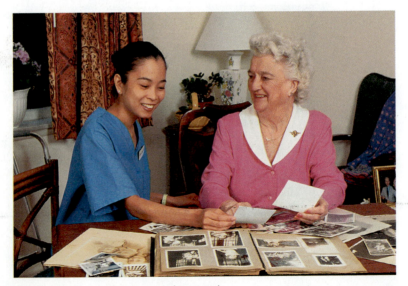

FIGURE 2.2 Communication is more than words.

Written Communication

Any time you write or draw, you communicate through writing. Each time a nurse leaves instructions for you in the home, or you write a note describing your observations regarding the patient, you exchange facts. The way in which you write tells a great deal about you and how you feel about the subject and your activity. The neatness, legibility, choice of words, and how you give the written work to the reader sets the scene for how it is received.

Nonverbal Communication

People have many ways of telling each other how they feel, that is, if they are happy or sad to be in a certain place or if they are doing a task willingly or unwillingly. One way is by saying what we feel. The other way is with our body, which is called body language (see Figure 2.3). No words are spoken, but the message is given and received by others. Pay attention to the way your body language is received by individuals within a certain culture. People in some cultures do not appreciate being touched unnecessarily. Some take it as a sign

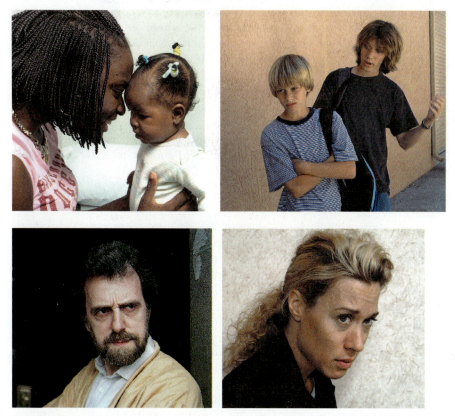

FIGURE 2.3 Nonverbal communication involves facial expressions that can indicate what an individual is feeling.

of caring. Some people expect you to address them by their last name; some do not care. It is always wise to discuss these fine points with the individual in which you are caring. Body language includes:

- The way we do or do not look at people
- The way we stand—with hands in pockets, on hips, or at our sides
- Where we stand—close to the person or far away
- What else we may be doing at the time—reading, folding laundry, or talking on the phone

As a caregiver, you will notice clues and other signals that tell how the individual you are caring for feels. These signs tell you a great deal about the person and the care you are providing. Be sure to report your observations to the other health care team members. Be alert to your body language! The patient will know how you feel about providing care by the way you carry yourself and by the way you interact.

Answering When the Client Calls

Every patient needs a way to signal other people. You will devise a system for your patient to call you. A hand bell, an intercom system, or voice signal are possible methods of signaling. Use whatever method is most appropriate in the house. Having a way to call for assistance helps the patient feel he is participating in his own care. He will know he is not alone and helpless.

Answer the patient's call as soon as you hear it. Every minute is important to the person waiting. When you are signaled, go to the person and ask in what way you can assist. Do what he asks as long as it is within your responsibilities and safe. If it is not within your responsibilities, be sure to inform the patient that you will communicate his needs to another member of the care-providing team.

Culture

We are a nation of ethnic diversity, and these differences are respected and celebrated. Each group of people has a culture of their own. That is, they share values, behaviors, and beliefs. These form the framework of their actions toward themselves and others, and influence their health care. When you enter a house, be alert and conscious of the culture within that home. You may be familiar with this culture, or you may find it different from your own. Showing respect by asking questions will indicate to the family and the patient that you wish to incorporate their culture into the care you provide.

Cultures communicate differently. Some cultures speak softly, others more loudly. Some use hand gestures; others do not. Some touch people to whom they are speaking; others consider this rude behavior. It is important to know what the client finds acceptable. After understanding how you usually communicate—your tone of voice, the speed at which you speak and your ability to make yourself understood—you can make changes to accommodate the patient. As you saw in the chapter-opening scenario, the daughter-in-law will need to learn how to communicate with Mrs. Garcia as well as learn the culture of Mrs. Garcia's home.

Patients who do not speak English have the right to safe, effective communication. These individuals feel safer when their caregivers speak their language.

- If you do not speak the same language as the person you are caring for, do not assume he or she does not understand your language. Do not say anything you would not want the patient or the family to understand.
- Maintain the level of formality in the house that is comfortable for the patient and his or her family.
- Speak in appropriate tones. Do not shout. Repeat yourself when necessary.

If necessary, you can use an interpreter to communicate. Just be sure the person approves of the interpreter and wants to share information with the person. You must be sure that having the interpreter does not violate the patient's confidentiality.

BASIC RULES FOR COMMUNICATING

BE A NONJUDGMENTAL OBSERVER AND LISTENER It is important to learn to receive information in a nonjudgmental way, that is, in an accepting manner without expressing your opinions. You must develop the skill of recognizing when your opinion is important and when you should not express it to show nonjudgement. Often, the patient, family member, or friend wants to express an opinion and have it accepted rather than have it commented upon (see Figure 2.4). When

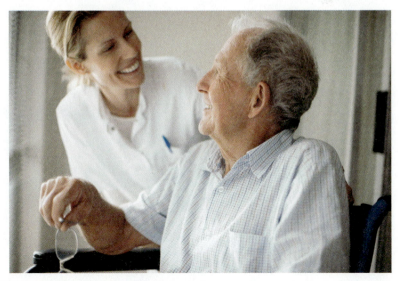

FIGURE 2.4 Listen without making judgment.

you work in a person's home, she may ask for your opinion. If you are unsure or think your opinion will upset her, you might say, "This is your house and here it is more important how you feel about this situation than how I feel."

BE A CAREFUL LISTENER Always listen when someone speaks to you. Listen to what the person says. Listen to what information is left out of the conversation. Listen for the speaker's tone of voice and breathing pattern. Is it fast? Is it slow and slurred? Do the words make sense? Is it appropriate to ask questions? Listen to what the speaker says, not what you think he or she says. Pay special attention when a complaint or problem is communicated. Sometimes it is helpful to write down important information as you hear it rather than trust your memory.

BE SENSITIVE Sometimes individuals don't want to talk. Respect these times of silence. Saying nothing may have more meaning than any words or facial expressions you convey. Sometimes, a pat on the shoulder or hand means more to a person than anything you could say. Simply being near the person in a moment of trouble may be the most comforting message of all (see Figure 2.5).

BE COURTEOUS AND TACTFUL Courtesy means being polite. Tact means being considerate of how communication will affect others. You should be courteous and tactful at all times. Never be critical or impolite in your contacts with others. If you feel like being impolite, try to understand why you are feeling or acting the way you are. By reviewing the situation, you may be able to prevent it from happening again. Both courtesy and tact are important in your relationships. The family and patient will be sharing information with

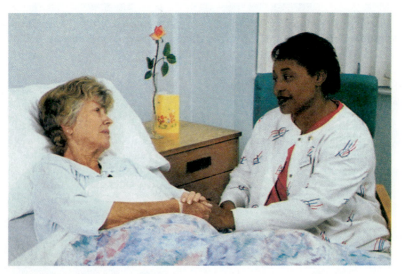

FIGURE 2.5 Be sensitive when listening.

you. Show them you are willing to hear what they have to say and then reply in a thoughtful manner.

If you are not clear about what you have heard, you can summarize what you think you heard and ask the speaker if you heard correctly. For example, "I heard you say that John was going to the store, then coming home and fixing you dinner before he goes to the doctor's. Is that correct?"

When the speaker is talking and you have nothing to add, but you think the speaker is not communicating clearly, try a technique called reflection. Reflection allows the person to know what you understand and provides an opportunity for him to clarify. For example, you might say, "You seem in pain today." The patient could then clarify, "I'm not, but it is cold in here."

USING THE TELEPHONE

The telephone is one way people communicate with others who are not in the immediate vicinity. Telephone communication may take the form of a cell phone or a land line attached to the house. Either way, you must remember that the phone is in the patient's house for her or his use and your emergency use, not for your personal calls (see Figure 2.6). As the caregiver, you should never ask to use the phone unless it is to place a call related to the patient's care or a personal emergency has occurred. Remember, the time you spend on the phone is time taken away from caring for your patient. You are in the house to do a job. This is not the appropriate time to take care of personal issues.

If you wear or carry a cell phone, put it on silent mode while you care for the person. If you receive a personal call, do not answer the phone. If time

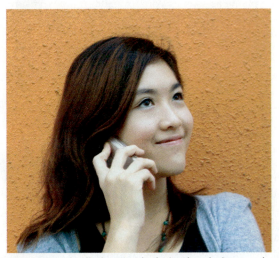

FIGURE 2.6 Use your personal cell phone only during break times and only if the call is important enough to make.

allows and the phone call is important to address, use your break time to call back. Never speak on your cell phone pertaining to personal issues while you are caring for the patient. Never take a patient's picture with your camera phone or discuss medical information with others. This is an unacceptable invasion of privacy. Remember that an answering machine or voicemail is considered private, and you should not listen to the messages unless you are asked to do so. If you are answering the patient's telephone, make sure that her wishes are followed in all of these situations: with whom she wants to talk, when she wants messages taken, and what information can be shared with callers. When you first arrive at the house, determine with the patient and the family if they wish you to answer the phone, let it ring, or if messages will go to an answering machine. See Procedure 2.1.

EMOTIONAL CONTROL

Sometimes the patient or a visitor can upset you. You may feel like making a rude or nasty remark. Don't do it! Remember that the patient is worried about himself, his illness, his family, or his job (see Figure 2.7).

PROCEDURE 2.1

Talking on the Telephone

Rationale

Speaking politely and clearly shows respect for the caller. It also presents a caring impression to the caller and provides an atmosphere in which information can be exchanged accurately.

1. Answer the phone as soon as you can get to it, making sure that the person you are caring for is safe when you do.
2. Identify yourself. "Hello, this is Harriett speaking."
3. Speak slowly, clearly, and courteously. Remember, your voice can display anger or acceptance. You do not want the caller to think it is too much trouble to answer the telephone.
4. Ask the caller's name: "Who is calling please?" If you do not understand the caller, ask him or her to please spell it.
5. Answer the caller's questions as best you can. If you cannot give the caller all the information, take a message, write the date and time of the call, the caller's name, and the message.
6. If the caller asks for information you cannot share, tell the caller politely that this is not information you are comfortable sharing and that he or she should speak with someone else in the family. Leave this as a message for the family.
7. End the conversation politely, saying "Thank you for calling," "Good-bye," or "Is there anything else I can help you with?"
8. Let the caller hang up first.
9. Leave the message in an agreed-upon place.

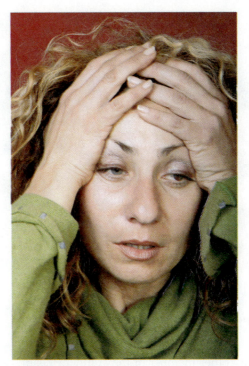

FIGURE 2.7 Don't let emotions get in the way.

A patient may be rude or difficult at times. Often, the individual is unable to determine exactly what is causing her to feel bad and act in a difficult or unpleasant manner. Tell her you know that she has many things on her mind. Offer to listen to her or bring another member of the health care team to listen to her problem. The patient's or family's stress levels may affect their ability to communicate and listen. Be sensitive to this. Speak in simple terms. Do not be upset if you have to repeat yourself several times. Be understanding if the patient or family member repeats the information numerous times.

Learn to take constructive criticism and accept suggestions from the individual you are caring for, from his or her family, and health care team members. You may feel angry when somebody tells you that you are wrong, but remember, everyone wants to make sure the best care is provided to the patient. If you do not agree with what is said to you, answer in a polite, courteous manner. Discuss the criticism, not the person giving it.

Be as tactful as you can. Being tactful means doing and saying the right thing at the right time. Before you make a remark to a patient or his family, think! Is this the right time? Is this the right word to use? What is the best way to express the idea to this person? Do not speak within hearing distance of the person if you do not want him to hear you, even if you think he is asleep, under the influence of medication, or unconscious.

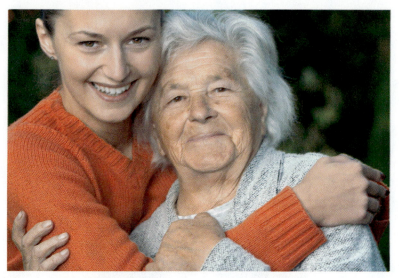

FIGURE 2.8   Visitors can make one's day!

RELATIONSHIPS WITH PATIENTS

You are important to the patient and the family. You may spend more time with the person than any other member of the family or health care team. You perform necessary personal tasks that permit the person to remain at home in a safe, comfortable, clean environment. These individuals come to depend on you and may share their feelings and thoughts. Often, you are the only person a patient will see all day.

The individual you are caring for may ask you a question about her doctor or her diagnosis. Do not lie! Do not tell her you do not know when you should be aware of the information. If you lie, the patient may find out and never trust you again. It is no shame to say you do not have the information readily at hand. But if you say you do not know, you close the conversation. Tell the patient you will find her an answer. Then call and talk to the other members of the family and/or members of the health care team. When you promise to find an answer, do it! Do not go back on your word!

FAMILY AND VISITORS   Visitors are often the highlight of the day for someone who must remain at home (see Figure 2.8). Patients usually feel better when they know family and friends are concerned and are making the effort to visit. Visitors may be worried and upset over your patient's illness. They, too, need kindness and patience. Pleasant comments, privacy, and polite, efficient manners will make them feel at ease. If it appears that visitors are upsetting or tiring your patient, you may have to suggest tactfully that they end the visit for a rest period. Remember, you are in the house to care for the patient, not to wait on or socialize with visitors. If they leave a mess or dirty dishes and expect you to clean up, it is appropriate to ask them to clean up after themselves.

You will find the following hints helpful to remember:

- Listen to visitors and family members. Whether it is a suggestion, a complaint, or a moment to pass the time of day, listen. Suggestions by visitors can be helpful. Some complaints may be valid; others may not be. When a complaint is first presented, you will need more information. You might ask, "Where did this happen?" or "What did you do?" Offer to bring the complaint to other members of the health care team.
- Try not to become involved in family affairs that are unrelated to you. Never take sides in a family quarrel.
- If visitors have questions about your patient and you are not sure you should answer, tell them you will find the information. Discuss these questions with your patient to be sure he wants the information given to his visitors.
- If a visitor or family member asks how he or she may help, give suggestions.
- Visitors may arrive at the house and give orders: "While I'm here to watch Mama, you clean the bathroom." Be open about the agreed-on responsibilities.
- It is important to use the talents and energy of family and friends in setting up a plan of care. Often, these family members must assume the patient's care when you are out of the house. Therefore, the more comfortable they feel with the care and the more they know, the better your patient will feel when you are gone.
- Be sure that all members of the health care team understand the roles family and visitors play in the life of your client. Report changes in family functions, relationships, and roles both as you observe them and as the patient relates them.

OBSERVING, REPORTING, AND RECORDING YOUR OBSERVATIONS

Get into the habit of observing the individual you are caring for during all of your contacts with this person. These contacts include bathing, bed making, mealtimes, and any other time when you are with him or her. Observation is a continuous process. Observation means more than just careful watching. It includes listening, talking, and asking questions. Be extra alert to anything unusual when you are with the patient. Changes in condition or appearance are most important. Watch also for changes in attitude or mood and the way in which the patient interacts with other people. Pay attention to complaints of pain or discomfort and to complaints that seem to have no reason. Be alert when the patient relates events that took place in your absence. Observation of the person's family and friends is also important and may have implications for the patient's future care.

You are the health care team member who will spend the most time with the patient. You will often be the first to notice a change in the patient's condition. This change may be for the better, or it may indicate a worsening of his condition. Observations are useful only if they contribute to the total care of the patient.

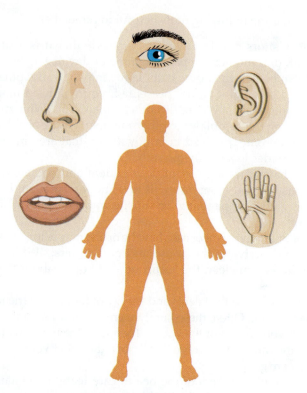

FIGURE 2.9 Use all of your senses to observe.

Therefore, it is an important part of your role to report these changes to appropriate health care team members. Then the patient's total care plan can be revised.

Methods of Observation

Use all of your senses to notice signs of change (see Figure 2.9):

- You can see some signs of changes in a patient's condition. By using your eyes, you can observe a skin rash or swelling of the feet.
- You can feel signs with your finger—a change in the patient's pulse rate, puffiness in the skin, or skin temperature.
- You can hear signs, such as a cough or wheezing sounds when the patient breathes.
- You can smell signs, such as an odor in the patient's urine.
- Listen to the patient talking to hear other changes in her condition. Some changes only the patient can feel and describe. Examples are pain, nausea, dizziness, a ringing in the ears, or a headache.

Making useful observations is one of the most important things you will do in your role as caregiver. Learning how to make useful observations will give you great satisfaction. Table 2.1 contains a summary of general observations you will make every day with the patient.

TABLE 2.1   General Patient Observations

Concern	Observations
General appearance	Has it changed? If so, in what way? Is there a noticeable odor or smell in the patient's room? Does she always complain about the heat or cold?
General mood	Describe the patient's actions rather than your interpretation of them. ("The patient threw a shoe at his daughter" rather than "The patient was angry at his daughter"). Has it changed? Does he talk a lot or a little? Does he make sense? Can he report things to you accurately? Does he hallucinate (see or hear things)? Is he oriented (know where he is, who he is, and who you are)? Is he anxious, calm, excited, or worried? Does he talk about pain? Does he speak rapidly or slowly? Does he look at you when he speaks? Can he be understood when he speaks? Can he remember? Is he confused or forgetful?
Sleeping habits	Have these changed? Is the patient a quiet or restless sleeper? Does she complain about lack of sleep? Does her report agree with your observations? How many pillows does she sleep with? How much does she sleep?
Pain	Where is the pain? How long does the patient say that he has had pain? Is it new pain? How does he describe it? Is it constant? Does it come and go? Is it sharp, dull, or aching? Has he had medicine for the pain? Does the patient say that the medicine relieves the pain? Is there any activity that brings on the pain?
Daily activities	Does the patient dress herself? Does the patient walk with or without help? If she walks with help, what kind of help does she use?
Personal care	Can the patient bathe himself? Can the patient brush his teeth, comb his hair, go to the bathroom, or wash his face? Does he ask for assistance?
Movements	Does the patient limp?
Skeletal system	Symptoms may include pain; limited movement; swelling in joints; warm, tender joints; unusual positioning of any body part.
Muscular system	Symptoms may include painful movement, swelling, limited movement, color of skin over painful areas. Does the patient lie still? Does she change position frequently? What is her favorite position?
Skin	Symptoms may include temperature, texture, moisture, bruises, healing of bruises, incision appearance, mouth condition. Has it changed? Is the patient's skin unusually

(continued)

Concern	Observations
TABLE 2.1 *(Continued)*	

Concern	Observations
	pale (pallor)? Is it flushed (red)? Are his lips or fingernails turning blue (cyanotic)? Is there noticeable swelling (edema)? Any reddened or tender areas? Where are they? Is the skin shiny? Any puffiness?
Circulatory system	Symptoms may include chest pain; swelling of fingers, toes, feet, ankles, around the eyes; pulse rate and quality; color of lips, nails, fingers, toes; headaches; pain in legs when walking.
Respiratory system	Symptoms may include pain while breathing, rate and quality of respirations, cough, sputum (color and consistency), wheezing, shortness of breath, color of fingers and toes.
Digestive system	Symptoms may include pain; appetite; flatus; vomiting (color of vomitus); feces (color, amount, frequency, odor); discomfort before or after eating. Can the patient control her bowels? Have her eating habits changed? Does she complain that she has no appetite? Does she dislike her food? What and how much does she eat? Is she always thirsty? Does she seldom ask for fluids? Is it difficult for her to eat or swallow?
Nervous system	Symptoms may include painful areas of the body, twitching, involuntary movement, inability to move, inability to feel stimuli.
Urinary system	Symptoms may include pain during urination; ability to control his urine; urine color, odor, amount, frequency; blood in urine; pain in kidney area.
Eyes	Symptoms may include pain, discharge, redness, sensitivity to light, vision change.
Ears	Symptoms may include pain, discharge, hearing change.
Nose	Symptoms may include pain, discharge, bleeding, change in sense of smell.
Female genitalia	Symptoms may include menstrual periods (frequency, amount of flow, pain), vaginal discharge (color, odor, amount), breasts (lumps), discharge, soreness, parasites, draining sores.
Male genitalia	Symptoms may include pain, discharge, parasites, draining sores.

Subjective and Objective Reporting

Subjective reporting means giving your opinion about something or stating what you think. You might report, for example, what you think is the cause of a change in a patient's condition or what might be the proper treatment. When you report your opinion to others, be sure you say that it is your opinion. Your opinion could be important to the care of your patient. An example of subjective reporting is, "Yesterday, Mrs. Garcia and her land-lady were talking in loud voices. I think they were fighting."

Objective reporting means reporting exactly what you observe—that is, reporting what you see, hear, feel, or smell. As a caregiver, always use objective reporting unless it is clear that the information is an opinion. Here are examples of objective reporting:

1. Mrs. Smith's breathing has changed since yesterday. She is breathing 20 times a minute and complaining of chest pain. Yesterday, she had no pain and her respirations were 12 times a minute.
2. Cindy Jones says that she has a pain in her right upper abdomen.
3. Every time John takes the pain pill, he gets very quiet and then reports seeing horses on the ceiling.

Reporting Observations

Each medical provider has a protocol for home health care aides to communicate observations of change. It is your responsibility to be familiar with these protocols and use them.

Does the protocol involve using the telephone? By calling the correct phone number and asking for the correct person, you will save time for yourself, the patient, and the health care team member. Does the protocol involve using the mail? By sending the correct information to the right person, you will save time and postage. You may be expected to make specific observations at a specific time of day. Be sure you know what to do with the information you collect.

When to Report

It is wise to ask the medical provider for the parameters of reporting information. Often after-care instructions will include the conditions for which the individual should be taken to the physician's office, call the office, or go to the emergency room. Keep these instructions in a communication notebook for future review.

What to Report

The importance of reporting the proper information at the proper time cannot be overemphasized. The health care team should establish protocols for what should be documented and what should be reported verbally. There are two types of patient information:

1. General observations: observations and information about visitors, family, and changes in the environment. General observations also include subjective information.

   Example: Mrs. Jones's sister came to visit for the first time. Her sister shared that Mrs. Jones was extremely thin compared to the last time she saw her. Mrs. Jones was saddened by the comment and cried after her sister left. Mrs. Jones seemed comforted by my explanation that it is normal to have weight loss after surgery because surgery can affect one's ability to eat normally.

2. Specific information: observations of particular patient behavior or other change. Members of the health care team will discuss this type of observation with you. They will explain to you what information is needed and when.

Example: When I changed Mrs. Brown's nightgown, I noticed some blood on the sleeve. I asked her where this blood came from, and she said, "Oh, you know how it is, I hit my hand." Then she pulled her hand away and said, "I don't think you have to report this." This was the first time this happened. She seemed upset. I can't figure out why.

In one situation, a reaction to medication may be important; another time, mental alertness may be the most important observation. Ask the health care team if any particular observations are important for you to note. In addition to any specific information, always report the total patient condition.

Where to Record Your Observations

It's important to communicate orally when you are able. It is just as important to be sure where to write your observations. Establish with the patient, family, and health care team where observations should be documented. A communication notebook (as discussed in Chapter 1), with contact information, current medication lists, and procedural protocols, can also include observations of changes in the patient's condition. When documenting be sure to date the entry, indicate the time of the entry, and sign your name after to the entry.

TEACHING

Teaching is an important part of your role as a caregiver. You will teach by example, by discussion, or by taking part in activities with patients. You will teach him new skills, help him relearn old skills, and help him gain independence in as many activities as possible. Everybody learns differently; therefore, you must have a teaching plan individualized to the person in which you are caring. Some people learn by reading or watching, some by listening, and some by practicing a skill.

The teaching plan is typically developed by the health care team. It is a cohesive document that provides guidance for various areas that must be addressed during care of the patient. The caregiver will be given areas for which the patient should be taught while under their care. It is necessary for you to be familiar with the teaching plan that the health care team has established for your patient. If you are not sure about your role, ask!

Reasons for Differences in Learning

As the health care team individualizes the patient's teaching plan, the following factors are taken into consideration:

- Life experiences
- Disease process
- Motivation for learning
- Family dynamics
- Language skills
- Past experiences with learning
- General abilities
- Teaching skills of the teacher
- Age
- Culture

When teaching, remember that methods should vary depending on the age of the individual. Adults can often read material and then discuss it. Adults can practice skills on their own. They can clearly relate learning a skill to achieving a certain outcome. For example, an adult who understands the reasons for keeping or maintaining a special diet will learn how to shop for and prepare special foods because he can understand that if he fails to follow this diet, he will become ill. A child, however, may not be able to think about the future and correlate the activity of eating to the deterioration of her general physical condition. So even though the outcome will be the same—learning the diet—the teaching method will be different.

People who are not fluent in English may need to learn with the help of a family member who speaks English and the language of the patient. When this occurs, be sure you confirm that involving another person is acceptable to the patient and the translator. Also, be sensitive in discussing personal information and/or activities (see Figure 2.10).

Points to Remember When Teaching

- Be sure the person is paying attention and is not distracted by television, a visitor, or other activities.
- Be sure the person wants to learn.
- Be familiar with the material you are teaching. Do not try to teach something you do not understand.
- Relate the teaching matter to the patient. For example, do not tell her the skill will help her become a faster runner if she has no interest in running.
- Speak slowly and clearly. Do not use baby talk, but do use words the person can understand.
- Remind the person of the purpose for each step of the lesson. This will help him understand that it is important to follow your example. It will also assure him that you are not wasting energy or time.

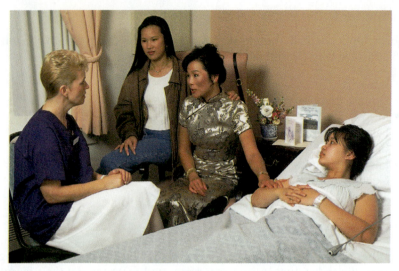

FIGURE 2.10 Teaching a non-English-speaking person may involve a translator or material written in their native language.

- Present one topic at a time. Everyone has a different attention span. People who are ill or who are taking certain medication often find it hard to concentrate for long periods. Plan your teaching sessions for short periods of time.
- Teach at the time of day most convenient for the patient. Some people learn better in the morning, some in the afternoon. Whenever possible, ask the patient which time she prefers.
- Use written material so the person will have something to refer back to when practicing alone.
- Show patience when you must repeat yourself or show an activity many times. When the patient demonstrates the skill to you, praise her and discuss the positive part of the demonstration before you show her corrections.

Summary

Communication is the essence of human interaction and is the foundation for lasting relationships. The caregiver should be able to communicate with professionals, family members, and the person for whom they are caring. Communication includes verbal, written, and nonverbal methods of trading information. To be successful as a caregiver, be an excellent listener and to adapt your communication style to meet the cultural and learning needs of the individual for whom you are caring. Recognizing individual needs through observation and in turn reporting such observations to other health care team members are essential elements in making the patient's care at home a success.

Chapter 3

Working with People

SCENARIO

Mr. Ricardo has been in this country 20 years. He worked in the flower business and until recently owned a small flower store in a strip mall, which he closed when a large chain store moved into the mall. He is outgoing, likes people, and speaks English well. His four children are all grown and live far away with families of their own. His wife of thirty-five years recently went back to their native country to care for her father. She hopes to return in three months. The house he has owned for twenty-five years is in a changing neighborhood. Most of his former neighbors have moved out, and younger people with small children have moved in. The house is far from the town center, and he must drive to the grocery store. Mr. Ricardo, a smoker since age fifteen, has difficulty breathing and has pain in his legs. He has not told anyone about his discomfort, but he walks more slowly each week and his legs hurt him (see Figure 3.1).

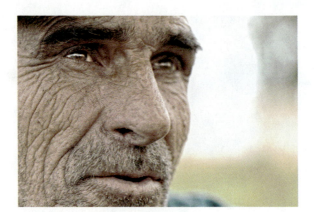

FIGURE 3.1

BASIC NEEDS

Every person has certain basic needs that must be met to survive. A need is a requirement for survival. Sometimes an individual can satisfy her own needs, and sometimes she requires help. A person becomes your patient when she is unable to satisfy all her needs herself. For example, a person may need help with meals or assistance with eating to meet her need for nourishment. As a caregiver, you will help your patient meet basic needs until she can meet them without your help.

It is important—and often difficult—to be sure the health care team actions are meeting the patient's needs. Your knowledge of these needs and your objective observations will help the health care team determine whether the plan of care meets all the needs of the patient.

Basic Physical and Psychological Needs

Not all needs must be met completely each day, but the more each person's needs are fulfilled, the better the quality of life (see Figure 3.2). Psychological needs must also be satisfied to have a healthy emotional and social outlook. As with physical needs, these do not have to be met totally each day. However, the more completely each need is met, the better the person's emotional state will be. Needs can be met by family members, by oneself, or by someone not a family member but available on an intermittent basis.

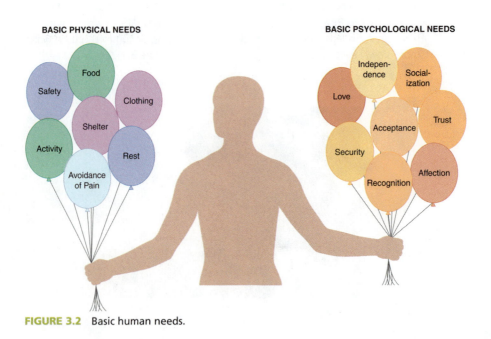

FIGURE 3.2 Basic human needs.

Balancing Needs

Children's needs are usually met by family members. During adult years, most people are expected to meet some or most of their own needs. Physical and psychological needs overlap and affect each other. Each person determines his or her particular balance. When one need is out of balance due to illness, the other needs are also affected. For example, when a person is ill requiring more rest, timing of food intake must meet this change in activity. Clothing needs change. Weight may change, and moods may alter. The person needing assistance is often the one who knows how to restore balance. In such a case, the patient might determine when to eat and what foods to decrease so that she does not gain weight. By consulting the patient, you will more likely meet the individual's actual needs. Needs can change, so be alert.

Several factors affect the way in which assist the patient in balancing needs:

- Patient knowledge
- Disease state
- Family support
- Mental state
- Age
- Available resources
- Culture
- Financial resources

The way in which these elements interact determines how the patient's needs are met and how all other family member needs are satisfied. Many things can change a person's behavior and attitude during an illness. The patient may be frightened, angry, or sad.

Family Needs

If your patient is part of a family unit, his change in status will affect all other members of the family (yourself included, if applicable). Remember that, although you are in the home primarily to meet the needs of the person needing care, your observations about the family are important. The family unit will continue providing support if and when you are no longer needed. Every member of the family has a set of basic needs, and these needs must continue to be met even though one of its members, the individual needing care, now has a changed status. Balancing all these requirements is difficult. Discuss this with the family and the health care team so a plan of care is established that is useful for the family and the individual requiring care (see Figure 3.3).

Your Needs as a Caregiver

Caregivers have the same basic needs as their patients. It is important that your needs are met, too, but not at the expense of the individual for whom you

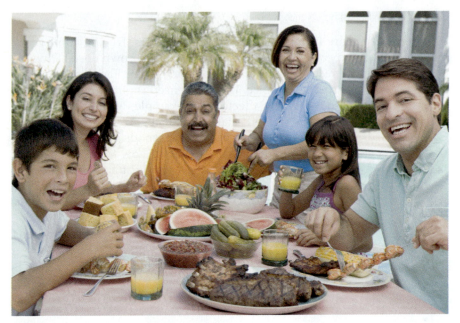

FIGURE 3.3 Families have strong traditions.

are providing care. Many times your needs will have to be put aside until you are done caring for the patient. Discuss with the family both your patient's needs and yours. Then a plan will be made so that the needs of the patient will be satisfied and you will not feel slighted. Caregivers must be alert to the reasons they do and say things. As you care for your patient, be alert and identify what basic need you are satisfying and whose need it is. Ask yourself these questions:

- Are you acting because the patient's needs must be met or because your needs must be met? For example, are you giving the patient a bath because she will feel better or because you will feel better having done it?
- Do you perform a procedure with the patient because he enjoys having you help him and shows improvement or because you feel that you must do it?
- Does helping the patient become independent (and thus no longer in need your help) make you feel good or useless?

Unmet Needs

When basic needs are not met, human beings react. If a physical need is not met, the reaction is usually obvious; for example, if the need for food is not met, the person might become irritable or weak. If an emotional need is not met, a person's reaction may be feelings of anxiety, depression, aggression, anger, or a physical ailment without apparent cause.

You will not always be able to decide why a person behaves in a certain manner. That is all right. It is necessary, however, for you to observe and, if appropriate, report these actions to the family or health care team. Often, by reviewing the patient's actions, others can help you determine if a need is unmet. Then, by altering the plan of care, the need will be fulfilled and undesired behavior will change.

Pain

The word *pain* means different things to different people. What is painful to one person may not be to another. It is important to find out how the person who you are caring for reacts to pain and how his family views pain. Many people think that pain is normal and must be tolerated; some believe it is a punishment; some do not want to complain; some people are afraid of medications; and some are afraid that, if they complain, their caregiver will leave them. Some people are afraid to discuss their pain with their physicians because they believe that if a physician could relieve the pain, she would do so without being asked.

People in pain often cannot participate in their care, relate to their families, or expend energy on the healing process. People in pain cannot have a good quality of life. Pain causes many reactions. Some you can see, and some you cannot see. Someone in pain may

- have a rapid pulse, and shallow and rapid breathing
- have increased fatigue
- have increased anxiety
- have increased stress
- withdraw and decrease communication
- decrease food and fluid intake
- grimace or make gestures with her or his hands
- moan, talk in baby talk, or cry
- demonstrate anger and even violent behavior

Different cultures treat pain in different ways. People of various cultures may hang a charm near the bed, say special prayers, burn candles, or dress the patient in special clothes. If these actions help the patient, support them even though they may seem unusual to you. Some people do not want to take medication. They are afraid they will become addicted, be questioned by the authorities, or bring shame to their family and to themselves. Encourage your patient to take medication as prescribed. If it does not have the expected result, report this immediately to the physician or nurse as appropriate. In the chapter-opening scenario, the reason Mr. Ricardo continues to be in pain may be related to a cultural belief that men shouldn't complain about pain. Health care teams are becoming more aware of the multiple, contributing factors to an individual's response to pain. Medication is becoming more acceptable and available to individuals who are in pain and are receiving care at home. (See Guideline 3.1.)

GUIDELINE 3.1

Alternative Pain Management Approaches

Along with or aside from pain medication, there are many alternative pain management approaches. Methods to address aches (such as sore muscles or swelling) include the application of cold and hot compresses. If there is no opening to the skin, simply wet a rag with warm water and apply for 15 minutes, then do the same thing with cool water for 15 minutes. Alternatively, you can use a heating pad and ice pack. If the compress causes any discomfort to the patient, discontinue use. For the actual procedures to follow for application of hot and cold compresses, see Chapter 17. Other alternative measures that can be used at home include rehabilitation (see Chapter 13), massage (see Chapter 12), and use of calming music.

YOUR ROLE AS A CAREGIVER

Your role as a caregiver is to help the patient and her family manage the pain. This can be done in many ways (see Clinical Alert 3.1):

- Ask the patient what usually decreases her pain. Do not change her routine if it decreases the pain!
- Try non-medication related pain management techniques such as deep breathing (see Chapter 17), massage (see Chapter 12), or positioning (see Chapter 11).
- Talk to the patient. Explain what you will do and how she may help.
- Allow the patient to move at his own pace. Do not rush him.
- Support the medication schedule. Encourage the patient to take medication before the pain becomes severe.
- Encourage the family to support the patient as he deals with pain.

CLINICAL ALERT 3.1

Understanding Pain Medications

When pain is caused by inflammation (i.e., a sprained ankle), it is more likely that an anti-inflammatory medication (i.e., over-the-counter ibuprofen or prescription celecoxig) will decrease the pain. If the pain is nerve-related (i.e., trigeminal neuralgia, or facial nerve pain), a prescription medication such as lioresal or carbamezepine would be most likely to help. If the pain is chronic, such as the pain that occurs with arthritis or fibromyalgia, a routine of over-the-counter acetominophen (which blocks the pain receptor from feeling the pain) may be followed. If the pain is severe, combinations of prescription opiate medications and acetominophen last longer and are stronger. It is important to ask your patient's physician which type of medication she or he recommends to avoid use of a type of medication that isn't as effective for the type of pain the patient is experiencing.

- Observe the patient for any increase of pain. Alter your care accordingly.
- Report to the physician or nurse if the patient's pain changes or if she does not respond to her medication.
- Encourage the patient to share her feelings about her pain.

Encourage family members to share their feelings about the patient's pain, the patient's reaction to the pain, and the effect of the patient's pain on the family members.

FAMILY

Most human beings live in some sort of family. It may be an extended family with several generations in the same house. It may be a single-parent family. It may be a unit made up of friends who live together and regard themselves as a family. Different cultures define family in different ways. In the broadest sense, a family is a unit bound together by common interests and working to maintain the well-being and meet the needs, of all members.

Needs and Rules of Families

Each family has needs and rules of its own. As you enter a caretaking role in a family unit, you become aware of how that household operates. Do the household members care for one another? Do they punish their members with violence? Do they speak lovingly to each other? Do they stop speaking to one member when they are angry? Do they tease members? As much as you can, it is your responsibility to care for your patient within the framework of her family. You are to follow the plan of care established by the patient, family members, and health care team. This ensures that the plan of care reflects the family's values. If there are activities in the home you do not understand, that make you uncomfortable, or that you consider dangerous, report them immediately to the appropriate individual on the health care team.

Culture and the Family

Many factors influence family function: size, economic resources, the needs of each member, the culture of the members and of the country in which they live. Sometimes, a family functions within the rules of their native country, even though its members live in the United States. This may cause conflict between family member roles and the health care team. In some families, the senior male makes decisions; in others, the mother-in-law makes the decisions. In some families, children are important, educated, and cared for; in others, they enter the workforce at a young age. The family culture has a great impact on its structure; decision-making pattern; and members' reactions to illness, pain, and healing. You must be sensitive to these issues because they will affect your patient. If you do not understand certain actions, decisions, or believe actions are not helping your client, discuss this with the appropriate individual on the health care team.

CLINICAL ALERT 3.2

Culture of People with Disabilities

Some people are born with disabilities and others acquire them as a result of illness, surgery, or accidents. Disabilities may be permanent or temporary. People with disabilities expect to be treated as a whole, functioning person, much as they would be treated without the disabilities. Always provide a safe and accepting environment. Respect the person and his or her wishes for assistance.

People taking on a caregiver role must be culturally competent, which means having basic knowledge and understanding about the culture of the person they will be caring for and of the family structure. If the family is multicultural (more than one culture), the caregiver must take all the cultures into consideration when planning and carrying out the care (see Clinical Alert 3.2).

Understanding a culture means understanding its members' basic ideas about themselves, their relationships to their family members, and their ideas about health care. Learning new skills and information is accomplished in different ways for different cultures. It is important that you are aware of how each person learns and obtains new knowledge.

Family Members and Roles

A role is the part a person has in his or her family or situation. Each member of a family has many roles. Sometimes these roles are learned from older members of the family; sometimes, if there is no role model, the role must be shaped to the best of the person's ability. Family members can have several roles; for example, a woman may be a mother, daughter, wife, and grandmother. Each role demands different behaviors and a different set of responsibilities. The important point is to balance these roles so that one does not conflict with another. This is difficult and often impossible. Family members who have difficulty balancing roles may need professional help to accomplish this task.

Middle Generation

In many homes, you may find a family member in the middle generation. This often is a woman about forty to fifty years old who cares for her mother or father (often seventy to seventy-five years old), and mothers her own children, often teenagers (see Figure 3.4). She may also work and have a husband. The caregiver in this generation may be in need of special understanding and assistance because she is balancing the needs of others in addition to trying to meet her own needs. In this special situation, it is important to understand family dynamics and work to maintain them so all members can have their needs met.

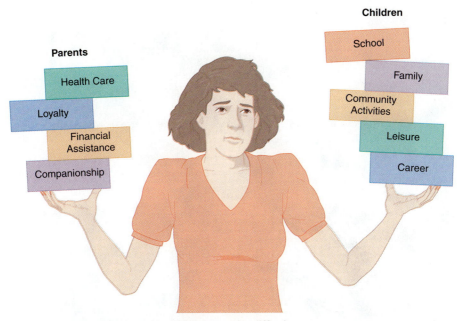

FIGURE 3.4   Balancing multiple priorities can be difficult.

In another scenario you may find a person who has raised a family and now cares for a parent. This requires an adjustment of resources, time, family responsibilities, and outlook. Your understanding of this process and ability to help the primary caregiver, family, and patient meet their needs is an important role. It is necessary to be nonjudgmental as family members learn new roles and readjust the ways in which their basic needs are met (see Figure 3.5).

Economics

All families have some money that they spend according to their own rules and beliefs based on family history, needs, culture, and severity of the patient's condition. Many families spend money on things of which you personally do not approve. You may be asked by one family member or another to comment on how money is spent; for example, "Do you think my son should have bought that car?" or "How could my daughter pay so much for that dress?"

If you are not directly part of the decision about spending money, it is important to act in a nonjudgmental way and not to inflict your opinions about money. All you need to say is "I'm not really in a position to comment on this situation. Why don't you talk to your son about how you feel?" If you believe that money is being spent in such a way that it will injure a family member or cause danger to the family, report your observations to the appropriate member of the health care team.

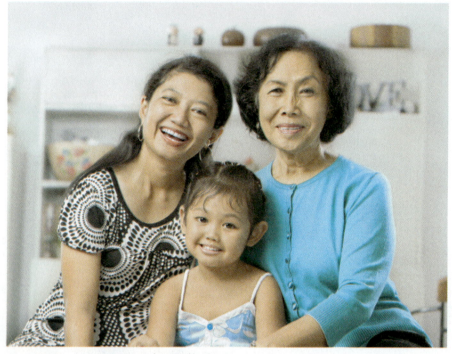

FIGURE 3.5 Care giving is multi-generational.

YOUR ROLE AS A CAREGIVER

As a caregiver, you may not be totally comfortable caring for the person who is the patient. These feelings may be due to the family or other situations. Ask yourself, Are you afraid? Do you understand what is happening? Do family members have values and actions of which you personally disapprove? It is important to recognize and be honest with yourself about your reactions to the patient and the family so that these feelings do not get in the way of your ability to provide care.

WORKING WITH SOMEONE WHO IS ILL OR HAS A DISABILITY

Every person reacts to illness, being disabled, and/or being dependent in a different way. Individual reactions are determined by age, family, culture, emotional health, and all the other parts that make up a particular person. Even though there are individual reactions, there are also certain common ways in which most people react to being ill or having a disability. As a caregiver, you must be aware of common behaviors so that you will know what to expect while caring for your patient.

It is important to remember that you bring your own feelings about illness with you when you care for a person who needs care at home. These feelings are part of you. Sometimes these feelings are helpful to you and the individual you are caring for; sometimes they are not. The important thing is to identify these feelings and not let them get in the way of your caretaking.

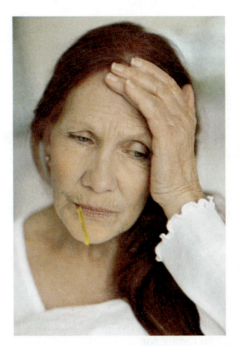

FIGURE 3.6

The most useful action you can take as a caregiver is to involve the patient and the family in the plan of care. By establishing a routine in which they take part, they can continue care of the person when you are gone.

THE DIFFERENCE BETWEEN ILLNESS AND DISABILITY An illness is the absence of good health (see Figure 3.6). An illness usually has pain and discomfort associated with it. This absence of health may be acute or it may be chronic. An acute illness starts suddenly and does not last long. A chronic illness continues for a long time, often for life.

A disability is a condition that produces a physical or mental limitation that may or may not respond to adaptive aids and/or medication (see Figure 3.7). Usually, a body function that we take for granted is impaired. A disability may be produced by an accident, illness, or birth defect. A chronic illness may cause a disability. For example, diabetes, a chronic illness, may cause a person to have poor eyesight, which can be considered a disability. A disability may or may not be painful or may or may not cause discomfort. The most important thing to remember about a disability is that it is usually permanent.

The National Organization on Disability estimates that at least 49 million Americans of all ages have disabilities. Some use assistive devices such as wheelchairs, canes, walkers, hearing aids, or glasses to help them in their daily activities. The way in which you interact with people with disabilities

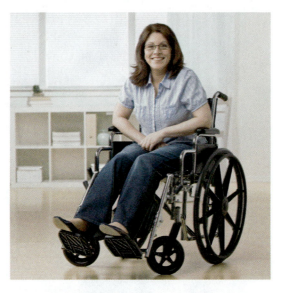

FIGURE 3.7

indicates the understanding and respect you have for them. Keep the following points in mind when caring for a person with a disability:

- Ask before you help a person. The person may not want or need your assistance. Do not assume that all people with disabilities require assistance.
- Speak directly to a person with a disability, not to her or his companion or sign language interpreter.
- Do not speak as though the person is not present.
- Be sensitive about physical contact. Some people require all their limbs for balance, and touching one limb may cause them to fall.
- Do not touch a person's assistive device. These devices are considered part of the person's personal space.
- Do not ask personal questions. Children may ask questions or act curious. Most people with disabilities do not mind this. Be sensitive to perceptions of rudeness.
- Do not lean over a client in a wheelchair to speak to or shake someone else's hand.
- Whenever possible, sit on a chair or stoop down to make eye contact when speaking to a person in a wheelchair. If this is impossible, stand a short distance away so she does not hurt her neck looking up at you.

Family Reactions to Illness and Disability

Reactions of family members to illness, disability, and crisis vary. The unique way in which family members function is called family dynamics. This method of functioning has been shaped over many years. Support systems are people or actions that help a person adjust to a new or difficult situation. Families may be able to make the necessary adjustments in their functions and rally to the short-term crisis or acute illness, but they may fail to adjust if the illness is a long-term or chronic situation. Other families make long-term adjustments. Still others fail to make any changes in their structure and fail to cope with any illness or disability.

Ideally, families choose support systems that allow them to continue functioning—even in time of crisis. You will recognize many kinds of support systems:

- *Informal systems:* People help one another because they want to; such systems include church groups, neighbors, and friends.
- *Formal systems:* People help because they are paid to do so by the government or health care agency.
- *Support groups:* People gather, usually with a leader or facilitator, to discuss and share similar problems, help each other, and gain knowledge from each other.

You, along with the family, the physician, and the patient, will work to set up an acceptable support system for the situation. As a sensitive member of the team, your observations about what works and what does not are important. Be sure to share your observations with the planning team.

Often, when the proper help is offered, a family in crisis can make necessary changes to cope with illness or disability. Remember, the family unit has set up patterns of coping over a long period of time. You must work with these patterns and help establish a support system that makes the family and patient secure and comfortable. If you are not comfortable with the support system or do not believe it will meet the client's needs, discuss this with the health care team.

Denial

Denial is used by some people in a situation with which they cannot cope at the time. They simply say, "This doesn't really exist; nothing is wrong." It is difficult to help a person who denies that a problem exists. Denial is a way people shield themselves from situations. A person may deny an event or situation and then come to accept it later when she is emotionally able to do so. Almost everyone uses denial at some point in their life. Patients may use denial to feel more acceptable to themselves and their families. Families use denial so they do not have to change their routines.

You will often be asked to take part in this process of denial. When a person has an illness, the family may wish to keep it from him. They will deny the problem and ask your help in keeping the secret. You must discuss this with the health care team and determine if the patient is his own responsible party. If the person is competent to make his own decisions, then the health care team cannot support keeping a condition a secret from him. If the patient isn't competent to make his own decisions, you must respect what the family chooses to tell the patient or not. By law, only a physician or court of law can deem a person incompetent to make his or her own decisions. Remember, the family and the patient have a right to deny a situation if that is their method of coping and the patient is not negatively affected. As the caregiver, you must deliver the best possible care within that situation.

Abusive Words and Difficult Behavior

Many patients can be impatient. A patient may show her impatience to members of the family or only to you. It is important to remain calm and not take the patient's words as a personal insult. Often, she is angry at the situation, not at you, but you are the closest person to whom she can react. A patient may complain that the medicine isn't working, that the exercises aren't working, and that she isn't getting better fast enough. She may complain that you are doing too much or not enough. She may become irritable due to pain, the general situation, or her feeling of helplessness. Remember, remain calm and put the patient's actions and words into perspective.

Patients may say things to you that they would not say to other people. They may use unpleasant, nasty, or abusive words. Why? If you are not a family member and therefore you do not have all the years of family relationship behind you, or you are paid to care for the patient, she may think that you will return even if she isn't nice because it is your job. A visiting family member that does not have to care for the patient may not return if the patient is unpleasant. Some patients may say and do things to test you and the limits of the situation. Often, patients will be nice to you but not to others, perhaps to make others jealous and show them that the patient is still in control of the situation. Patients may do or say unpleasant things but are not aware that their behavior is a problem to anyone. If you tell a patient that something she does makes you uncomfortable, she will often stop that behavior.

Working with an unpleasant patient is difficult. Remember that there is a reason for such behavior. Abusive words may indicate many things about the family dynamics. It is important to explore these. Do not assume this behavior is temporary or done only when you are present. If you are really uncomfortable, utilize the social worker or nurse on the health care team to process these feelings.

Goals to Keep in Mind as You Provide Care

All patients, whether they are ill, disabled, have a chronic condition, or are having an acute attack, will have a plan of care. As the homemaker/caregiver, you will be asked to follow this plan of care. A plan of care is created either by the physician or a health care team made up of a nurse, therapists, and possibly a social worker who care for the patient. This plan is formulated to meet both short- and long-term patient needs. Your maintenance of this routine is important. Your careful observation and reporting to the health care team are also important.

The goal of the patient's care plan will be established by the professionals and the patient. The plan is made in coordination with you and the family. It is essential that the patient and his caregivers share the same goals and that they all work toward the same end. Although each patient has his individual care plan, certain broad goals are present in all care plans:

- Promote self-care
- Promote self-respect
- Promote behavior appropriate to the client's condition and age
- Promote a safe, clean environment

ADVANCE DIRECTIVES FOR HOME HEALTH CARE DECISIONS   Each patient has the right to determine the kind of health care he wants if and when he cannot actively make the decision. This document, often called a living will, indicates to others the person's wishes concerning heroic measures, accepting or refusing treatment, and/or withdrawing life support. It is always a good idea to discuss the presence or absence of a living will before you accept the responsibility of being a caregiver. The contents of an individual's living will influence the plan of care and your activities in the home. If a patient tells you that he is interested in making a living will, contact the appropriate person in the health care team to assist the patient in having this accomplished.

MENTAL HEALTH AND MENTAL ILLNESS

Mental health is the ability to function effectively and satisfactorily in society. Mental health is a condition of the whole person. It reflects how a person deals with daily life and crises. Our mental health is the basis for our behavior and relationships with others. Mental health is also a matter of degree. At times, everyone shows behavior that may be judged unusual. The difference between a mentally healthy person and one with a mental disability is that the person who is mentally disabled adopts characteristics or behaviors that no longer enable him to function safely within society. Mentally healthy people can:

- adapt to change
- give and receive affection and love
- tolerate stress to varying degrees
- accept responsibility for their own feelings and actions
- distinguish between reality and non-reality
- form and maintain relationships with people

Not long ago, mental illness was thought to be a punishment or a curse. Many people thought mental illnesses were contagious and could be spread. People who had mental illnesses were put into institutions so that the rest of society would not catch their disease. We now know that mental illnesses are not contagious and that mental illnesses and socially unacceptable behaviors have many different causes. Not all mental illness is permanent. With treatment and medication, many people recover and lead productive lives.

Mental illness often starts slowly, and people cannot tell you when the problem started. They can say, however, when the behavior became unacceptable. There are many types of mental dysfunctions. Individuals with a mental dysfunction should be respected and provided support like any other individual. Chapters 4 and 18 include additional information about mental dysfunctions related to Alzheimer's and other dementias.

Common causes of mental dysfunction include the following:

- Genetics
- Reaction to a medication or illicit drug
- High fevers
- Environmental factors
- Chronic, uncontrolled stress
- Alcohol and/or substance abuse
- Specific traumatic event(s)

Besides reacting to illness and disability in physical ways, people also have mental and emotional reactions. Some people become mentally ill as a result of a physical ailment. In these cases, caring for the patient's mental illness is an added component to caring for his physical condition.

People show their dysfunction in different ways. One classic symptom is a marked change in behavior patterns. If you notice any change in the person you are caring for, or her family tells you that your patient's behavior has changed, report it immediately to the appropriate team member. After a careful assessment, the health care team members may determine there is a need to change the patient's plan of care to reflect her mental needs. Other symptoms of mental illness include:

- Hallucinations (hearing voices or seeing people and/or things that aren't really there)
- Sleeplessness or sleeping the majority of the day without cause
- Unrealistic fears or beliefs that people are out to hurt her
- Nervousness or unusual, repetitive movements without cause
- Disorientation or unusual difficulty concentrating
- Excessive worry or crying
- Withdrawal or isolation
- Mood swings

DEFENSE MECHANISMS   A person who experiences stress reacts with certain defenses. Such reactions are normal. When defense mechanisms are used to such an extent that a person loses touch with reality, he is said to be mentally ill or has a personality disorder. Here are the most common defense mechanisms:

- *Denial:* "It's not happening."
- *Self-pity:* "It's no use. It's hopeless."

- *Displacement:* Attributing uncomfortable emotions to someone or something else. "The dog is mad at you."
- *Regression:* Acting like a child or becoming very dependent.
- *Repression:* Forgetting about the situation and/or putting it out of the mind.
- *Projection:* "It's not my fault but the fault of the medical people."
- *Rationalization:* Explaining how one's behavior is acceptable even though it isn't.
- *Aggression:* Behavior that attacks everyone regardless of cause.
- *Learned helplessness:* Taking no responsibility for personal decisions; relying on others for all needs.

The two the most common forms of mental dysfunction are depression and learned helplessness.

DEPRESSION   Depression may be due to low levels of a brain chemical, a way in which a person deals with illness or trauma, the result of an illness, or a side effect of medication. The primary sign of depression is lack of interest in the present situation and environment. Other signs of depression include the following:

- Poor appetite or severe overeating
- Disinterest in people and activities previously of interest
- Feelings of worthlessness ("I'm not up to that" and "What does it matter anyway?")
- Sleeplessness or sleeping most of the day without cause
- Withdrawing or isolating oneself
- Lack of expression in face or voice (or inconsolable sadness and/or crying)
- Obsession with death and dying

Allow the person you are caring for to take part in as much of his care as he wants and which he is able. Point out the decisions he can make. Consult the patient whenever you can. Encourage his decisions and opinions. Try to establish routines that are good for the patient and have a high rate of success. For example, it may be more convenient for you to help the patient exercise before his bath. But the patient may want to do his exercises after his bath, and he participates easily at that time. It would be appropriate for you to alter your schedule and do the exercises when the patient feels they are most helpful. You must remember that some patients remain depressed no matter what you do. Do not become discouraged. Continue to try to interest them in meaningful activities. If the symptoms are significant or the patient talks about wanting to hurt or kill themselves, report your observations to the health care team or emergency medical services immediately. Never leave a patient alone who is thinking about suicide. Elderly men with depression have the highest success rate of suicide of any age group. Taking threats of suicide seriously is critical (see Clinical Alert 3.3).

CLINICAL ALERT 3.3

Suicide Prevention

Any time a patient talks about wanting to hurt themselves or commit suicide, you should take him or her to the emergency room or call emergency medical services (911). If a patient becomes violent or threatening and you feel you or others are in danger, call the police or 911.

LEARNED HELPLESSNESS   Some people adopt learned helplessness because they have learned it brings them rewards. Some cannot function any other way.

When people realize they are no longer in total charge of their situation, as with the new diagnosis of a chronic disease, they may fail to adjust to this change. Instead, they become totally dependent on others and take no responsibility for their care. When a patient refuses the responsibility he is able to take, he is said to be acting in learned helplessness. It is important to assist the patient in assuming, at his own pace, the role of accepting assistance, while continuing to be responsible for himself when possible. No matter how ill he is, a patient still may take some part in his care. Remember that most of the time, though, patients will assume their independence when they are ready to meet their own needs. Until then, it is your responsibility to assume the care. If, however, you are guided by the physician to perform only certain tasks for a person so he will be forced to be independent in others, follow the physician's instructions. This may be a recommendation from a physician when the patient is using learned helplessness to remain dependent upon a caregiver.

MENTAL ILLNESS AND YOUR ROLE AS A CAREGIVER

As society recognizes the causes of and develops better treatments for mental illness, more people are returning to the community after hospitalization. Communities have set up clinics, foster homes, day care programs, and halfway houses to help these formerly institutionalized patients adjust to community life.

You may be caring for an individual with a mental illness or you may be in a home where a family member is disabled. Be sure you understand your responsibility to the person. The plan of care will be your guide to both the physical and emotional care of the person. One of the most important parts of your care will be to support the patient and the family. Encourage family members to discuss their feelings and concerns with the physician. For the patient to reach her maximum ability, she needs an accepting environment. Keep the following points in mind:

- Your observations of the patient and family are important.
- Report your observations objectively.

- Your friendly, understanding manner will show how you feel about the patient and will encourage others to feel positively about the individual.
- Be aware of the message your body language is communicating.
- Encourage the patient to take part in his own care as is appropriate.

If, at any time, you need assistance or resources to continue in your role as a caregiver, contact the members of the health care team and they will have suggestions for support.

SUBSTANCE ABUSE

The definition of substance abuse is the continued use of a substance despite adverse consequences that affect major life areas and alter the ability to interact in society. There are many types of substance abuse. A person can abuse prescribed medications, illicit drugs, alcohol, or a combination (see Figure 3.8). Substance abuse is seen in all ages and in all economic levels. Abuse may be obvious or subtle. Some people think altering the way they feel through the use of alcohol or drugs is a way of escaping their problems. Some people do it because their friends do it. Others start using drugs to help them with an illness and then are unable to stop. Still others start using alcohol slowly and do not realize they are in trouble until it is too late. The term *substance abuse* means that a person uses a drug or alcohol to excess and that his or her behavior is altered due to the abuse. In the past, most people believed that no one could help someone who abuses substances. We know now that is not the case. Many receive treatment and return to living useful and productive lives.

General Misconceptions About Substance Abuse

"EVERYONE DOES IT." This statement is not true. We read many stories in the newspapers about famous people who use drugs, and we read about everyday

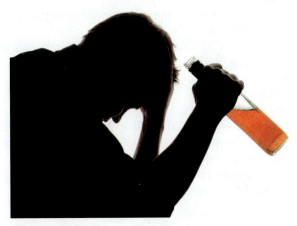

FIGURE 3.8 Substance abuse.

people who try them. This leads some readers to believe that everyone is doing it. Actually, nobody knows how many people really abuse drugs and alcohol, and although the number certainly seems to be growing, "everyone" does not abuse drugs and/or alcohol!

"I CAN CONTROL IT." Wrong! The body may become used to the substance and then no longer reacts to the usual amount that is taken. Therefore, the person must increase the "dose" to achieve the same feeling. As the dose increases, so does the price. There has never been an addicted person who could control it. Sooner or later, the habit controls the person.

"NO ONE WILL KNOW." It is entirely possible that when the user starts, no one will know. But as the body accustoms itself to the foreign substance, there are definite changes in behavior. Soon, employers know. Families can no longer deny the problem. Finally, somebody must confront the user.

"IT MAKES ME FEEL GOOD." A person who starts to use drugs or alcohol may do so to get "high." But this state does not last long. Some people may enjoy this feeling because they feel they are avoiding their real problems. When they are no longer high, however, they do not feel good, and their problems are still present.

General Signals of Substance Abuse

Many signs are associated with abuse of specific substances. The most important sign is a change in the person's behavior. Some general signals include the following:

1. Personality changes, such as mood swings, bizarre activities, or change of friends; disinterest in familiar activities
2. Change in the way money is spent
3. Change in employment or in the relationship with present employer
4. Change in school habits
5. Alteration in physical appearance, such as weight gain or loss, reddened eyes, dilated pupils, nausea, and vomiting
6. Change in eating habits or consumption of fluids
7. Change in sleep habits
8. Liquor is missing
9. Unusual breath odor, unusual smell on clothing
10. Change in gait; change in sense of smell, vision, or hearing
11. Change in breathing pattern
12. Continued discussion about drugs or alcohol
13. Phone calls at odd hours

SUBSTANCE ABUSE AND YOUR ROLE AS A CAREGIVER

You may be assigned to care for an individual who is in a house with some-one who abuses substances. First, you must be sure your patient is in no danger and that the abuser cannot harm your patient—or you. Discuss the situation with the health care team so that a plan can be made to offer help to the abuser. Do not try to obtain help on your own. Offering help to a long-time substance abuser can be a complicated affair and must be care-fully planned. It is important that the correct help be offered and that the most appropriate community resource be utilized. The health care team will know how to plan this.

Do not tell the abuser he must stop. The chances are he would if he could but is unable to do so without help.

Do not make family members feel guilty that they have permitted the situ-ation to continue. They may not know what to do. With your help and support and that of outside professionals, a plan can be made. Families of substance abusers need a great deal of support. Your understanding and demonstration of nonjudgmental behavior will be important.

If you are taking care of an individual who is presently under treatment for having been an abuser, you should act in the manner we have already discussed. You must be observant to detect if the individual you are caring for has reverted back to previous habits of abuse. Report to the health care team any actions that suggest the patient is not drug- or alcohol-free. Follow the care plan carefully and support the patient. Recovery from drug or alcohol abuse is not easy. With your presence and support, it can be made easier.

Summary

Caring for people, regardless of illness, disability, or dysfunction, is a vital role in families and society. There is support for caregivers within the community, health care system, and other agencies. The health care team can give you sug-gestions for obtaining additional support or you can search the Internet for caregiver support groups that relate to what you are experiencing. Know the warning signs of a patient's condition worsening. Reach out for help when needed to keep you and your patient safe.

Chapter 4

Caring for an Elderly Patient

SCENARIO

Mrs. Lee lives in a small apartment in the center of town with her daughter, Naomi Lee. Naomi is an engineer who is used to giving directions and working with Americans. Mrs. Lee speaks no English and has never become accustomed to the American culture. Naomi works six days a week and is seldom home before 10 P.M. She attends church, but her mother does not join her. Mrs. Lee continues to wear her native dress and cooks her native foods. She continually chastises her daughter for not doing the same. While Naomi works, her mother cleans the apartment, cooks the meals, and does all the laundry. There are no visitors to the apartment, and the two women do not take part in any local activities together. When Mrs. Lee must visit the doctor, Naomi takes time off from work. They also consult a native herbalist who prescribes teas, which Mrs. Lee prefers to her western medication (see Figure 4.1)

THE ELDERLY POPULATION

The elderly population is growing faster than any other segment of our society. Here are some interesting facts:

- On January 1, 2006, the first baby boomer turned 60.
- Women who are currently 50 have a life expectancy of 82.5 years.
- Men who are currently 50 have a life expectancy of 78.5 years.
- In 2010, there were 78 million baby boomers, and there are almost as many men as women.
- Women over 65 are twice as likely to live below the poverty line than are men of the same age. Women ages 75 years and up are over three times as likely to be living in poverty as men in the same age range. Only 416,000 men in this age range live at or below the poverty line, while over 1.3 million women ages 75 years and up are poor.

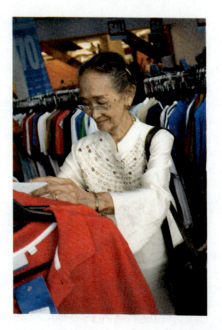

FIGURE 4.1

- One of the main sources of income for the elderly is Social Security; however, it is estimated that in 2020 there will no longer be Social Security for all the baby boomers who are eligible to collect Social Security.
- Half of the people over 65 work part-time, although they have at least one chronic disease.

Although about 5 percent of the elderly live in nursing homes, the rest live in the community. About 15 percent live in some type of assisted-living arrangement where they receive some help with cooking, housekeeping, or medical care. It is expected that as medicine, nutrition, and the general standard of life improve, the number of aged will increase. As this happens, more people who remain at home will need assistance. The home health care system is changing to meet the needs of these people. Many people who are aged will require assistance so they can remain in their own homes with as much independence as possible along with self-respect. Some people will need minimal assistance; others will need maximum assistance. It is important that individuals receive the type of help most appropriate for their individual needs.

There are many different types of living arrangements for the elderly. Some live in their own homes; some live in supervised homes with several others; and some live in communities with various levels of assistance, such as meals, medical supervision, and/or home health care services provided by professional caregivers. The world has changed so much in the past fifty years that the aging population is often unfamiliar with the technology that now exists. It is not that they cannot learn about new machines or new systems, but rather that few people take the time to teach them. They often find themselves in a strange world. Adjustment to change is often difficult for the elderly and their families. Although many families have a well-tested and strong system of coping that enables them to adjust to changes and new roles, many elderly are unable to cope with all the changes. With people living longer than they did even ten years ago, and the ratio of people getting older to those being born is reversing (there will be more elderly than people in other age groups), home care is going to be utilized more and more.

The term *geriatrics* refers to the knowledge and care of the elderly. As a caregiver, you will use this specialized knowledge for the individual for whom you are providing care.

Aging

Aging is universal and starts the moment we are born. The way in which society views the aging citizen varies. In some cultures, the aged are of no value and are often neglected because they are unable to contribute to society. In other cultures and some professions, the elderly are well respected and cared for, and are given a place of honor. American society often appears to value youth for its beauty and to not value the contributions of its elderly citizens (see Figure 4.2) It does seem, however, that society is also gaining a greater understanding of the aged. There are many signs that U.S. society is coming to see all ages as valuable. More advertisements for products of interest to the elderly are appearing. Community programs designed for the elderly are gaining popularity. We are also seeing laws passed that meet the concerns of

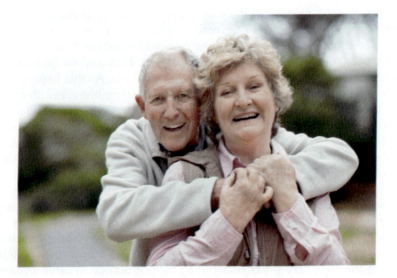

FIGURE 4.2 Aging happily.

our older citizens and that protect them. U.S. society is coming to the conclusion that, although youth has its value, age has its value, too.

When caring for elderly people, the following facts are important for you to remember:

- They usually want to remain independent.
- They can still enjoy sexual relationships.
- They can maintain good health.
- Memory loss is not the same as old age.
- They usually want to be contributing members of society.
- They can still learn new things.

Feelings About the Elderly

Everyone has feelings about the aged. Some people are afraid of them, or feel sorry for them, and others avoid them because they are a reminder of what may happen when they age. Think about the following statements regarding the elderly and learn more about the feelings you have toward the elderly. Ask yourself, Which of these statements are true? Are they true about all older people?

1. Old people are untidy and messy.
2. Old people tend to worry about financial matters.
3. It is normal for the elderly to withdraw from society.
4. Old people prefer to be with people their own age.
5. Old people have no friends.
6. Old people live in the past, and that is boring.
7. Old people only talk about death and are afraid of dying.
8. Old age is a problem for poor people, but not for rich people.
9. Old people prefer to be waited on hand and foot.
10. Old people remind us of what is in store for us when we age.

The aging process has many phases (see Figure 4.3). The exact combination of physical, mental, and social changes vary from person to person. Changes may be obvious or not. Some changes are more easily acceptable than others. There are several theories about aging, but the results of aging are the same.

As people age, they have the same needs as they did when they were younger. The main difference is that the needs of an older person are often met in a different way than are the needs of a younger person.

Physical Changes as We Age

As we age, visible changes occur in the body, including how it functions (see Table 4.1). It may take longer to walk a certain distance, longer to make decisions, and longer to execute a task. The physical changes of aging are the most obvious, and for some, the most difficult to accept. These changes occur at different rates and at different ages. Every individual has a unique

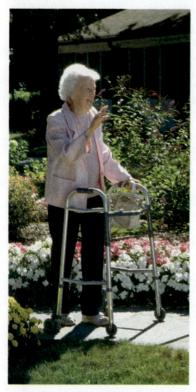

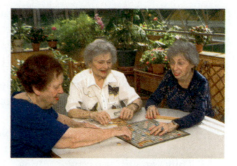

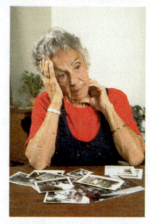

FIGURE 4.3 Putting the many phases of the aging process into perspective is the best way to ensure a well-balanced life.

TABLE 4.1	Physical Changes of Aging	
Body System or Organ	**"Normal" Aging Change**	**Possible Problems or Consequence**
Skin	Decreased response to pain sensation, temperature changes, and vibration.	Accidents; inability to feel hot and/or cold objects, weather changes, injury, and/or pain.
	Loss of fat under the skin (subcutaneous fat) and fatty padding over bony prominences (i.e., hips); change in number of blood vessels.	Veins appear more prominent; wrinkles, especially facial, and folds in skin appear; occurrence of pressure sores (bedsores); slower healing; loss of hair; fluid balance of skin is difficult to maintain.
	Decrease in number of sweat glands.	Difficulty in regulating body temperature.
	Decrease in oil production.	Dry skin, itching, easily injured.
	Formation of pigment cell clusters.	Moles and "old-age spots" (liver spots), graying of hair.

TABLE 4.1 *(Continued)*

Body System or Organ	"Normal" Aging Change	Possible Problems or Consequence
Eyes	Clouding of lenses.	Development of cataracts.
	Decrease in ability to focus.	Difficulty seeing at night or in fluorescent lighting.
	Decrease in production of tears.	Dry eyes.
	Inability to blink as quickly.	Easier to get a foreign body in the eye.
	Muscle degeneration in 50 percent of people over age seventy.	Central vision loss.
	Less light reaching the retina.	Need for adequate lighting.
	Eyelids tend to evert or invert.	Irritation.
Ear	Decrease in ability to hear high-frequency sounds (presbycusis).	Hearing loss; distortion of sound and pain if volume is too high.
	Stiffness and inflexibility of ear structure.	
Sense of taste	Decrease in number of taste buds.	Food may become tasteless.
	Salty taste decreases the most, sweet next.	Use of salt and sugar.
Sense of smell	Generally declines.	Difficulty smelling smoke, gas, etc., or enjoying pleasant odors.
Mouth and teeth	Loss of gum and bone structure around teeth.	Periodontal disease, loss of teeth.
Brain	Change in reaction time and in verbal and vocabulary skills.	Slowed reactions and reflexes; inability to learn quickly.
	Memory loss may occur after age fifty.	Recall, recognition may slow slightly (i.e., "Where are my keys?").
	Decrease in deep sleep.	Periods of wakefulness during sleep hours.
	Decrease in need for sleep.	Hours of sleep may change.
Lungs and chest	Stiffness of respiratory muscles.	Expansion of the lungs becomes more difficult.
	Decrease in elasticity of rib cage.	Mild barrel chest due to structural changes.
	Decrease in area for oxygen and carbon dioxide exchange.	Less oxygen available during physical exercise and activity.
	Diminished activity of cilia (help to clean lung) and diminished cough reflex.	Difficulty coughing and eliminating foreign particles from lung; incidence of bronchitis and pneumonia.

(continued)

TABLE 4.1 *(Continued)*

Body System or Organ	"Normal" Aging Change	Possible Problems or Consequence
Heart and circulatory system	Decrease in cardiac muscle strength.	Cardiac output is decreased.
	Narrowing of arteries and veins.	Blood pressure is increased.
Musculoskeletal system	Decrease in absorption of calcium.	Osteoporosis (thinning of bone).
	Decrease in bone replacement.	Incidence of fractures increases.
	Loss of muscle mass and tone.	Fatigue and weakness.
Balance	Less-efficient balancing mechanisms and reactions.	Incidence of falls increases; standing position tends to be with flexed hip and knees
Gastrointestinal system	Decrease in esophageal muscle action.	Indigestion is more frequent, slower.
	Decrease in large bowel mobility, nervous stimulation.	Constipation, diminished frequency of bowel movements (BM)s, incomplete emptying of the bowel.
	Decreased sensitivity to thirst.	Dehydration.
Renal system	Decrease in size of urinary bladder,	Increased frequency of urination,
	Decrease in kidney size, slowing of filtration, blood flow to kidney.	Increased sensitivity to medications, decreased ability to eliminate toxic wastes.
Genitalia	**Men**	
	Enlarged prostate gland.	Urinary system obstruction.
	Increased time needed to urinate.	Increased urinary retention, frequency, and infections.
	Full erections may be more difficult to achieve.	Decreased ability to delay ejaculation.
	Women	
	Decreased vaginal and cervical secretions, thinning of vaginal walls.	Uncomfortable intercourse, longer time to experience orgasm.
	Changes in estrogen after menopause.	Changes in secondary sexual characteristics.
Hormones	Decreased insulin response	Blood sugar elevation

schedule. Physical changes that eventually occur in everyone include the following:

- Reflexes are slower.
- Circulation becomes less efficient.
- Hair turns gray and may change in texture.
- Bodily processes slow.
- Skin loses elasticity and underlying fat and becomes thin and more fragile.
- Senses become less acute and aids, such as glasses or hearing aids, are sometimes needed.
- Posture becomes more stooped, and walking becomes more difficult.
- Muscles lose strength, and familiar tasks become more difficult.
- Sensing the temperature of water and air becomes less accurate.
- Healing takes longer.
- Short-term memory often decreases so directions have to be repeated often.

Cognitive Changes

It was once thought that all older people became senile. This is a myth. Not all older people become confused, forgetful, and dependent. Those who do must be treated carefully, just as you would treat any other impaired person, not as an object of pity or as a child.

Decreased circulation and therefore oxygen to the brain can cause mental changes. Medications can cause mental changes. Some changes are temporary, and some are permanent. Obvious changes in brain function are forgetfulness, disorientation, and irritability. A physical change may also cause mental changes. Other mental changes are brought about as a reaction to social changes.

Dementia is the gradual decrease in a person's ability to make judgments. This is not a normal part of the aging process. The presence of dementia and the type of dementia can be diagnosed only by a physician. Dementia used to be called senility.

The two main categories of dementia are the reversible dementias and those that are not reversible. Reversible dementia is often caused by a physical, social, or chemical stimulus. When that stimulus is removed, the person reverts to his pre-dementia status. Irreversible dementias can be caused by small portions of the brain losing function due to strokes, formation of lesions or plaque on the brain, or deterioration of the brain from chronic disease. These conditions lead to confusion, decreased mental acuity, decreased physical abilities, and decreased ability to make judgments. The patient may not have the same problems all the time; he may have good days and bad days. One type of irreversible dementia is Alzheimer's. (See Chapter 18 for additional information on Alzheimer's.)

When a patient exhibits questionable behavior, it is important for you to discuss with the health care team the causes of the behavior. Knowing why people act in a certain way will help you in caring for them. Aged people who are confused and forgetful require special precautions. It may be necessary to remind them where they are, who they are, and who you are. Safety is the key to the care of these individuals because they may be unable to make judgments on their own.

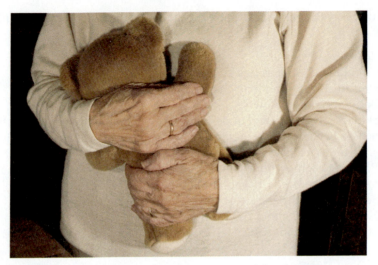

FIGURE 4.4 Elder with dementia, clutches a stuffed animal for comfort.

Caring for people with dementia takes time, understanding, and patience. It can be tiring for you to spend long periods with a cognitively impaired person. When you feel overwhelmed by your patient, call for reinforcement. Use the support system discussed in Chapter 1 to have regular breaks from caretaking.

Families of elderly people are often stressed. Caring for an elderly relative brings with it several responsibilities. Caring for an elderly person with dementia requires an additional set of skills. If necessary, encourage your patient's family to discuss their feelings with professionals.

Social Changes

Many social changes affect the elderly. Some are the result of physical changes, some are brought about by society, and some just happen. Changes include the following:

- Retirement
- Change in income
- Change in level of activity
- Fear of illness
- Isolation from friends and family
- Death of a spouse
- Change in housing
- Increased dependence on others

One or two of these changes may not cause any change in your patient's behavior. Several of these changes, however, can cause a person to change his usual behavior patterns because he will no longer be able to cope with the situation. Your patient's reaction to change depends on his usual coping ability and the result of the changes. He may become anxious, depressed, or with-drawn, or he may increase his activity. His eating habits, sleeping habits, or memory may change. He may no longer show interest in activities he used to enjoy. He may suddenly develop an interest in activities he always disliked. If you notice any of these changes in your patient's behavior, report them im-mediately to the appropriate member on the health care team.

YOUR ROLE AS A CAREGIVER

The needs of the aged are the same as the needs of all other people. It will be your responsibility to help meet these needs. By giving necessary assistance in a safe, warm, understanding manner, you help the person you are caring for remain at home in familiar surroundings and be as independent as possible. The following tips can help you when caring for the elderly:

- Assist with all phases of personal care. For example, although a complete bath may not be necessary every day, many people have dry, flaky, fragile skin requiring lotion or oil daily. Lubricate the skin with lotion or oil as the patient wishes. Expensive lotions are not necessary, but lubrication is.
- Observe the patient for nonhealing irritation, redness, or bruises on the body and report them to the health care team.
- Teach the patient without dementia how to maintain her own personal hygiene when you are not in the home. Provide an environment for safe, simple exercise, such as walking up stairs or moving from room to room.
- Plan your care around the patient's usual household schedule and eth-nic customs.
- Provide for warmth and ventilation in the home. Elderly people often react to temperature differently than do younger people. They often wear sweaters in the summer. Dress and groom them in what makes them comfortable and is appropriate for their age.
- Protect them from extreme heat or cold.
- Do not disturb personal belongings, letters, pictures, and so on. You may suggest moving them, however, to another obvious place where the patient can still enjoy them so that you can provide better care.
- Do not use baby talk with the individual to whom you are providing care.
- Do not speak about the patient to others as though he or she is not there.
- Be patient!

AREAS OF SPECIAL CONCERN AS YOU CARE FOR AN ELDER

Although caring for an elderly person is much the same as caring for a younger person, you must be aware that the elderly often need special atten-tion in certain aspects of their care. You will have to be extra alert in the areas of safety, exercise, and in assisting them with medication. In addition, because an elderly person often is unable to report abuse or find someone to talk to outside his home, you will have to be his voice. This is an important role.

Because you may be the only person who sees the patient regularly, you will develop a special relationship with her and will be able to notice changes in mood and activity. Report to the health care team every change, no matter how slight, so that your patient's status can be assessed and monitored. Remember, your overall goal as a caregiver is to preserve the individual's independence, self-worth, and safety.

Safety

Safety for the elderly is always a prime concern. As their activity level changes, so do places and objects that are considered safe (see Figure 4.5). A situation that at one time was considered safe may become a hazard as a person ages. Poor eyesight, decreased reflexes, and poor hearing can all contribute to accidents. In addition, many elderly attempt tasks they cannot execute and thus cause themselves harm. In an effort to be independent, an elderly person may take unnecessary risks.

As people age, their ability to sense and then react to hot water is decreased. Many elderly are severely burned each year because they cannot feel that water is too hot. Teach your patient to test his washing and bathing water *before* he uses it. If hot water has been run through a faucet, the faucet itself may be hot enough to cause burns should someone touch it. Briefly running cold water through the faucet after the hot water will cool the metal and prevent such burns (see Clinical Alert 4.1).

It is easier to prevent accidents than it is to heal injuries. People who fall and break bones take months to heal and then may never regain full use of the limbs. The elderly heal slower than younger people do, so fall prevention is even more important for elderly patients than it is for younger patients. Safety

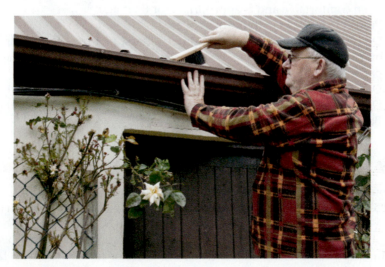

FIGURE 4.5 Safety first.

CLINICAL ALERT 4.1

Although independence is the goal, safety in meal preparation should be a consideration. Metal of any kind placed accidentally in a microwave will start a fire; leaning on a stove top that has been left on will cause severe burns. Electrical switches can be installed and secured so that the stove or microwave is operable only when the caregiver unlocks the security box and turns the switch on.

remains one of your primary responsibilities as a caregiver. Help your patient maintain a safe environment in the following ways:

- Encourage your patient to discuss her capabilities realistically.
- Help provide good lighting with switches that are easy to operate.
- Encourage the use of banisters and properly installed grab bars.
- Encourage safe practices in the kitchen. Never let your patient wear long or flowing sleeves while cooking.
- Set the thermostat on the water heater at a safe temperature (under 110°F is best).
- Plan emergency exits.
- Help install and test smoke detectors according to package instructions. If you do not feel comfortable installing the smoke detectors or if the package recommends professional installation, contact the recommended professional.
- Encourage your patient to discuss her driving capabilities with her physician.

It is important to discuss with the health care team and the family members any unsafe practices you observe while caring for the patient. If you find yourself in an unsafe situation, you and/or members of the health care team or family may have to confront the patient. Although we can never forget that the patient has the right to act in any way he wants in his own house, it is not part of your role to remain anywhere that is unsafe. It is also important to determine if the patient is acting in such a way that it will cause harm to others. For example, does he smoke in bed? In this case, you will have to keep cigarettes and lighting materials away from the individual. If the person you are caring for needs structural changes in the house, the health care team, most likely the occupational therapist, should be able to arrange for a reputable person to perform this work. Often community groups do such work for minimal pay.

Exercise

Health professionals now believe that planned exercise is important for everyone (see Figure 4.6) The benefits are many:

- A feeling of well-being
- Increased strength of bones

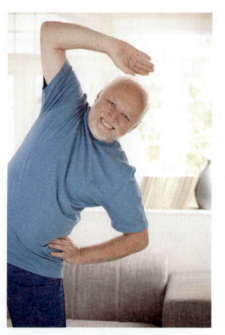

FIGURE 4.6   Exercise is essential to the health of seniors.

- Increased cardiac and respiratory capacity
- Increased strength and tone of muscles
- Decreased weight
- Decreased blood pressure
- Decreased anxiety
- Better sleep habits

All individuals should consult with their physician before they start an exercise regime. There are many considerations before the proper regime is chosen, and only a physician can make the most informed decision. Be sure to report any change in a patient's level of exercise or if you notice that she is experiencing difficulty while exercising.

Sleep Changes

Many elderly people experience changes in their sleep patterns. Among the changes may be the total hours of sleep per night, the time of sleep, and the effect of medications. Before you suggest changes to your patient's routine, try to determine what the routine was before her illness. In that way, you can compare her former activity with her present activity. Consider the following suggestions as you discuss the sleep regime that is best for the individual for whom you are providing care (involve the health care team as needed):

- Limit caffeinated drinks.
- Create a relaxing, pleasant atmosphere before going to sleep.

- Develop a regular sleep schedule.
- Limit naps and time spent without activity.
- Create a regular exercise routine.
- Review medications for side effects of sedation or sleeplessness.

Sleep is necessary to the body for optimum function. A rested individual is better able to take an active part in his care and interact with others in an alert and calm manner. If your patient is unable to create a regular, healthful sleep routine, discuss this with the health care team.

Medications

Elderly people may react to medications differently from younger people. Elderly individuals often have several diseases and disabilities and take several medications for each one. The interaction of these medications often results in unexpected side effects (see Figure 4.7). The following can also be problems:

- The older body retains medications at a rate different from a younger body.
- Elderly individuals may stop taking medications for financial reasons, because they forget, or because they read or hear negative news about the drug and its potential side effects.
- The kidneys and liver of an older person removes waste products more slowly than do those of a younger person.
- Older individuals may forget they have taken medications and take them again.

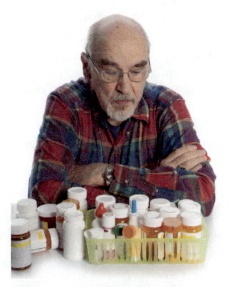

FIGURE 4.7 Numerous medications can make appropriate use difficult.

- Some people tend to save medications that become outdated and then start retaking them.
- Elderly individuals may have several physicians, each of whom may not be aware of all the medications that have been prescribed by other physicians.
- Some individuals may not discuss their reactions to medications with their physician because they believe the physician will be disappointed in their inability to take the drug.

Your role as a caregiver is to assist the person you are caring for with a safe medication schedule. Help your patient maintain a foolproof, organized method of taking medications. This method should be established by a nurse on the health care team, with input from you and the patient. Be sure all your patient's medications are prescribed for him. Borrowing medications can be dangerous! Report all side effects, no matter how slight, to the nurse or physician on the health care team.

Be sure your patient knows why he is taking his medication and the possible side effects. Talk to the nurse if you think your patient is unaware or confused about this. When your patient visits his physician, encourage him to take all his medications with him. Using this strategy, the physician will have a clear picture of the medications the individual is taking and can prescribe new ones accordingly.

Encourage your patient to throw out old, expired medications and to get rid of any medications that are not his.

Many medications are now packaged in childproof bottles. These bottles are difficult for the older individual to open. Help the person you are caring for order his medications packaged in containers that are easy for him to open and close. Elderly people often fail to take their medication because they cannot open the bottle (see Clinical Alert 4.2).

Accompanying a Patient to the Doctor

You may be asked to accompany your patient to a physician's office. Prior to taking the individual, it is important that you discuss your role with the family and health care team. Be sure you are comfortable in the role and that you understand exactly what is expected of you. Questions to consider regarding your role include the following:

- Are you going to ensure the patient's safety?
- Are you expected to discuss the patient's status and care?

CLINICAL ALERT 4.2

If the patient has cognitive loss or memory problems requiring you to assist her in taking her medication, the medication should be secured and placed somewhere out of the elder's reach. A box or filing cabinet that locks is often helpful for storing these medications securely.

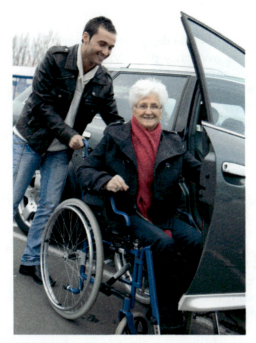

FIGURE 4.8 Learn to transfer your patient safely to and from a car.

- Are you expected to relate to the family changes in the individual's medication, exercise level, or medical regime?
- What should you bring with you?

Transportation to the doctor's office can be by car or other arranged medical transportation method depending on the ability of the person to walk, sit, and/or transfer to and from a vehicle (see Figure 4.8). Contact the health care team if you need resources for transportation or to teach you to transfer your patient safely. At the doctor's office, it is important that the patient feels in control. Give the patient and the physician privacy if the patient requests. Allow the patient to speak directly to the physician whenever possible. If the information the patient gives is incorrect, find a respectful way to communicate this to the physician. If the physician gives you instructions or changes medication, be sure you have these changes in writing.

When you return from the doctor's visit, document the entire experience, including the time you left the house and the time you returned. Include the following details:

- Mode of transportation
- The patient's reaction to the whole experience
- Information or instructions you received from the physician and what you did with them

Sexuality

The need for intimacy does not disappear with age, although sexual response gradually slows and frequency of activity may decrease. Sex and the desire for closeness, companionship, and touching are the same. Sexual performance may decrease, but the desire for human companionship does not. Sexual desire, response, and activity also are often affected by medications. Therefore, any change in sexual activity or any concern expressed by the person you are caring for should be referred to the nurse or physician on the health care team.

Some medications can affect sexual desire and performance. When this happens, the individual may stop the medications rather than discuss the problem with her physician. Often, the medications can be changed, and desire and performance will return. Some diseases affect sexual performance and desire. This situation should be discussed with the patient so that she is aware of this possibility. If you are uncomfortable discussing this or do not have the answers to her questions, refer the individual to the nurse, physician, or social worker on the health care team. Do not forget about them. The fact that the patient has discussed this with you indicates this is of great concern to her (see Figure 4.9).

You may have preconceived notions and feelings about sexual activity between older people. It is important for you to prevent these ideas from interfering with your relationship with the person for whom you are providing care. Patients may have sexual practices unfamiliar to you. Remember to

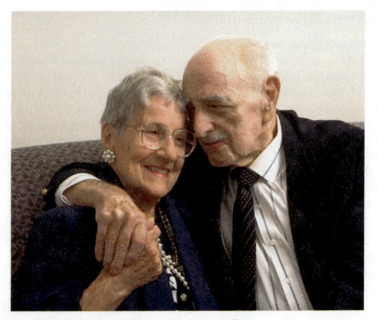

FIGURE 4.9 Closeness and sexuality are necessary at all ages.

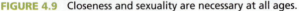

remain nonjudgmental and give privacy as requested. If you have concerns or questions, talk to other members of the health care team.

Abuse

Abuse is any act that causes another person harm. Abuse is a disturbing situation. Abuse of the elderly is especially disturbing because the abused are often helpless to fight back or call for help. Today, health professionals are seeing more cases of the elderly being physically and emotionally abused and neglected. There may be many reasons for abuse, but the result is always the same: an elderly person is hurt or in danger. As you work in your patient's home, you will be privileged to see and hear activities that no one else sees or hears. Be alert for signs of abuse or neglect, and look for the following common signs:

- Bruises on a patient that are hard to explain
- Fear of one particular person
- A request from the patient not to be left alone with a particular person
- Conflicting stories from family members
- A "feeling" that things are not right
- Lack of nourishment or care for the patient
- Lack of family concern for the safety of the patient
- Exchange of abusive words between family members
- Unexpected deterioration of the patient's health
- A drastic change in behavior when certain family members are present

The accusation that a person is abusing an elderly person is serious. Do not take it lightly. Report immediately all activities you see that indicate the possibility of abuse. Most states require that any case of suspected elder abuse be reported. It is your responsibility to become familiar with the laws of your state and the proper reporting agency in your area. Remember, most abuse is inflicted by a family member. Be alert!

Summary

Care of the elderly can be very rewarding. It takes patience, understanding, and continued learning about the patient and his or her medical condition(s). When patients age at home, they are able to remain independent longer, continue life-long routines, and maintain relationships important to social and mental health. The caregiver plays a pivotal role in keeping the health care team and family informed of changes in physical and cognitive abilities so that the plan of care can be adjusted accordingly. Enjoy your work with elderly patients, listen to their life experiences, and cherish the time you have with them.

Chapter 5

Working with Children

SCENARIO

Janet is the youngest of five children. Although she is seven years old, she still sleeps in a crib and has just learned to walk. Janet has Down syndrome, a common developmental disability. She is quiet and does not talk unless the speaker is directly in front of her and speaks slowly. Janet smiles and laughs a lot, but she is developmentally behind others in her age group so she is made fun of at school. Due to her impulsivity, Janet requires extra supervision to ensure her safety (see Figure 5.1).

CARING FOR CHILDREN

An individual may become a caregiver for a child for many reasons, including:

- The primary caregiver becomes ill or suffers a disability.
- The primary caregiver needs a rest from or assistance with the care of a child with an illness or disability.

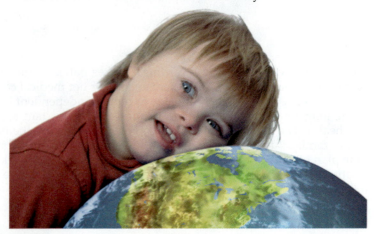

FIGURE 5.1

- The primary caregiver must be taught, by your example, how to care for the child.
- The primary caregiver must leave the house to work.
- Child abuse or neglect has been reported or suspected in the home.

When caring for a child, it is important to know what your relationship is with the child and his parent(s) or guardian. When meeting a child for the first time, bend down so you are at eye level. If the child is your patient, it is important to work immediately on developing rapport. If possible, spend a few minutes alone with the child. This will signal the child's importance and allow both of you to get to know each other. You will also be able to learn about any special concerns or questions the child may have.

Working with children can also occur when a caregiver who is caring for an adult patient finds that she needs to relate to the children of the individual who is requiring care. This interaction calls for a different relationship than when the child is your patient. Understanding the basic needs of children will assist the caregiver in being successful in addressing these needs.

Basic Needs of Children

Children have many of the same physical and emotional needs as adults (see Figure 5.2). They often depend on adults, however, for fulfillment of these needs. Just as adult needs change in importance and fulfillment, so do the needs of children. The age of the child may make certain needs more

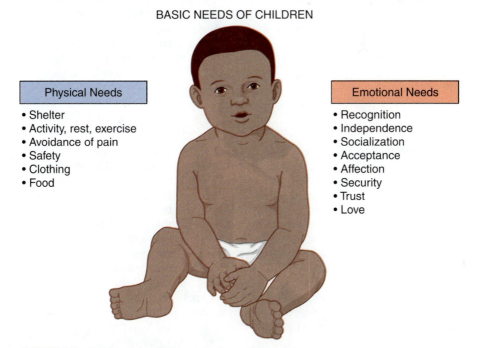

BASIC NEEDS OF CHILDREN

Physical Needs

- Shelter
- Activity, rest, exercise
- Avoidance of pain
- Safety
- Clothing
- Food

Emotional Needs

- Recognition
- Independence
- Socialization
- Acceptance
- Affection
- Security
- Trust
- Love

FIGURE 5.2 Children have the same basic needs as adults.

important. Children are not little adults. Their reactions and needs are based on their experiences as children. Researchers believe that a child must meet specific needs successfully at a certain age before he or she can mature. Often, when the child is ill or a family member is ill, meeting these needs completely is difficult. That is your most important role—to meet the needs of the child (see Table 5.1).

Congenital Anomalies—Birth Defects

A congenital anomaly is any abnormal organ or part of an organ present at birth, even though it may not be noted at that time. Such conditions may result from a genetic disorder or from external factors, such as exposure to toxic substances, drug use, or alcohol abuse during pregnancy. Congenital anomalies may be visible, such as a child born with a shorter arm or one born with no fingers, or they may be invisible, such as a child with a malformation of the heart.

TABLE 5.1   Stages of Childhood from Birth to Adolescence

Stage of Development	Age	Key Characteristics or Tasks of the Age	Guidelines for Activities
Infancy	Birth to 1 year	Rapid growth; totally dependent on adults; experiences first relationship; starts to distinguish the world through her senses.	Provide calm routine, taking into account infant's schedule; encourage family to participate in care; stimulation includes brightly colored objects held high or tied to crib, music, different shapes and textures, swings, carriages, rockers, toys she can put into larger containers, smooth objects that do not injure.
Training period	1 to 3 years	Attachment to mother and regular caregivers is strong; begins independence and exploration; learns to say no; puts everything in mouth; shows food likes and dislikes; frightened of loud noises and absence of primary caregiver; can understand simple honest explanation; may or may not share; usually starts to toilet train by age 3.	Tell familiar stories again and again; do not lie because the child does not know fact from fiction; help child become familiar with objects that are part of his care; help with toilet training as the family wishes without punishment but with positive reinforcement; provide pull toys, balls, stackable objects, mirrors, threads, large beads, wind-up toys.

(continued)

TABLE 1.2	(Continued)		
Stage of Development	**Age**	**Key Characteristics or Tasks of the Age**	**Guidelines for Activities**
Independence and initiation	3 to 5 years	Girls mature more quickly; discovers sharing of friends and parents; affection and jealousy apparent; imitation; attempts to please; assumes some of his own personal care; assists with simple household chores; vivid imagination leads to stories; likes to use familiar objects over and over; approval of family important; older children like to take active part in care.	Activities with hands and crayons, simple puzzles; simple ball games, and tag; always give simple reasons for activities.
Middle childhood	6 to 12 years	Peer acceptance important; easily embarrassed; asserts independence and makes friendships; secretive; argues with adults; growth spurts; 10 to 12 years: sexual curiosity.	Reasons for actions important; explain; give timeframe for schedule; provide scientific play, jigsaw puzzles, table games, board games, electronic and video games, music, puppets, sewing, crafts, and model building.
Adolescence	13 to 18 years	Rapid change physically and emotionally; sexual development; mood changes; relationship sensitive; need for privacy; peer relationships important; independence important; enjoys reading, use of telephone, music; may reject familiar objects or foods; exerts opinions, may reject suggestions from parents or caregivers but accept them from strangers; idol worship is common; concern for appearance and virility.	Respect need for privacy; sexual concerns; explain all actions logically and honestly; encourage teen to express his or her desires and interests.

When you work in a home with a child who has a congenital anomaly, you will assist family members as they learn to cope with the situation and the way it will affect the whole family. It is not unusual for family members to experience anger, guilt, denial, and emotional difficulties as they learn to care for this child. You must show accepting behavior and encourage the family to seek help and support. Further information and resources on this topic are provided on the Resource Page at the end of this book.

Discuss your feelings with the nurse or social worker on the health care team so that your actions will complement the plan of care for the whole family. Do not be surprised if you need support during this time. This situation may evoke feelings in you that you may need help to understand. As you work in this type of situation, be alert to the need for separating your feelings from those of the family.

Developmental Disabilities

A developmental disability is any condition that interferes with the proper development of a person. Developmentally disabled people were once put into institutions and not taught to be part of society. The most familiar developmental disabilities are mental retardation and cerebral palsy (see Figure 5.3), which interfere with the way in which a person speaks, learns, and performs activities of daily living. Although these conditions are permanent, with

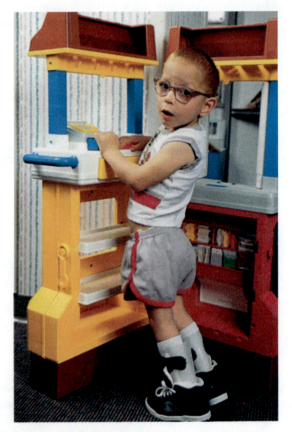

FIGURE 5.3 Child with cerebral palsy.

proper care and teaching, individuals with these conditions can live productive and happy lives.

The exact reason people are born with developmental disabilities is not known. However, we do know that these conditions are not contagious. Here are four reasons that are known to cause developmental disabilities:

1. Deficiency during the development of the fetus (i.e., Down syndrome, as is shown in Figure 5.1 is believed to occur at this early time of development)
2. Infection or injury during fetus development or birth
3. Accident during developmental stages of childhood
4. Heredity

YOUR ROLE AS A CAREGIVER

As you care for children who have developmental disabilities, remember that they have the same needs as other children. As they become adults, they are expected to meet more needs for themselves. If your patient cannot meet all her needs, you or another adult will have to continue to help her meet her needs throughout her life.

Your feelings as you care for your patient are important. Do you feel as though you are doing a worthwhile activity? Do you feel as though you are contributing to the family life of your patient? Do you feel that your activities are a waste of time? If you feel uncomfortable or negative about your care of the patient, discuss your feelings with the health care team so that you can put your activities into perspective.

As you care for your patient, the plan of care will be determined by what your patient can do presently and what is expected of him in the future. The health care team can instruct you in ways to feed, carry, and/or help the child with mobility issues. It is important that each step be carefully planned so that the patient does not get discouraged or attempt an activity that is dangerous for her. In addition, it is necessary to establish a plan the family can follow when you are not in the home and they must assume the care of the individual.

Stimulation of the patient is an important activity of the caregiver. You may "play" with the patient. Do not neglect this activity because it is necessary for proper development of the senses. However, different activities are appropriate for different ages and stages of development, so do not assume an activity is correct until you are directed by the health care team. All of your activities will fall into one of these categories:

• Supporting the family in the form of demonstration, respite, or discussion
• Encouraging independence up to the ability of the patient
• Providing physical and emotional care for the patient
• Providing a safe general environment, in particular with feeding, bathing, and ambulation

As you care for the child in the home, observe the family dynamics. How do the members of the family interact with each other and with the patient?

Do they consider her a part of the family or merely an imposition? Are family members following the agreed-upon plan when you are not in the home? The care of a developmentally disabled child can be a draining experience on all family members. Each one is affected in a different way. It is your role to observe and report family interactions that may affect the care and safety of your patient. With prompt reporting, the health care team can intervene and provide support, counseling, or other aid to the family.

Children Under Stress

Everyone reacts to stress and change differently. Children are especially sensitive to threats to their security and familiar routines. This is true both of children who are ill and those who are in homes where there is illness. You may notice a child behave in a manner that is unusual, offensive, and difficult to explain. You may notice:

- refusal to follow familiar household routines
- shyness, fear, withdrawal
- aggressive behavior
- jealousy
- nightmares and fears
- denial of the condition
- being overly dependent
- bed wetting
- regression

When illness is present in a home, many factors can affect the child. Here are a few examples:

- noise restrictions
- attention restrictions
- financial conditions
- family fears
- activity restrictions

Discipline and Punishment

You may be faced with the subject of discipline or punishment—and there is a difference. Remember, if you are not the parent or guardian but the caregiver in the home, your role will be different. Discipline is a set of rules that govern conduct and actions, resulting in orderly behavior. Discipline can be strict or loose. The rules can be well known or not well known. Discipline can be accepted or just followed for fear of punishment. Punishment is a harsh act imposed as a result of an offense or wrong doing, as when a rule or discipline is broken.

The goal of directing children is to teach them behavior that is accepted by society and will foster self-reliance and independence. Children must feel good about themselves and their actions. They should not act because it will prevent punishment. Self-esteem is developed early in a child's life and is directly related to the way in which behavior is taught and reinforced.

Your role is usually to maintain the discipline already in the home. If you are going to set up new rules in the house, be sure and discuss the rules with the household members and if necessary the health care team before implementing them. Remember, if you leave this house, the other people will still be present. You must set up rules they can live with when you are gone. If the current discipline seems unusually harsh or punishment seems severe, report this with objective data to the social worker on the health care team. Punishment is not within your role as a caregiver. As you work with children, remember the following points:

- Treat each child as an individual.
- Discuss with the child the expectations related to his behavior or a particular task. "I expect ____. Do you understand?"
- Encourage and praise children whenever possible.
- Use positive suggestions. Avoid saying "Don't." Instead, say, "Please make your bed," or "Please lower the television because it is disturbing your grandfather and he needs to sleep now. Thank you."
- Explain the limits set on the behavior before the child makes a mistake. "You may play outside until it is dark. Then you are to come in. Do you understand?"
- Make mealtime a pleasure.
- Prepare food the child enjoys.
- Encourage parents to take an active part in making decisions.
- Do not take sides in arguments.
- Suggest that people separate during an argument before harsh words are said or physical punishment takes place.
- Do not be judgmental.
- Report changes in family members.
- Report changes in family activities.
- Report feelings or suggestions and the objective happenings that lead you to your suspicions.
- Report child abuse or neglect.

YOUR ROLE AS A CAREGIVER

Your role in the family will be different when you are a caregiver. Be sure you discuss your role with the family and the health care team so you understand exactly what is expected of you. Usually, you will be expected to assume one or more of the following roles:

- Teacher
- Primary caregiver
- Observer
- Stabilizer
- Assistant caregiver

Try to maintain the routine familiar to the family. If things are working for the household, the fewer changes, the better. Familiarity maintains a feeling of security. If a child has always been involved in household tasks, it would be best to continue this practice. However, if the child has never taken an active part in the house or its care, this time of illness might not be the best time to start. On the other hand, it might. Use your judgment.

Report all your observations of behavior changes in the child and the adults of the house. You may notice many changes or few. When caring for children, remember that they are part of a unit and depend on that unit. Therefore, the behavior of other family members is important.

Be alert for observations concerning behavior in the home when you are not there. What does the child say? Do your observations agree with the child's report or the adult's report? Your personal opinions about the responsibilities children are not important at this time. The most important point is what works for this household!

CHILD ABUSE

Abuse is any act considered improper and that usually causes harm or pain to another person. No one knows exactly how many children are harmed, and no one knows why some people abuse children. Many possible reasons for abuse have been explored. Abuse may be linked to increased stress in a house and may happen only once in a while. Even if it only occurs occasionally or just once, it must be reported to protect the child and help the family as a whole (see Clinical Alert 5.1).

No matter what the reasons for abuse of children, all of them result in children being either physically or emotionally traumatized. Sometimes the children report these events, but most often, they do not (see Figure 5.4). Thus, your role in reporting child abuse is important for children's safety.

Some Reasons for Abuse

- The abuser was also abused and is repeating this learned behavior.
- The abuser cannot cope with the stress of having children or a child who is ill or disabled.
- The abuser is not the parent, but the parent is unable to stop the event.

CLINICAL ALERT 5.1

Observations About Children

Whether a child is your patient or not, if you witness, hear about, or find out about something hurtful, cruel, or dangerous to a child, you must report this immediately to the appropriate member on the health care team. Different cultures treat children in different ways, but *all* children in the United States are entitled to be safe and free from harm, regardless of the culture in which they live. This is one time when cultural differences are not acceptable and abuse should be reported.

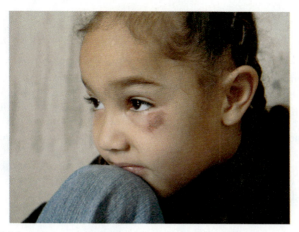

FIGURE 5.4 Child abuse is a serious problem that must be reported.

Reasons Children Do Not Report Abuse

- They are ashamed, believing some action on their part caused the abuse.
- They do not know whom to tell.
- They do not know any other type of behavior, so being abused is the norm.
- They are afraid the abuse will increase.
- They believe they deserve it.
- They don't think anyone will believe them if they tell.
- The abuser has threatened to harm others (for example, a cherished pet) if they tell.

Types of Abuse

There are three main types of child abuse:

1. *Physical:* This form of abuse is seen when a child is beaten, tied up, and/or burned. Evidence of this abuse is usually visible, except in the case of broken bones, when the evidence must be verified by X-ray (see Clinical Alert 5.2).
2. *Emotional:* This form of abuse is seen when a child is scared, neglected, screamed at, called names, not permitted to feel safe, or is confined.
3. *Sexual:* This form of abuse exists when a child is forced to submit to sexual acts because of fear of either physical or emotional harm or because the child cannot prevent it.

Your Feelings About Child Abuse

Many people have strong feelings about child abuse and the punishments they feel are appropriate for abusers. Some people think children should be removed from the house where they were abused. Some people feel the

CLINICAL ALERT 5.2

Shaken Baby Syndrome

Shaking an infant or child can never be justified. Shaking a baby usually occurs when the caregiver is stressed by the infant's or child's crying or other behavior that doesn't change when the caregiver tries other techniques. In an adult brain, there is a fluid that cushions the brain from trauma or sudden impact against the skull. In children, however, this cushion and the skull are not fully developed, and shaking can cause a lack of oxygen to the brain, brain cell damage, and even death. The best way to prevent a child from being shaken is to intervene or ask for help when a behavior is distressing the caregiver. Even a small break from a crying baby can make all the difference.

abusers should be put in jail. It is important to think about your feelings on this subject. It is also important to be able to care for a patient in a home where there has been abuse without judging the people. For example, as a caregiver your responsibility will be to care for the child in the family without punishing the parent or family member who is the abuser. If at any time you feel unable to be in the role of caregiver in this home where abuse has occurred, call a member of the patient's health care team.

Your Role as a Caregiver

As a caregiver, your role will be determined in part by the home situation. For instance, the courts will sometimes insist that a caregiver be in the home. In this case, the parents may feel you are acting as "the police." Your main role is to provide a safe environment for the child and to support the parent in learning to cope with the problem. Learning new behavior is difficult, and your support is crucial in this situation. Be calm and nonjudgmental, and demonstrate the proper way to interact with the child.

In some cases, the parent is removed from the house and you will be the primary caregiver instead. In this case, act in a supportive way to the child and provide a safe, calm environment.

It is possible you will be caring for a member of the family where abuse is taking place. In this case, you may have come by this information by accident. No matter how you obtained this information, it is important to report it immediately! In some states, it is a crime *not* to report such information.

No matter what the case, if you are in a home where child abuse has taken place, here are some general guidelines:

- Do not be judgmental. Do not compare their lives with yours. Be supportive to the parents.
- Be observant! Observe the family dynamics. How do the people in the family interact? Do they scream? Do they tease? Do they talk nicely to one member and in a hostile tone to another?

- Are there any signs of further abuse? Do the children have marks on them? Are they fed? Is there food in the house? Do they have a place to sleep? Are they clean? Do they laugh? Do they play? Do they seem afraid?
- Have you noticed any unusual behavior?

Your feelings are important in these cases. If you suspect something wrong in the family dynamics, report your feelings and objective observations to the health care team immediately. Do not wait! Children cannot always protect themselves. They need adults to do it for them.

NEWBORN AND INFANT CARE

You may be caring directly for a child or you may be caring for the mother and other family members may care for the child. Or you may be caring for both mother and child. Reasons you may care for an infant include the following:

- The mother is recovering from surgery.
- The mother is unable emotionally to assume the care of the child alone.
- There are many other children in the house that need the mother's attention.
- The infant is ill.
- The infant has been abused.

The most important part of your role in this house is to teach by example. You may not be in this home forever, and it is important that others can take over when you leave. One of the tasks you will teach is how to hold the baby comfortably and safely.

Most infants are fed six times a day or about every three to four hours. Nursing babies, however, may be fed as often as every two hours. It is important to remember that some will eat more often and some less. Stick to the schedule already in place in the home. If the mother is breastfeeding her baby, it may be your responsibility to bring the baby to her when it is time for feeding. If the baby is being bottle-fed, you may need to prepare the formula. Your role will be established by the family and health care team if applicable. If you have any questions, ask.

The Postpartum Period

The first several weeks after childbirth are considered the postpartum period, the time when a woman is getting used to being a mother for the first time or getting used to this baby. She is bonding with the child and getting acquainted with it. Her body is changing rapidly. Women also experience emotional changes as their role changes, as their hormones change, and as their bodies return to their pre-pregnancy state (see Clinical Alert 5.3). For more information on postpartum care, see the Resource Page at the end of this book.

CLINICAL ALERT 5.3

Postpartum Care

Call the physician if:

- the patient experiences a high temperature and/or chills.
- there is any discomfort, pain, or discoloration of the limbs or abdomen.
- there is any difficulty breathing or speaking, or general anxiety.
- the lochia is excessive and/or foul-smelling.
- the patient has difficulty urinating or voiding is painful.
- there is a sudden change in the patient's condition.
- if the breasts develop a red area that is hard, warm, or unusually painful.

Families react to the addition of a new child in many ways. Families have cultural practices that dictate how they react to the new mother. Some families react differently when the child is a girl or when the child is a boy. Some families lavish gifts and attention on the child. Some lavish gifts and attention on the mother. Some do neither.

Changes for Family Members

Changes affect all members of the family. Husbands or significant others either become fathers for the first time or learn to balance emotions for one more children. Sometimes, the new responsibility is assumed with ease. Sometimes, the man becomes frightened and does not know how to respond. It takes time to learn the role of father. Be patient. Refer to role models the man may have had as he grew up. He will be able to identify those behaviors he liked as a child and those he did not. Thinking about those details will help him pattern his behavior to support his child.

Learning to relate to a woman who has become a mother also takes time. Encourage the new mother and father to talk about their needs and feelings with each other. If they need professional assistance, contact the physician for a referral.

Children need to adjust to a new sibling, too. The presence of a new brother or sister can affect each child differently. Respect each child's way of adjusting to the new family member. If you have any questions about the meaning of behaviors, discuss it with your supervisor. Remember, children are all individuals. Do not compare one child with another.

- Some children assume extra responsibility.
- Some children return to childish behaviors such as baby talk, thumb sucking, or even bed wetting.
- Some children may refuse to go to school, leave their house, or leave their parents.
- Some children ignore the new baby.
- Some children are anxious to take part in the care of the new baby.

Emotional Changes for the New Mother

It is difficult to predict how a woman will react to a new baby. Each woman is different, and each birth experience is different. Usually, however, there are several shared experiences. When emotional concerns prevent the woman from taking part in the care of the new baby or from having any interest in her family, report this to the physician or nurse so that a complete assessment can be made and a plan of care formulated that will help the mother through this difficult time.

- Women usually experience mood swings, which result from the hormonal changes and the fact that the woman is assessing her new role and planning how to adjust. Some women are weepy. Some are euphoric and have a great deal of energy.
- Women may want friends around or they may want to be alone. Be sensitive to the wish of your patient. If she wants to be alone, gently tell friends and family members that perhaps they should call before coming to visit or they should come and stay for short periods of time. Designating a time to visit is helpful so that the patient and the visitor know the time frame set for the visit.
- Getting used to a body that is continuously changing is difficult for some women. It takes about six weeks until the internal organs return to prenatal status. It may take six months for the woman to lose weight and regain her prenatal appearance. Support her as she tries to exercise, change her diet, and become familiar with her changing needs. Encourage her to discuss exercise regimes with her physician before any new activity is started.

Physical Changes

During the first six weeks after birth, a woman's body is continuously changing. During the first two to three days, a reddish, bloody discharge from the vagina is to be expected. About the fourth day, this discharge, called locia, changes to yellow and continues for another week. Usually, all discharge stops about the twenty-first day. The discharge is normal, and the woman should wear whatever peripads she wishes. It is usually recommended that they be deodorant-free. Tampons are not to be worn. Dispose of the used pads as you would any dressing in a paper or plastic bag. The perineum should be cleaned and washed with warm soapy water after each bowel movement and voiding. The peripads should be changed at that time, too.

Usually, the woman loses the fluid she accumulates during pregnancy between the second and fifth day postpartum. Encourage her to continue to drink fluids throughout this period as water and fruit juices will help with the process and prevent dehydration.

It is important that bowel function be regular during this time. Because the perineal area may be sore, bowel movements may be uncomfortable. If this is the case, encourage your patient to discuss this with her physician so that stool softeners can be prescribed. A diet that has sufficient fiber and fluid usually prevents most discomfort. If you have concerns that regular bowel function is not occurring, discuss this with your supervisor. If hemorrhoids are present, a sitz bath (warm water with Epsom salts) or an over-the-counter product can ease the swelling. A doughnut-shaped pillow will also relieve the pressure from the hemorrhoids.

Diet

During this period, a balanced diet is important. It helps with maintaining a feeling of well-being, regulating bowel and bladder function, and helping the body return to prenatal status. A woman who is nursing requires additional calories and fluids. During the postpartum period, a woman should be encouraged to eat regularly and enjoy her food. This is not the time to start crash diets or decrease fluids in an attempt to lose weight.

Contraception

Sexual relations following the birth of a child are a deeply personal activity. Sometimes, a change occurs in the pattern of sexual activity. This change will be discussed between the patient and her partner. Often, if questions or concerns remain, she should be encouraged to discuss these with her physician.

Remind your patient that pregnancy can occur shortly after the birth of a child. Pregnancy can also occur while a woman is nursing a child and before normal menstrual periods have resumed. Contraception or abstinence is recommended if another pregnancy is to be avoided.

Breast Care

The decision to breastfeed a baby is a personal one. If your patient has made a decision different from the one you would have made, respect her decision and support her. Sometimes, even when a woman decides not to breastfeed, her breasts fill with milk. Encourage her to call her physician if this happens. Breasts should always be supported with a good bra until they return to prenatal size. They should be kept clean at all times.

Carrying an Infant

Carrying an infant is a big responsibility. It is important to pay close attention to many details and safety factors.

- Always support the child's head (see Figure 5.5).
- Hold the infant close to you.
- Do not carry other objects while you are carrying a baby.
- Do not hold an infant while you are talking on the phone or cooking at the stove.
- Do not carry a baby into a dark room. Turn on the light before you enter.
- Be alert to basic household hazards such as liquid spills, shoes, clothing on the floor, and loose rugs.

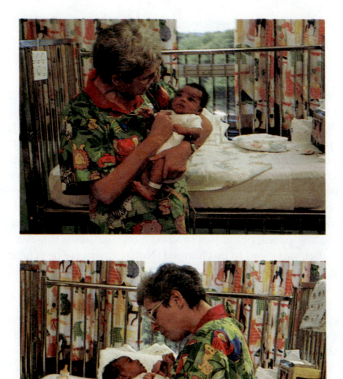

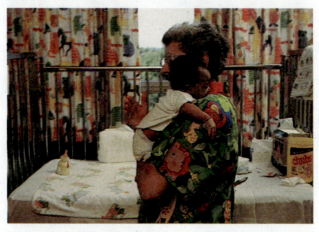

FIGURE 5.5 Support the baby in a comfortable manner so you can see where you are going and the baby is still safe and secure.

- Be alert while carrying a baby up and down stairs.
- Wear good supporting shoes with nonskid soles while you are carrying a baby.

Chidren's Diets

Children's diets vary. Different pediatricians add cereal to diets at different ages. Some pediatricians encourage breastfeeding; some do not. It is important to support the family members as they learn to follow the diet their physician has prescribed. Although you may have definite feelings about the manner in which the child's diet has been ordered, do not change it. Do not change a diet or routine without discussing it with the physician and the parent(s).

Observe the pediatric patient for her acceptance of the diet. If you notice the child has a great deal of gas following a meal, cries a great deal, has diarrhea or is constipated, or refuses food on a regular basis, this is a sign something in the diet may need to be changed. Notify the nurse or physician on the health care team if these conditions continue. Remember, the child is unable to ask for help herself. She needs you to report her distress.

BREASTFEEDING As a caregiver, your responsibilities may include assisting in the feeding of an infant or in the training of a new mother to breastfeed a newborn. Breastfeeding is a natural act. Most babies and mothers learn how to do this while the mother is still in the hospital. By the time they come home, the mother will probably have had an opportunity to learn basic breastfeeding skills. If further training is necessary, providing more materials on the topic may be helpful. Ask the nurse on the health care team for this information (see Guideline 5.1).

GUIDELINE 5.1

Assisting with Breastfeeding

1. Remind the mother to wash her hands before each feeding. Hands should be washed with a mild soap. Nipples are usually washed with mild soapy water or plain water and rinsed thoroughly during daily bathing. Washing the nipples before each feeding is not usually necessary. The mother should use circular motions, from the nipple outward, when she washes.
2. Assist the mother with nursing aids such as breast shields or pumps.
3. The decision to stop nursing is a personal one and will affect both mother and child. Suggest to the mother that she discuss this decision with her physician before any decision is made.
4. Assist the mother in positioning the baby into a comfortable position (see Figure 5.6).
5. If the baby does not take the breast, have the mother stroke the cheek closest to the breast with her nipple. This will cause the child to turn toward the breast.
6. Support the mother as she learns the skill of breastfeeding. Provide quiet time between feedings so the mother can rest.

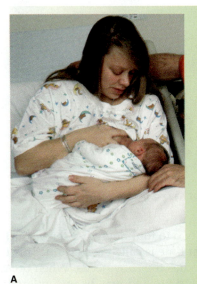
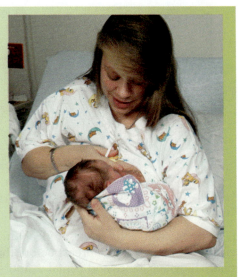

A

B

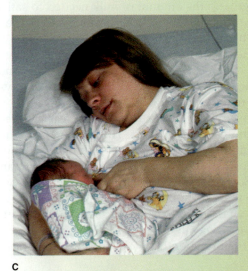

C

FIGURE 5.6 Various positions the mother can use when nursing Cradle Hold **(A)**, Upright Position **(B)**, Football Hold **(C)**.

7. While the nipple is in the baby's mouth, remind the mother to keep the breast tissue away from the baby's nose with one or two fingers (see Figure 5.7).

8. If milk drips from the breast not being sucked, clean the breast. This is normal.

9. To remove the nipple from the baby's mouth, the mother should break the suction by either inserting her little finger in the corner of the baby's mouth or pushing on her breast tissue near the baby's mouth.

10. The feeding routine and length of nursing will vary and should be decided by the mother.

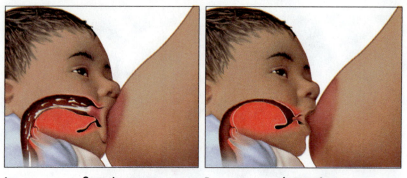

A   **Correct**   B   **Incorrect**

FIGURE 5.7 The correct and incorrect position of having the baby latch on.

The female body makes milk about two to four days after the birth. The clear yellow fluid in the breast before that time is called colostrum. This is a nourishing substance and contains antibodies the baby needs. When breasts start to fill with milk, they become hard and full and may be uncomfortable. As the baby nurses, the body regulates the amount of milk needed to satisfy the baby, the discomfort disappears, and the breasts become soft. As the baby grows and needs more milk, the body adjusts the supply.

During the first few days after birth, nursing may stimulate the mother's uterus to contract. Sometimes this is uncomfortable, and sometimes it is not. Encourage the new mother to discuss any discomfort with her nurse or physician before she takes medication to relieve the pain.

Most experts recommend feeding the baby from both breasts at each feeding—usually six to eight minutes at each breast. The mother's nutrition greatly influences the quality of milk the body produces. The mother should eat a balanced diet, take vitamins if the physician recommends them, and increase calorie intake slightly. Some medications, alcohol, and caffeine will pass through the bloodstream to the milk and to the baby. It is generally advised to avoid these substances while nursing. The nursing mother should drink six to eight glasses of fluid each day. If the baby sleeps well and nurses seven to ten times a day during the first months of life, the milk is sufficient and the baby is nursing well.

Some families feel comfortable with having a mother feed her baby while other family members are present. Some women prefer privacy. Support the mother and the family in their decision. You may be asked to help the mother ready herself to breastfeed, which may involve assisting the mother in getting comfortable; removing distractions; or bringing the baby, after you have changed the diaper, to the mother. Some women nurse sitting up; others lie on their side, which allows the infant to lay on its side facing the mother.

The mother may have questions about the timing of the feeding, ways in which to interest the baby in feeding, her diet, or care of her breasts. Assist the mother in reading the material provided to her. This material includes advice on whether to feed from both breasts in one feeding, how long to nurse, and how to supplement feedings if necessary. If this material does not answer her questions or if you have questions, contact the nurse or physician for further information.

BOTTLE FEEDING The decision to bottle-feed an infant or to supplement breast-feeding with formula is made by the mother and her physician. Choosing the type of formula is also made with medical advice. Your role is to support the mother and the family with their decision. In some cases, the mother will use a special pump to remove her breast milk and put it in a bottle for use later.

Sterilizing Bottles and Nipples

Bottles and nipples are sterilized to destroy bacteria that might cause illness. There are many opinions as to the age when sterilizing bottles is no longer necessary. Some physicians do not require sterilizing bottles for newborns. Follow the instructions from the hospital and/or physician. If you do not agree or have questions, ask for an explanation. Do not alter the procedure without the nurse or physician recommending the change.

Some people sterilize bottles and bottle nipples in the dishwasher. Others use microwave ovens. The most common method of sterilizing bottles and nipples, however, is on the stove by placing them in boiling water for one to two minutes (see Procedure 5.1).

PROCEDURE 5.1

Sterilizing Bottles

Rationale
Removing bacteria from baby bottles is a major factor in decreasing the possibility of infection and disease in an infant.

1. Assemble your equipment: bottles, nipples, caps, jar, bottle brush, dish detergent, large pot with cover or a special sterilizing pot for baby bottles, small towel, tap water, stove or heat source for cooking, timer or watch, tongs.
2. Wash your hands.
3. Scrub bottles, nipples, and caps with hot soapy water. Use the bottle brush to clean inside the bottles. Always squirt hot soapy water through the holes in the nipples to clean out any dried-on formula.
4. Rinse thoroughly with hot water.
5. If you do not have a bottle rack for the pan, fold a small towel to fit in the bottom of the pot and lay the bottle on the towel. This will prevent the bottles from breaking.
6. Stand the washed bottles on the towel in a circle around the inside of the pot (see Figure 5.8).
7. Place the caps and nipples into the clean, empty jar. Place into the pot at the center of the bottles.
8. Pour water into and around the bottles and into the jar with the nipples until two-thirds of each bottle is under water.

(continued)

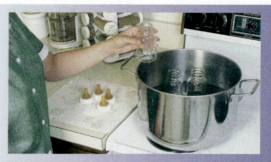

FIGURE 5.8 Sterilizing bottles on the stove.

9. Cover the pot.
10. Place the pot on the stove burner and turn on the burner to the high or full setting.
11. When the water comes to a full boil, begin timing. Allow the water to remain at a full boil for twenty-five minutes.
12. Remove the jar with the nipples and caps ten to fifteen minutes after the full boil begins. With the nipples still inside the jar, stand the jar on the table to cool.
13. Turn off the burner.
14. Take the cover off the pot and allow it to cool.
15. Remove the sterile bottles from the pot with sterile tongs.
16. Empty the water out of the pot. The pot is now sterilized, so you can use it for mixing the formula.
17. Wash your hands.

Types of Formula

READY-TO-FEED FORMULA (PREPARED FORMULA) The can or bottle of formula does not need to be refrigerated before it is opened. Wash all cans and bottles before opening. This type of formula needs no preparation. Remember to shake it before opening. Open the can with a sterilized can opener and pour the contents into sterile bottles. Open the bottle of ready-to-feed formula by unscrewing the cap. All you need to do now is screw a sterilized standard nipple right on the bottle the formula came in and feed the baby. Once opened, this formula must be kept refrigerated.

POWDERED FORMULA Powdered formula costs less per serving than ready-to-feed formula. The powdered formula comes in regular cans or in cardboard boxes. If the formula is in a can, wash and dry all cans before opening. Some cans will need to be opened with a sterilized can opener; others have a plastic lid with an inside cover to seal the powered milk for freshness. Carefully follow the instructions on the label about the amounts of powder and sterile water to mix together. Be sure to mix the powder with water that you have boiled or to use purified water. Mix the powder and boiled water in sterile bottles, a sterile pitcher, or a sterile pot. Once mixed, this formula must be kept refrigerated (see Clinical Alert 5.4; Guidelines 5.2 and 5.3; and Figures 5.9, 5.10, and 5.11).

CLINICAL ALERT 5.4
Feeding Safety

When feeding an infant with a bottle, be sure the formula or breast milk is not too hot. Test the milk by dripping some onto your wrist; it should be lukewarm, no more than 98.6°F, which is what temperature the milk is when it comes from the breast. If you start feeding an infant, and the infant starts to cry or moves its head away from the nipple of the bottle, it could be that the milk is too hot or too cold.

GUIDELINE 5.2
Assisting with Bottle-Feeding Using Formula

1. Make sure that the formula is fresh and the bottles have been properly stored.
2. Follow the mother's wishes about the temperature of the bottles when the baby is fed. However, always check the temperature of the formula before you feed the baby.
3. Babies should be held while they are given bottles. Do not prop bottles. Do not leave babies unattended while they are drinking from a bottle.
4. Hold the bottle so that the nipple is full of formula and the baby does not suck air.

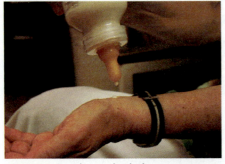

FIGURE 5.9 Always check the temperature of the milk before feeding it to the baby.

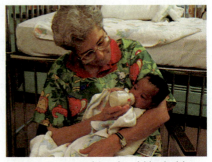

FIGURE 5.10 Babies should be held during bottle feeding.

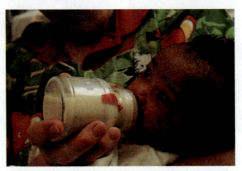

FIGURE 5.11 The nipple should be full of milk to avoid the baby sucking and swallowing air.

GUIDELINE 5.3

Storing Formula

1. Any opened container of formula can be refrigerated for two days without spoiling. After two days, it must be thrown away. If you do not know how long formula has been in the refrigerator, discard it. Mark the new can with the date when you open it.
2. Prepared formula will begin to spoil within two hours when left at room temperature. Keep the bottle refrigerated until ten minutes before the feeding.

CONCENTRATED LIQUID FORMULA Concentrated liquid is the least expensive type of formula and requires water to be added prior to feeding. Shake and wash all cans before opening. Use a sterilized can opener. Be sure to mix the formula according to the directions on the container. *Dilute by adding the exact amount of water as directed.* Once mixed, this formula must be kept refrigerated.

Burping the Infant

Most infants, especially those who are bottle-fed, swallow some air while drinking. Air in the gastrointestinal tract can cause vomiting and abdominal pain. You can prevent a buildup of air by feeding the infant slowly and stopping after every two ounces to burp the baby. Burping helps the baby get rid of this excess air. There are two methods for burping a baby:

> *Method A:* Cover your shoulder with a clean cloth. This could be a small towel or a cloth diaper. Hold the baby in a vertical position so his head is resting on your shoulder. Gently rub and/or pat the infant's back until you hear the burp (see Figure 5.12).

> *Method B:* Sit the infant on your leg so her feet are dangling on your side. Put one of your hands on the infant's chest, and lean the baby over so your hand supports her. Gently rub and pat the baby's back with your other hand until you hear the burp (see Figure 5.13).

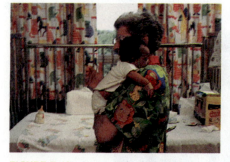 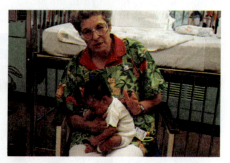

FIGURE 5.12 Support the baby against your shoulder as you gently pat his back.

FIGURE 5.13 Support the baby and his head by placing your hand on the chest and under the chin as you gently pat his back.

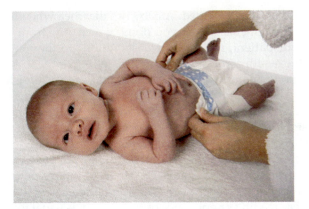

FIGURE 5.14

Diapers

Diapers are used to catch the urine and stool babies expel. By using diapers, you help keep the babies and their environment clean and free of waste material. The methods used to diaper a baby and the types of diaper used vary from house to house (see Figure 5.14). It is important for you to try and follow the wishes of the family as you care for the baby (see Guideline 5.4).

Observing the Infant's Stool

You will need to observe the infant's stool or bowel movement at each diaper change to detect constipation or diarrhea. A baby is constipated when

GUIDELINE 5.4

Changing Diapers

1. Change the diapers often to decrease odor and irritation of the baby's skin.
2. Clean the baby's genital area each time you change the diaper. Cleanse from front to back. Apply lotion or cream as you have been instructed.
3. If you use cloth diapers, rinse the stool from them in the toilet before you put them into a diaper pail.
4. If you use rubber pants on top of cloth diapers, be sure the elastic is loose enough to allow air to circulate in the pants.
5. Do not use rubber pants over disposable diapers because they already have moisture-proof protection.
6. Do not flush disposable diapers down a toilet. Dispose of them in a covered trash bin.
7. Observe the baby's skin each time you change the diaper for color, texture, and discharge.

the stool is hard and well formed. A baby has diarrhea when he has frequent watery bowel movements. When you observe a change from what has been normal for your patient, report your observations to the mother and other members of the health care team as appropriate.

The bottle-fed infant will have stools that are yellowish or mustard-colored. They will be lumpy, but soft. One to three bowel movements each day is normal for an infant who is bottle-fed every three to four hours. It is not unusual for the stools of bottle-fed babies to look as if there are tiny seeds in them.

The breast-fed infant will have stools that are yellowish or mustard-colored, but the color may change slightly and may appear to have a greenish tint, depending on the mother's diet. The stools of infants who are breast-fed will be looser and smoother than those of bottle-fed infants. A bowel movement after every feeding or only once or twice a day is usual for an infant who is breast-fed every three to four hours.

Diarrhea in infants can be a serious problem and requires immediate attention. An infant with diarrhea can become dehydrated within two days. You will see a change in the infant's elimination pattern and in the color and consistency of the stools when an infant has diarrhea. The stools may appear green and watery, running right out of the diaper. There may be a foul odor, and stool frequency will increase as compared to the infant's normal habit. Report to the physician at the first sign of diarrhea, or encourage the mother to call the physician.

Diarrhea has many causes in infants. It may be caused by equipment that is not sterilized properly, by carelessly prepared or spoiled formula, or by allergies. Much diarrhea is caused by passing bacteria to the infant from the hands of those who handle her. This is the reason proper handwashing is essential when caring for an infant. Encourage everyone who handles the infant to wash their hands frequently and certainly before handling the baby or equipment used in her care. Be sure to explain why you are asking them to do this to avoid offending anyone.

Care of the Umbilical Cord

Before birth, the umbilical cord serves as a lifeline, connecting the fetus with the mother's placenta. All nourishment is passed from mother to fetus through the umbilical cord. At the time of delivery, the cord is clamped and cut, and the healing process of the umbilicus begins. Within five to ten days, the part of the cord that is still attached to the baby will become dry, turn black, and eventually fall off, forming the umbilicus. This does not hurt the baby. As the caregiver, you may be asked to clean around the area where the umbilical cord was clamped, but it is important to let the cord piece fall off on its own (see Guideline 5.5).

Bathing the Infant

Sponge baths with warm water or baby lotion can be given daily until the umbilical cord falls off. More frequent bathing is usually unnecessary. A tub

GUIDELINE 5.5
Care of the Umbilical Cord

1. Keep the diaper folded down away from the cord. A wet diaper on top of the cord could cause an infection.
2. At every diaper change, wash the cord according to physician's recommendations. Never pull on the cord. Let it fall off by itself. Laying the infant on his abdomen will not hurt the cord. Binders or belly bands are not advised.
3. Never give the infant a tub bath until the cord has fallen off.

bath is not permitted until the cord has fallen off. Sponge bathing an infant means gently washing each part of the baby's body with mild soap and warm water, not submerging the infant in water. A safe table or counter is a convenient place to give a sponge bath. Clear off the counter and wash it well. Spread a towel on the counter to make a soft warm place on which to place the baby. Prepare warm water, mild soap, washcloth, blankets, and towels before bringing the baby to the counter. Only one part of the body is washed at a time. Wash, rinse, and dry each body part or area well. Then cover the body part right away with a towel or blanket. The safety of the infant is most important. Whenever in doubt about anything, call the appropriate member of the health care team who can provide you further instruction.

TUB BATHS Tub baths are allowed after the cord has fallen off. You can use the tub or a baby bathtub. Be sure to clean the tub by scrubbing with a cleanser and rinsing it thoroughly. Assemble your equipment before you begin so you will not need to leave the room for something you may have forgotten. Lock the front door so no one can come in and distract you or the infant's mother. Taking the phone off the hook, if the mother agrees, will prevent it from ringing during the bath. You cannot leave the infant in the tub or on the counter while you answer the phone or the doorbell.

Bath time should be a pleasant and enjoyable time for the mother and baby. Try to involve the mother as much as she is able, and take the opportunity to teach her how to care for the baby. The infant's safety is your first responsibility. Keep your hands and eyes on the baby throughout the bath (see Procedure 5.2).

Infant Safety

When you care for an infant, you must take special precautions to protect the baby from preventable accidents and infection. Even if an infant has not yet learned to roll over, he can wiggle and kick until he falls off beds, chairs, tables, or counters. Never leave an infant unattended on any of these surfaces. If you are far from the infant's crib and you must leave him unattended for a few seconds, put him on the floor. The safest place for an infant is in his crib with the side rails up. It is important to make sure a baby is sleeping on his or her back

PROCEDURE 5.2

Giving an Infant a Tub Bath

Rationale

Bathing an infant removes bacteria, increases circulation, and allows close interaction between you and the infant.

1. Assemble your equipment: infant tub or sink, two bath towels (soft), cotton balls, washcloth, warm water, baby soap, baby shampoo (optional), baby powder, lotion or cream, diaper, and clean clothes.
2. Wash your hands.
3. Wash the sink or tub with a disinfectant cleanser and rinse thoroughly.
4. Line the sink or tub with a bath towel.
5. Place a towel on the counter next to the sink or tub because you may want to lay the infant down to dry him.
6. Fill the tub or sink with one to two inches of warm water (warm to the touch of the elbow).
7. Undress the infant, wrap him in a towel or blanket, and bring him to the tub or sink.
8. Using a cotton ball moistened with warm water and squeezed out, gently wipe the infant's eyes from the nose toward the ears. Use a clean cotton ball for each wipe of the eye.
9. To wash the hair, hold the infant in the football hold, with the baby's head over the sink or tub. This will free your other arm to wet the hair, apply a small amount of shampoo, and rinse the hair.
10. Dry the infant's head with a towel.
11. Unwrap the infant, and gently place him on the towel in the sink or tub. One of your hands should always be holding the baby. Never let go, not even for a second.
12. Wash the infant's body with the soap and the washcloth, being careful to wash between the folds (creases) of the skin (see Figure 5.15).

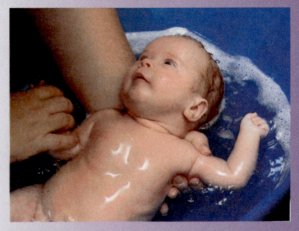

FIGURE 5.15 Tub baths are fun.

13. If the infant is female, always wash the perineal area from front to back.
14. If the infant is male, gently clean the penis. Be careful to follow the physician's orders regarding circumcision, if applicable.
15. Rinse the infant thoroughly with warm water.
16. Lift the infant out of the water and onto the towel you laid out on the counter.
17. Dry the infant well, being careful to dry between folds of skin.
18. Now you can apply powder, lotion, or cream to the infant. When applying lotion or cream, apply to your hands and then to the infant.
19. Diaper and dress the infant.
20. Place the infant in his crib, or hold him.
21. Clean and return equipment and supplies to their proper place.
22. Clean the area where the bath was given.
23. Wash your hands.

with few extra covers or toys in the crib. Too many items in the crib can provide the opportunity for the baby to get trapped or even suffocate. This is one of the leading theories on what causes sudden infant death syndrome (SIDS). Some people keep babies in a baby carrier or bassinet because they do not have a crib. Here are other ways you can prevent accidents when caring for an infant:

- Wash your hands before caring for the infant or handling supplies used to care for the infant.
- Place the infant on her side after feeding to prevent aspiration.
- Keep the crib rails in the up position when the infant is sleeping or playing.
- Use only one to two inches of bath water, and never leave the infant alone in the water.
- Never place an infant in an infant seat on tables, chairs, beds, or counters.
- Keep all medications and cleaning solutions out of the reach of all children.

Circumcision

Circumcision is the surgical removal of the loose piece of skin, the prepuce (foreskin), from the end of the penis (see Figure 5.16). Circumcision can be done in the operating room before the baby comes home. It is always a voluntary procedure. That means that the mother of the baby must give her permission to have it done. In the Jewish faith, there is a ritual circumcision on the seventh day after birth. This ritual is performed either in the hospital or at home.

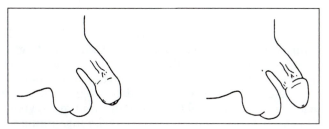

FIGURE 5.16 Uncircumcised vs. circumcised.

GUIDELINE 5.6

Care After a Circumcision

1. Keep the penis protected from rubbing on a diaper. The pediatrician will leave instructions.
2. Keep the penis clean and free of fecal matter.
3. Observe for bleeding, drainage, and/or infection. Report any signs of these conditions to the physician.

The physician will give the mother special instructions about the care of the penis. Be sure to follow these instructions carefully to prevent complications. The after-care instructions will include signs and symptoms that indicate when the physician should be contacted (see Guideline 5.6).

Assisting with Medication

A child you are caring for may require medication. Although you may assist, you may not necessarily be the person who assumes the responsibility of giving the medication. The family may take responsibility for giving the medication. See Chapter 17 for additional discussion on giving medication. In either case, part of your role is to observe the child after she has received medication. If you notice any change in her behavior, call the physician or 911 immediately. Common changes that should be reported are the following:

- Rash or any change in the skin color or texture
- Irritability, confusion, or unusual fussiness
- Change in sleep pattern
- Pain that persists and is not removed by the medication
- Vomiting, diarrhea, or constipation
- Change in breathing pattern
- Confusion
- Seizures

Summary

Working with children can be very rewarding. Caring for a child with an illness or disability can also be very challenging. Understanding the development, cognitive functioning, and activities that can be used when caring for a child can contribute to the caregiver's success. The most important thing you can do is keep the child safe. Safe not only from injury but safe from illness caused by lack of infection control (i.e., washing equipment, your hands, and the hands of visitors). Finally, support the family by integrating your caregiving style into their family culture and support the routines in place.

Chapter 6

Care of the Dying in the Home

SCENARIO

Mrs. Bell is eighty-six years old and lives with her husband of sixty years. She has just been told she has advanced breast cancer. Mr. and Mrs. Bell have decided that she will be cared for at home without any treatment or heroic measures to prolong her life, and they will face this as they have faced everything, together. Mr. Bell has learned how to manage the pain medication, and by working with the nurses and volunteers, he cares for his beloved wife. He will accept help only once in a while from you, Mrs. Bell's health aide and granddaughter. Mrs. Bell eats small amounts of puréed food and drinks little. The three children and ten other grandchildren visit and help with the shopping, laundry, cooking, and cleaning. They update their grandparents on their activities, and the little children draw them pictures, which hang around the bedroom. Your aunts and uncles confide in you that they do not know how their father will manage when their mother dies. When they try to talk to their father, he says, "Don't worry. It will work out" (see Figure 6.1).

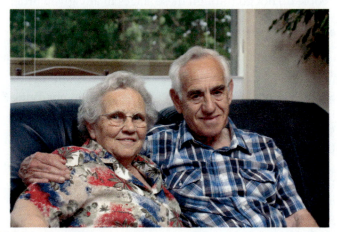

FIGURE 6.1

97

M any of us feel uncomfortable when we are around a person who is dying. We may not know how to act or what to say to him. We may feel sad or helpless or angry. These feelings may be strong indeed if the person is the same age we are or a member of our family. Sometimes, we deal with our feelings by avoiding caring for the person who is dying, or we rush through our tasks as quickly as possible so that we can leave the room. This often leaves the dying person feeling isolated, lonely, or deserted.

To prevent negative feelings and repercussions, as a caregiver, no matter your relationship with the family, it is your responsibility to help meet the special needs of the dying person and the family. Do not be frightened by the thought of helping a person who is dying. As with any person, it is important to be caring and to show consideration and understanding to the individual who is dying.

Delivering the news to a patient that he or she is dying should be done by a family member or physician. If a family decides not to tell the incompetent patient that he or she is dying, you are obligated to carry out the family's wishes even though, at times, keeping up this charade is difficult.

THE DYING PROCESS

Dr. Elisabeth Kübler-Ross spent many years talking with the dying and studying how people die. She found certain stages are involved. It is important to remember the following:

- All people are different.
- The family of the person who is dying may also go through all or some of these stages.
- Everyone may not experience every stage
- Patients and families can go from stage to stage at any time for any length of time.
- People do not go through these stages in any given order.

Stages of Grieving

The following are the stages Dr. Kubler Ross found to be consistent with the grieving process.

Stage 1: Denial/ Shock—"I don't believe it, I am not dying."
Underlying this denial is a feeling of numbness.

Stage 2: Anger—"Why me? It isn't fair."
Underlying the anger is a feeling of helplessness.

Stage 3: Bargaining—"If I do . . . , then maybe I won't die."
Underlying this attempt at bargaining is a feeling of hope. This bargaining is often done with God.

Stage 4: Depression—Mourning past and future losses.
Underlying this depression is a feeling of sadness.

Stage 5: Acceptance—"I am dying."
Underlying the admission of imminent death is a feeling of peace or contentment.

Emotional Needs of the Dying

People who are dying are still living people and have the same needs as you, including:

- *The need to be normal:* Patients need to know that their thoughts and feelings are like those of others in their situation.
- *The need for meaningful relationships:* Patients need a chance to talk to friends and family members on a meaningful level.
- *The need for love:* Patients need to feel that they are the object of someone's love (couples may have sexual exchanges).
- *The need for recreation:* Patients need ways to pass the time. These types of activities may include knitting, playing cards, watching TV, reading books, or talking to loved ones.
- *The need for safety and security:* Patients need to know that they will be cared for carefully up until the moment of death. Most patients worry about pain management.

Understanding Your Feelings About Death

To work effectively with someone in the end stages of life, it is important to explore your own feelings about death. When was the first time you experienced death? What do you believe about the dying process? What are your wishes for your end of life? For most people, their first exposure to death (usually as a child) affects how they will react to death for the rest of their lives. The time, place, and manner of death we experience may be different, but the feelings are the same. Often, people think differently when they experience a death of a baby or young person versus an older or terminally ill person. Some people feel differently about the death of a person when it occurs unexpectedly. Explore your beliefs and feelings to process any uncomfortable feelings you have in discussing death or being around people who are dying. To process these feelings, you may want to share these feelings with a close friend, member of the clergy, or someone else you trust. There is no right or wrong way to feel about death or to react to death. It is an individual experience.

YOUR ROLE AS A CAREGIVER

When a person suspects that she is going to die, she may react in various ways:

- She may ask everyone about her chances for recovery.
- She may be afraid to be alone and want a lot of attention.
- She may ask a lot of questions.

- She may seem to complain constantly.
- She may make requests that seem unreasonable.

Usually, when a patient asks questions of caregivers, she is sending a signal that she wants information. Many times, you may not have all the information needed to answer the questions. Assure the individual that you will either find the information or provide someone who will be able to help. Here are guidelines that you, as a caregiver, may wish to follow when talking with a patient who is dying:

1. *Be honest.* If you don't know, be honest and say so. The individual probably does not expect you to know everything about his condition anyway.
2. *Do not offer false hope or reassurance.* By telling a dying person that she will be better soon, the caregiver is proving she cannot be trusted. Offer realistic short-term goals or say nothing.
3. *Do not say too much.* Listening with a caring look, an unhurried manner, a nod, or word at the right time tells the person that you care. Example: "I understand how you feel. I think I would feel the same way" (see Figure 6.2).
4. *Let the patient take the lead.* Often, a question represents a fear or concern of the patient. He may feel relieved if you allow him to express the concern. Example: "I don't know when you'll die. Why do you ask?"
5. *Do not destroy hope.* If the patient really believes that she will recover, even if you know she won't, do not destroy this hope. Hope is an important part of life. The patient who has hope usually lives longer than the patient who does not. Example: "I'm happy to hear of your plans to go on a trip next year."

Many areas of the country have hospice programs. Hospice programs are organized systems of professional care that help families care for individuals

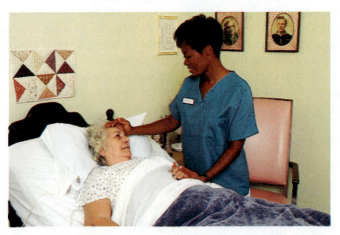

FIGURE 6.2 Show the patient that you care by listening.

CLINICAL ALERT 6.1

Palliative Care

The principles of palliative care can be applied to all patients. The way in which different cultures and individuals view pain and medication is important when creating a focus of care. Be aware of your personal views because they may unconsciously influence the way in which you approach providing care. Always report your observations of the patient, his or her family, and the effects of medication and other therapies in a timely and objective manner to the physician so any needed changes can be made.

at home up to and including the time of death. An individual typically begins care with hospice if the life expectancy is no longer than six months. The hospice concept is not appropriate for everyone because not everyone is able to die at home without any heroic methods. You can apply many principles of hospice care to your daily tasks even without actually having a hospice program in place.

Most hospice patients do not wish any treatment except to remain comfortable and pain-free. This is often difficult for families to accept. These programs support and help the dying person and his family without the use of curative methods. Palliative care is a multidisciplinary approach to managing pain and caring for a patient and family when the individual is seriously ill, suffers from a chronic illness, or is dying. Individuals who have palliative care programs may not be expected to die within six months and need not forego curative medical treatments (see Clinical Alert 6.1).

The primary goal of palliative care is to give the client the best possible life during the illness, through pain and symptom management, as well as patient and family support. Support and/or physical care may last a short time or an extended time, such as months or years.

Hospice and palliative care programs share many elements, including philosophy and caregivers, but the requirements of each program may differ. It is important for the family and patient to understand all elements of the program in which they enroll. As a caregiver, your role does not change much whether the person you are caring for is receiving palliative care or hospice care. The caregiver's responsibilities for either program include the following:

- Treating the patient and family as a unit of care.
- Allowing the patient and family as much choice as possible in determining care in the home.
- Making use of health care team professionals experienced in home health care.
- Supporting the family through the dying process.
- Supporting family members after the death of their loved one.

Both programs use trained volunteers to help with transportation, shopping, and assisting the patient with hobbies and other important activities that paid employees seldom have time to do. Program volunteer training sessions prepare community members to work with the dying and their families.

If you find yourself caring for a patient who has refused aggressive treatment and has decided to die, this may be hard for you to accept no matter your relationship with the individual. Remember, this is the patient's decision and you must accept it. You may also go through a grieving process. To learn more about hospice and death and dying, see the Resource Page at the end of this book.

ADVANCE DIRECTIVES FOR HEALTH CARE

All Americans have the fundamental right to make choices about their health care treatment. They can accept or refuse treatments as long as they are able to understand the consequences of those choices. However, when patients suffer from a disease or injury that takes away their ability to understand and make decisions about health care, they often suffer through treatments that they may not have wanted. Family members often consent to treatments for their loved one because they do not know what the patient wants and they are afraid to withhold any treatments. Such treatments may include ventilators, feeding tubes, dialysis, and other aggressive, life-prolonging interventions.

Laws have been created in all states to allow competent adults to create a document that indicates their choices about life-sustaining and life-prolonging treatments before an illness or injury strikes and before they may lose the capacity to make decisions for themselves. These documents are called advance directives for health care, commonly called living wills. The document is created by someone who has decision-making capacity and can describe her wishes with regard to future health care treatment choices. The document may also name a health-care proxy, whom they designate to make treatment choices for them in the event they become unable to do so. Each state has specific requirements for the advance directive to be valid. Therefore, the document should be tailored to the state in which the individual lives. Many states are incorporating documents such as a Medical Order for Scope of Treatment (MOST), which addresses the following issues:

- Do you want cardiopulmonary resuscitation (CPR) or not if your heart stops?
- What medical interventions do you want (comfort measures only, limited additional interventions, or full treatment)?
- Use of antibiotics or not and in which situations?
- Use of artificial nutrition and hydration or not and in which situations?
- Who was present when these issues were determined?

The Five Wishes document is another guide one can use in making end-of-life decisions (for more information or to obtain this document visit www.agingwithdignity.com). The Five Wishes document guides the doctor in following your wishes because you have answered the following questions:

- Who do you want to make health care decisions for you when you can't make them?
- What kind of medical treatment do you want or don't want?
- How comfortable do you want to be?
- How do you want people to treat you?
- What do you want your loved ones to know?

Some states require a specific form to validate a person's wishes to be a DNR (do not resuscitate), which means that if the individual's heart stops, he or she does not want CPR performed in order to stop him or her from dying.

It is important to know if the person you are caring for has an advance directive and whether the doctor and the health care team are aware of it. A copy should also be on the medical chart. Some individuals keep advance directives in a drawer or file, and no one knows where it is or even where to look for it. Unless everyone is aware of it, the advance directive cannot be followed in the event the person loses his or her ability to make decisions. As long as a patient can understand and make choices, the advance directive is *not* necessary. It is implemented only if the individual loses the capacity to make his own health care decisions.

Advance directives regarding resuscitation or DNR become operative in a medical emergency setting. If a call for emergency medical services (EMS) is placed, the EMS providers may not take time to read all the advance directives, but they will make decisions as indicated by a DNR document. Advance directives are often confused with DNR orders, but they are *not* the same. Persons who have advance directives do not necessarily have DNR orders; and individuals with DNR orders do not necessarily have advance directives. For a sample advance directive form, see Figure 6.3.

Do Not Resuscitate Orders

No CPR should be initiated for patients who have DNR orders. This DNR order may be indicated by a special bracelet or a special DNR document located in a prominent place. DNR orders must always be written by the person's physician (or in some states by an advanced practice nurse). A decision to write a DNR order for a setting other than a hospital is always discussed with the patient and/or the patient's surrogate decision maker (family or guardian) prior to writing the DNR. A DNR order may be rescinded by the patient or by the patient's surrogate/guardian. In all other cases, it should be respected and honored by all health care providers and EMS professionals.

Different states have different DNR rules when the patient is outside the hospital and it is important that the caregiver is familiar with the practice and the forms used in the state where he or she is providing care. It is also important to know if the EMS organization in your area will honor these DNR orders when their providers are called to a person's home.

Sample Advance Directive Form

This form is a combined durable power of attorney for health care and a living will (in some jurisdictions). With this form, you can name someone to make medical decisions for you if in the future you are unable to make those decisions yourself. You can also say what medical treatments you want and what medical treatments you do not want if in the future you are unable to make your wishes known.

Instructions

Read each section carefully. Before you fill out the form talk to the person you want to name, to make sure that he or she understands your wishes and is willing to take the responsibility. Write your initials in the blank spaces before the choices you want to make. Write your initials only beside the choices you want under Parts 1, 2, and 3 of this form. Your advance directive should be valid for whatever part(s) you fill in, as long as it is properly signed.

Add any special instructions in the blank spaces provided. You can write additional comments on a separate sheet of paper but you should write on this form that there are additional pages to your advance directive. Sign the form and have it witnessed. Give copies to your doctor, your nurse, the person you name to make your medical decisions for you, people in your family and anyone else who might be involved in your care. Discuss your advance directive with them.

Understand that you may change or cancel this document at any time.

Definitions to *Know*

Advance directive—A written document (form) that tells what a person wants or does not want if he or she in the future cannot make his or her wishes known about medical treatment.

Artificial nutrition and hydration—When food and water are fed to a person through a tube.

Autopsy—An examination done on a dead body to determine the cause of death.

Comfort care—Care that helps to keep a person comfortable but does not make him or her get well. Bathing, turning, and keeping a person's lips moist are types of comfort care.

CPR (cardiopulmonary resuscitation)—Treatment to try to restart a person's breathing or heartbeat. CPR may be done by pushing on the chest, by putting a tube down the throat, or by other treatment.

Durable power of attorney for health care—An advance directive that names someone to make medical decisions for a person if in the future he or she cannot make his or her own medical decisions.

Life-sustaining treatment—Any medical treatment that is used to keep a person from dying. A breathing machine, CPR, and artificial nutrition and hydration are examples of life-sustaining treatments.

Living will—An advance directive that tells what medical treatment a person does or does not want if he or she is not able to make his or her wishes known.

Organ and tissue donation—When a person permits his or her organs (such as the eyes or kidneys) and other parts of the body (such as the skin) to be removed after death to be transplanted for use by another person or to be used for experimental purposes.

Persistent vegetative state—When a person is unconscious unlikely to regain consciousness even with medical treatment. The body may move and the eyes may be open, but as far as anyone can tell the person cannot think or respond.

FIGURE 6.3 Sample advance directive.

Terminal condition—An ongoing condition caused by injury or illness that has no cure and from which doctors expect the person to die even with medical treatment. Life-sustaining treatments will only prolong the dying process if the person is suffering from a terminal condition.

Complete this portion of the advance directive form

I, _____,

write this document as a directive regarding my medical care.

In the following sections, put the initials of your name in the blank spaces by the choices you want.

PART 1. My Durable Power of Attorney for Health Care

_____ I appoint this person to make decisions about my medical care if there ever comes a time when I cannot make those decisions myself. I want the person I have appointed, my doctors, my family, and others to be guided by the decisions I have made in the parts of the form that follow.

Name: _____

Home telephone: _____

Work telephone: _____

Address: _____

If the person cited above cannot or will not make decisions for me, I appoint this person:

Name: _____

Home telephone: _____

Work telephone: _____

Address: _____

_____ I have not appointed anyone to make health care decisions for me in this or any other document.

PART 2. My Living Will

These are my wishes for my future medical care if there ever comes a time when I cannot make these decisions for myself.

A. These are my wishes if I have a terminal condition.

Life-Sustaining Treatments

_____ I do not want life-sustaining treatment (including CPR) started. If life-sustaining treatments are started, I want them stopped.

_____ I want the life-sustaining treatments that my doctors think are best for me.

_____ Other wishes

_____

Artificial Nutrition and Hydration

_____ I do not want artificial nutrition and hydration started if they would be the main treatments keeping me alive. If artificial nutrition and hydration are started, I want them stopped.

FIGURE 6.3 (continued)

_____ I want artificial nutrition and hydration even if they are the main treatments keeping me alive.

_____ Other wishes

_____

Comfort Care

_____ I want to be kept as comfortable and free of pain as possible, even if such care prolongs my dying or shortens my life.

_____ Other wishes

_____

B. These are my wishes if I am ever in a persistent vegetative state.

Life-Sustaining Treatments

_____ I do not want life-sustaining treatment (including CPR) started. If life-sustaining treatments are started, I want them stopped.

_____ I want the life-sustaining treatments that my doctors think are best for me.

_____ Other wishes

_____

Artificial Nutrition and Hydration

_____ I do not want artificial nutrition and hydration started if they would be the main treatments keeping me alive. If artificial nutrition and hydration are started, I want them stopped.

_____ I want artificial nutrition and hydration even if they are the main treatments keeping me alive.

_____ Other wishes

_____

Comfort Care

_____ I want to be kept as comfortable and free of pain as possible, even if such care prolongs my dying or shortens my life.

_____ Other wishes

_____

C. Other directives

You have the right to be involved in all decisions about your medical care, even those not dealing with terminal conditions or persistent vegetative states. If you have wishes not covered in other parts of this document, please indicate them below.

_____

_____

_____

_____

_____

_____

_____

FIGURE 6.3 _(continued)_

PART 3. Other Wishes

A. Organ donation

_____ I do not wish to donate any of my organs or tissues.

_____ I want to donate all of my organs and tissues.

_____ I only want to donate these organs and tissues:

_____

_____ Other wishes

_____

B. Autopsy

_____ I do not want an autopsy.

_____ I agree to an autopsy if my doctors wish it.

_____ Other wishes

C. Other statements about your medical care

If you wish to say more about any of the choices you have made or if you have any other statements to make about your medical care, you may do so on a separate piece of paper. If you do so, put here the number of pages you are adding: _____

PART 4. Signatures

You and two witnesses must sign this document before it will be legal.

A. Your signature

By my signature below, I show that I understand the purpose and the effect of this document.

Signature:_____ Date:_____

Address: _____

B. Your witnesses' signatures

I believe the person who has signed this advance directive to be of sound mind, that he or she signed or acknowledged this advance directive in my presence, and that he or she appears not to be acting under pressure, attempt to fraud, or undue influence. I am not related to the person making this advance directive by blood, marriage, or other kinship. To the best of my knowledge, am I not named in this will. I am not the person appointed in this advance directive. I am not a health care provider or an employee of a health care provider who is now, or has been in the past, responsible for the care of the person making this advance directive.

Witness #1

Signature: _____ Date: _____

Address: _____

Witness #2

Signature: _____ Date: _____

Address: _____

Adapted with permission from the District of Columbia Hospital Association, 1250 Eye St., N.W., Suite 700, Washington, DC 20005.

FIGURE 6.3

CPR and resuscitation attempts at the end of life for patients for whom death is expected are not appropriate interventions. DNR orders are meant to allow death to occur naturally and with respect for the patient's dignity.

Dying and Culture

Most cultures have traditions and rituals around death and dying. Learn the expectations of the patient and family members regarding the dying process. You can explore these wishes with a patient through the use of the five wishes document. Or you can discuss with the patient what to expect during the end-of-life process and what the patient's desires are during this process. Additional areas to explore include the following:

- Who, if anyone, does the patient want present when they are dying?
- Are there any personal items such as a rosary or other significant religious item that the patient wants near?
- Is there any specific music, clothing, or other environmental enhancements the person would like to have nearby when he or she is dying?

PHYSICAL CARE OF THE DYING

The patient who is dying usually needs assistance with his physical needs. As the caregiver, you will be attending to many needs that the person used to attend to himself. Allow the patient to do as much as possible for himself. This permits him to be independent for as long as he is able. Discuss with the health care team, family members, and the patient the responsibilities that each member of the health care team will be assuming to ensure that the patient receives the needed care (see Procedure 6.1).

THE MOMENT OF DEATH

Many people now choose to die at home rather than return to the hospital. Usually, the nurse of the home health team (or hospice agency) has prepared the family for the moment of death and related events. Many patients die as they have lived: the fearful die in fear, the angry die in anger, and the peaceful die in peace. Some simply slip into an unconscious state for days before death, and others cling constantly to a loved one's hand.

Dying is a spiritual process for some people. Many patients and families ask to see a priest, minister, rabbi, or person who shares the same concept of spirituality. As the time of death nears, services or prayer rituals may be held at the bedside, and privacy may be requested. Breathing may become irregular and stop for periods of up to 30 seconds or more. This breathing is called Cheyne-Stokes breathing. Although it may be upsetting to the family, it is a usual occurrence. As death approaches, the gurgling breathing called the death rattle may begin. At this time, the person is usually unconscious, so it

PROCEDURE 6.1

Physical Care of the Dying

Rationale

The dying body is fragile and can be in pain. Using proper care techniques allows the patient to be as comfortable as possible. Follow these steps:

1. **Assemble your equipment:** Bed bath supplies, loose clothing, pillows and towels for repositioning, patient preferred foods, glycerine toothettes, lotion, water, suction machine, and any other items requested by the patient.
2. **Skin care:** Bathe as needed with partial bathing as necessary. The skin may be fragile, so wash gently with mild soap. Apply lotion to bony prominences.
3. **Clothing:** Do not use tight clothing, stockings, garters, or tight bed linens. Use pillows and rolled blankets for careful positioning. Change the person's position often, at least every 1½ to 2 hours. Change soiled linens and protective pads. Change nonsterile dressings when soiled. Reinforce sterile dressings.
4. **Mouth care:** Cleanse teeth and mouth at least twice daily. Remove dentures, or brush teeth. Cleanse mucous membranes and teeth if the patient is not alert with glycerine swabs (toothettes) as needed. *Note:* Mouth care is important as people often get upper respiratory infections from bacteria in the mouth.
5. **Bowel movements:** Keep a careful record of bowel movements, and notify the nurse or physician if the client has not had a bowel movement in seventy-two hours. Most palliative and hospice programs will prescribe a bowel regime to prevent or address constipation. Remember, most pain medications can cause constipation.
6. **Circulation:** The circulation slows as death approaches, and the arms and legs may feel cold and look ashen. Elevate the limbs as needed to aid blood return and avoid having the limbs in a pressure position for more than one hour.
7. **Food/water:** Assist the patient to a comfortable position and cleanse the mouth. Wash his or her hands, and refresh the linen. Ask the patient and his or her family about food choices and seek as much variety as possible. Offer small portions of food and frequent sips of water to avoid tiring the patient with long meals (see Figure 6.4), Arrange portions in a neat, appetizing manner according to the patient's preferences.
8. **Breathing:** Remove secretions from the mouth as necessary with a suction machine or washcloth. Urge the patient with a wet cough to cough up mucous for as long as possible. Elevate the head of the bed or prop the patient on pillows if this makes breathing easier.

does not bother her, but it may be distressing to the family. Notify the nurse when it begins.

Talk openly and in a comforting manner to the patient, even when she is seemingly unconscious. Hearing is the last sense to be lost, and loving words from a loved one, up until the moment of death, are comforting. Because it

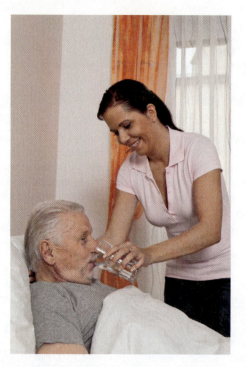

FIGURE 6.4

may be difficult for patients and families to deal with death and associated relationship changes among the family, it is best to plan with the family and health care team exactly what you will be expected to do when the death occurs. Whom should you call? What should you do?

Usually, caregivers feel sadness and loss when a patient dies no matter their relationship with the individual. This is normal. The hospice agency or your health care team may hold special support sessions for aides and nurses who have had a patient die so that they can discuss their feelings and help each other.

POSTMORTEM CARE IN THE HOME

Care of the body after death is called postmortem care. Most of the time when death occurs at home, the family has been prepared for what to do by the patient's doctor and nurse. Usually, the patient's doctor, the nurse from the home health agency, and the funeral director/mortician are notified. Check with the hospice or home care agency for their preferred policies to be followed at the time of death.

Regardless of the procedures, the body must be prepared for removal. After death occurs, the family may sit at the bedside and say their final good-byes. Families handle grief in many ways, and they should have time and privacy as they need it. Be sure to inquire about specific religious practices that should be observed at this time.

Judaism and Death

In a traditional Jewish death, the following should be honored:

- The body is laid on the floor and candles lit near the body.
- The body is never left alone until after burial.
- The people watching the body do not eat or drink because the deceased can no longer do these things. Eating and drinking in front of the dead is seen as mocking the dead.
- The body is cleaned and wrapped in a simple plain linen shroud.
- Anyone who has been guarding the body washes her or his hands before entering her or his own home.
- Be sure to find out ahead of time what the family wishes to occur when the patient dies.

Buddhist Death Rituals

When a Buddhist knows that death is near, he or she may request that a monk be present during the death. This monk(s) will likely read prayers and chant to assist the person in avoiding fear of death and dying in peace. To keep the spirit in a peaceful space after death, the body is not touched for three to eight hours to allow the spirit to transition without influence from the corpse. Honor these rituals as you have learned from the patient and/or family prior to the death.

Christian Death Rituals

The Christian religion has many sects, and thus many Christian traditions related to death and dying exist. A Catholic for example, may ask for last rites from a priest, where the person dying is able to confess her or her sins and be forgiven prior to death. If this is a wish of your patient, obtain the contact phone numbers prior to the time of dying so that you can contact the priest for the patient.

   If no instructions are given from the patient or family, follow the list of instructions in Procedure 6.2. After the body is removed from the home, strip the bed and air the room. Remove any equipment. Check with the family regarding the proper disposal of these items. Place personal items carefully at the bedside so family members can remove them at the appropriate time. If the patient is a family member, other health care providers may take care of the body and removal for you so that you may spend time with other grieving family members. If you are not part of the family, you may offer to help the family by answering phone calls from friends and neighbors, providing refreshments, or sitting with grieving family members. Ask the family how you can help, and try to do whatever is necessary to help them through this difficult time (see Figure 6.5).

PROCEDURE 6.2

Care of the Body After Death

Rationale

Following a predetermined set of steps in quickly caring for a body after death prevents problems for morticians and/or families. When appropriate, prepare the body in the following manner:

1. Assemble your equipment: towels, washcloths, water and other bathing equipment for a bedside bath, trash bags to cover soiled equipment or carry soiled linens.
2. Remove all pillows except one under the head.
3. Bathe the body, removing secretions and reinforce dressings.
4. Place dentures in the mouth if possible.
5. Close the eyes, but do not press on the eyeballs.
6. Keep the body flat on its back, straightening the arms and legs.
7. Move the body gently to avoid bruising.
8. Check with the family regarding any jewelry the client may be wearing.
9. Fold the arms over the abdomen.
10. Remove any tube according to the hospice agency's policy. Usually, you will not be asked to remove a tube after death if you did not care for it when the patient was alive.

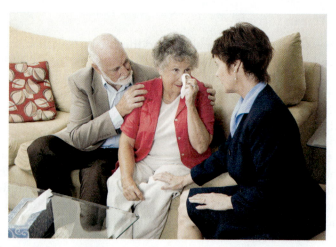

FIGURE 6.5 Healthcare professionals can help people through the loss.

Summary

The chapter-opening scenario is an example of the intricacies found in families caring for loved ones who are dying at home. The amount of help a family member is capable and/or willing to provide will vary. The caregiver needs to be flexible in providing the amount of care necessary at any given time. This type of care takes patience and listening to the patient and family throughout the dying process. Death and dying can be the most difficult time in providing care for someone at home. Allow yourself to grieve at your own pace, and do the same for the patient.

Chapter 7

Infection Control in the Home

SCENARIO

Mrs. Day lives alone in her own home. She has not changed anything in the past twenty-five years, saying that it was fine when her husband was alive so everything is fine now. Although she has never worked, she is financially secure. She has managed to keep up the house and the garden. She admits to being somewhat forgetful and finding physical work a challenge. This bothers her; however, she rejects help in the house, memory aids, or other minor assistance with her daily activities. The house is tidy but has not had a thorough cleaning in a while. It is dark and the windows are seldom opened. She eats three regular meals, which she prepares herself. To save water, Mrs. Day washes her dishes once a day. Her three children are attentive, calling frequently. Only one daughter lives close by, and she is the primary caretaker; the other children only visit or call on special occasions.

INFECTION CONTROL

The Importance of Handwashing

When caring for others, you will use your hands constantly. You will touch patients. You will handle supplies and equipment used in the treatment and care of patients. Microorganisms will get on your hands. They will come from the individual you are caring for or from the things they have touched. Your hands can carry these microorganisms to other persons and places. They can be moved to your face and mouth. Washing your hands frequently with antibacterial soap and warm water is the best way to prevent the transfer of microorganisms that could lead to infection or disease (see Guideline 7.1 and Procedure 7.1).

GUIDELINE 7.1

Handwashing

- Wash your hands before and after each task and before and after direct patient contact.
- The water faucet is always considered dirty, which means it may harbor pathogens. Use paper towels to turn the faucet on and off.
- If your hands accidentally touch the inside of the sink, start over. Do the whole procedure again.
- Take soap from a dispenser, if possible, rather than using bar soap. Bar soap leaves pools of soapy water in the soap dish, which is considered contaminated.
- Wash your hands before you put on gloves for a procedure and again after you remove the gloves.

PROCEDURE 7.1

Handwashing

Rationale

Proper handwashing technique is the most effective way to prevent the spread of disease.

1. Assemble your equipment: Soap in liquid soap dispenser, nail brush, paper towels, warm running water, wastepaper basket.
2. Remove any jewelry. Artificial nails are discouraged due to their tendency to provide a place for bacteria to grow.
3. Use a clean paper towel to turn on the faucet. Adjust the water to a comfortable temperature.
4. Discard the paper towel in the wastepaper basket.
5. Completely wet your hands and wrists under the running water. Keep your fingertips pointed downward. Hold your hands lower than your elbows while washing. This is to prevent microorganisms from contaminating your arms. Holding your hands down prevents backflow over unwashed skin. Apply soap.
6. Work up a good lather. Spread it over the entire area of your hands and wrists, Get soap under your nails and between your fingers for at least fifteen to thirty seconds.
7. Use the nail brush to scrub under your fingernails at the start of each day and anytime hands are heavily soiled.
8. Rinse under running water with your fingertips pointed down (see Figure 7.1). Be careful not to touch the faucet or other parts of the sink.
9. If hands are heavily soiled, reapply soap and wash them again.
10. Dry thoroughly with paper towels.
11. Use a clean paper towel to turn off the faucet. Never touch the faucet with your hands after washing.
12. Throw the paper towel into the wastepaper basket. Do not touch the basket.

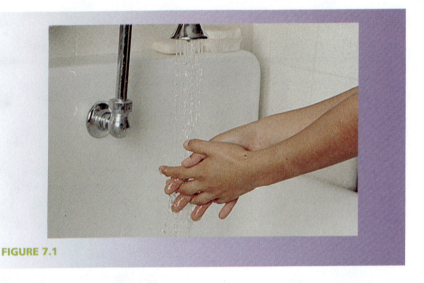

FIGURE 7.1

Disinfection and Sterilization in the Home

While you care for an individual, it is important to prevent the spread of path-ogens. Pathogens can grow in several ways. Despite our best efforts, harm-ful microorganisms are always present. Microorganisms can be made harm-less, however, by simple cleanliness procedures. We keep ourselves clean by bathing and frequent handwashing. We keep the environment and equip-ment clean with soap, water, and solutions that assist in decreasing bacterial growth (see Guideline 7.2).

One way to control the spread of disease is to have designated clean areas in the house and dirty areas. The kitchen is considered clean, the toilet is considered dirty; the area of dishwashing is considered clean, and the area of toileting is considered dirty.

Clean: Uncontaminated referring to articles and places from which disease cannot be spread. Clean areas contain food, dishes, and clean equipment. No waste material is ever brought into this area.

Dirty: Refers to areas that have come in contact with disease-causing or -carrying agents. In the home, there are degrees of dirty. We make a distinc-tion between items that are dirty with human waste, such as wound drainage or fecal matter, and bed sheets that are soiled. Articles that are dirty with po-tentially infectious material are brought into the dirty area for initial cleaning or disposal. This includes linen, bath water, or equipment. Articles that are soiled without potentially infectious waste are cleaned like regular laundry.

Two important methods for killing microorganisms are:

1. **Disinfection:** The process of destroying as many harmful organisms as possible, slowing down the growth and activity of organisms that cannot be destroyed.

GUIDELINE 7.2
Aseptic Techniques

- Wash your hands after using the bathroom or blowing your nose, before handling food, after caring for the patient, before any procedure, and before/after meals.
- Practice good personal hygiene.
- Cover your nose and mouth when you sneeze or cough. Turn your face to the side when you cough. Wash your hands after you cough into your hands.
- Clean wastebaskets often.
- Wash, dry, and put away all patient-related equipment after each use.
- Dispose of contaminated articles in the proper way.
- If you have an open area on your skin, cover it with a waterproof bandage and wear gloves when performing patient care.
- Wash your hands before you put on gloves and after you take them off.

2. **Sterilization:** The process of killing all microorganisms, including spores, in a certain area.

Spores are bacteria that form hard shells around themselves as a defense. These shells are like a protective suit of armor. Spores are difficult to kill. Some can even live in boiling water. Sterilization is necessary if the article comes in direct contact with a wound, as in the case of surgical instruments; solutions used for cleaning a wound; or wound dressing. Supplies and equipment used for these processes come in sterilized packages. If these presterilized supplies are not available, use wet-heat or dry-heat sterilization techniques (see Procedures 7.2 and 7.3).

Care of Persons with Transmittable Diseases

The discovery of certain diseases within the past fifteen years has alerted health care workers to the need to lower the chance of transmission of these diseases from patient to caregiver. These diseases are spread through exposure to blood and body fluids and are called blood-borne pathogens. Two of these diseases are AIDS (acquired immunodeficiency syndrome) and hepatitis B. The human immunodeficiency virus (HIV) causes AIDS. Hepatitis B virus (HBV) causes hepatitis B. Both diseases are spread through sexual contact, shared intravenous needles, and the exchange of blood and/or body fluids. AIDS may awaken negative feelings because of fear or because some victims may have an unfamiliar lifestyle. The physician will determine if isolation precautions should be instituted for a particular patient. Remember, not all individuals with AIDS and hepatitis B need to be on isolation precautions. However, standard precaution with any person receiving care should be observed. The chance of transmitting a disease such as AIDS or hepatitis from any patient to a caregiver is small if caregivers follow current regulations from the U.S. Centers for Disease Control and Prevention (CDC) and the Occupational Safety and Health Administration (OSHA).

PROCEDURE 7.2

Wet-Heat Sterilization

Rationale

Removing pathogens from instruments decreases one cause of disease.

1. Assemble your equipment: Items to be sterilized, cleaned, and dried; clean, covered pot large enough to hold items; cold water to cover the items in the pot; timer or clock; sterilized tongs; potholder; and stove.
2. Wash your hands.
3. Place the equipment in the pot so that water touches all parts of it. If there are glass parts, put a clean piece of cloth in the bottom of the pot to protect them.
4. Cover the contents of the pot with cold water. Be sure to leave headroom in the pot.
5. Put the pot on a source of heat big enough to heat it. Turn handles away from the edge of the stove.
6. Bring water to a boil. Do not open the pot. Note when steam escapes under the cover.
7. Boil the contents undisturbed and covered for twenty minutes.
8. Turn off the heat.
9. Allow the contents to cool undisturbed. Leave the equipment in the pot until you are ready to use it.
10. Use sterilized tongs to remove the contents to a sterilized holder.

Viral hepatitis, an inflammation of the liver caused by a virus, has three types. Although no vaccine against hepatitis C is available, a vaccine against type A and B is available. You may elect to receive such a vaccine or you may refuse it. The best way to prevent transmission of this disease remains the use

PROCEDURE 7.3

Dry-Heat Sterilization

Rationale

The removal of pathogens from cloth used for dressings is one way to decrease the spread of pathogens.

1. Assemble your equipment: Pie tin, dressing or cloth to be sterilized, oven, potholder.
2. Wash your hands.
3. Place the clean dressings wrapped in a clean cloth in the pie tin.
4. Place the pie tin in an oven at 350°F. Allow the dressings to bake for one hour. Allow them to cool.
5. Unwrap carefully. Do not touch the dressings; they are now considered sterile.

Note: A hot iron held on dressings for several seconds also sterilizes them; however, the oven method is preferred.

TABLE 7.1   Different Types of Hepatitis

Type of Hepatitis	Transmission	Complications	Risk to Health Care Workers	Vaccine	Prevention
Type A	Oral-fecal; poor sanitation; contaminated water or food; sexual contact.	Rare	Poor hand-washing.	Available	Handwashing; avoid contaminated food and water; cook all food.
Type B	Body fluids; sexual contact; blood-to-blood contact; contaminated needles.	Cirrhosis; cancer	Contact with bodily fluids into open skin; needle sticks.	Available	Standard precautions; safe sex; do not share personal items with people you don't know well.
Type C	Direct blood-to-blood contact; sexual contact.	Cirrhosis, cancer	Needle sticks.	None	Standard precautions; safe sex; do not share personal items with people you don't know well.

of standard precautions; you may not know who has this disease and who does not (see Table 7.1).

Methicillin-resistant staphylococcus aureus (MRSA) is the staph bacterium strain resistant to usual antibiotics. It can pass from person to person through direct contact or droplet transmission. This infection is often found in hospitals or other health care facilities. The best way to prevent giving or getting this infection is to practice good hygiene and standard precautions. Washing hands frequently and disposing of used tissues and soiled dressings is important. If you care for a patient who has been diagnosed with MRSA, the physician will institute isolation precautions. You will be instructed on how to work safely in this atmosphere. If your immune system is suppressed or you are pregnant, discuss this situation with the physician in charge.

STANDARD PRECAUTIONS

Medical tests and careful medical history are often not enough to identify patients who have blood-borne pathogens (see Guideline 7.3). Therefore, the CDC prescribes precautions to decrease the risks of being exposed to blood-borne pathogens found in all body fluids except sweat. These basic activities are called standard precautions. An important point to remember is that

GUIDELINE 7.3

CDC Standard Precautions

- *Disposable gloves:* Disposable gloves must be worn when contact is possible with blood, all body fluids except sweat (whether or not they contain blood you can see), skin that has breaks in it, and all mucous membranes. Contact includes activities during direct care and care of equipment.
- *Gowns or aprons:* Gowns or aprons must be worn during procedures or situations when there may be an exposure to blood, body fluids (except sweat), draining wounds, or mucous membranes.
- *Masks, face shields, or goggles:* Masks, face shields, or goggles must be worn during procedures that are likely to generate droplets of blood or body fluids (except sweat), or when the patient is coughing excessively.
- *Handwashing:* Hands must be washed before gloving and after gloves are removed. Hands and other skin surfaces must be washed immediately and thoroughly if contaminated with blood or body fluids (*except sweat*) and after all patient care activities. If you have open cuts, sores, or dermatitis on your hands, wear gloves for all patient contact.
- *Transportation:* When transporting (moving) any patient who may have an infection, ensure that care is taken to use standard precautions to minimize the risk of transmission of microorganisms to others and to limit the contamination of environmental surfaces or equipment.
- *Resuscitation:* Use resuscitation devices as alternatives to mouth-to-mouth resuscitation.

standard precautions are actions taken universally for all patients and are designed to protect you against transmission of microorganisms through body fluids. It is the law that standard precautions be incorporated into the routine tasks of all health care workers. In addition to standard precautions, if a definite diagnosis is made, specific types of isolation, called transmission-based precautions, will be added to the patient's plan of care.

Standard precautions include the use of protective barriers. Protective barriers are the types of equipment that protect you from splashes, spills, droplets, or other sources of contamination. Protective barriers include gloves, gowns, aprons, masks, face shields, and goggles. You can purchase this equipment at any medical supply store. If you do not have a medical supply store nearby, be sure to ask the patient's physician for resources (see also the Resource Page at the end of this book).

Using Nonsterile Gloves

Gloves protect you and the patient. Use gloves whenever there is a chance you will touch body fluids other than sweat. Follow these guidelines (see also Procedure 7.4):

- Wash your hands before and after you use gloves.
- Always dispose of gloves in the area you are working. Wearing gloves from one room to another leaves potential for transmission of germs.

PROCEDURE 7.4

Putting on Nonsterile Gloves

Rationale

Gloves provide a barrier between you and potential contamination.

1. Assemble equipment: nonsterile gloves, trash can in which to dispose of the gloves, a place or method of washing your hands.
2. Wash your hands.
3. Select a clean pair of gloves in your size (see Figure 7.2). Hold a glove at the wrist opening and insert fingers, pulling the glove up to the wrist.

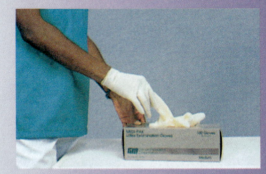

FIGURE 7.2

4. Apply the second glove in same manner
5. Check both gloves for holes and other flaws. If there are any flaws, discard that glove (see Figure 7.3).

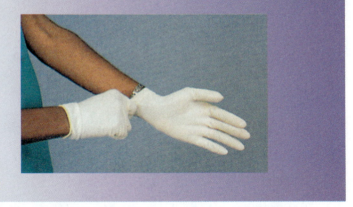

FIGURE 7.3

- Put on a new set of gloves each time you need to use gloves. Do not reuse gloves.

  Note: Once the gloves are *on*, the outside of the glove is considered dirty and the inside is considered clean. The outside of the gloves should not touch any of your skin surfaces (see Procedure 7.5).

PROCEDURE 7.5

Removing Nonsterile Used Gloves

Rationale

Removing gloves correctly will decrease the chance of contamination.

1. Assemble your equipment: trash can in which to dispose of the gloves, a place or method of washing your hands.
2. Grasp the glove at the palm of your hand with the other gloved hand and pull it away (see Figure 7.4).

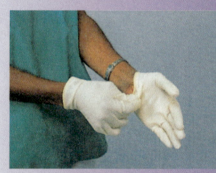

FIGURE 7.4

3. Continue holding the removed glove with the gloved hand (see Figure 7.5).

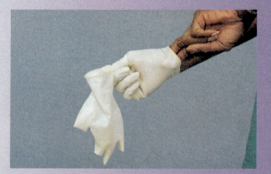

FIGURE 7.5

4. Place the index and middle finger of the ungloved hand inside the cuff of the remaining glove and peel it down inverting over the other glove (see Figure 7.6).
5. Discard the gloves in the trash (not your pocket).
6. Wash your hands.

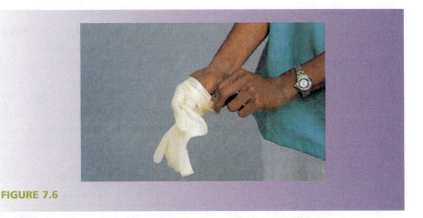

FIGURE 7.6

Using the Standard Precautions Guidelines

Standard precautions are commonsense guidelines. Wear gloves whenever exposure to body fluids (except sweat) may occur. Patients often feel uncomfortable being cared for by somebody wearing gloves. Explain to them that this is to protect both you and the patient. If you cut or stick yourself while caring for a patient, seek medical evaluation and tell the physician the condition of your patient. If you have any cuts or injuries on your hands or body, cover them with a waterproof bandage and wear gloves while giving care. Follow these guidelines:

- *Exposure to body fluids or blood:* Wear gloves if a chance exists for contamination. If splattering is possible, wear a gown or protective apron and mask. Flush waste products down the toilet. Spills should be wiped up with soap and water by a person wearing disposable gloves, then wiped with a solution of 1 part household bleach to 10 parts water. The rag should be thrown out. Change gloves frequently. When removing gloves, do not touch the outside of the gloves.
- *Personal items:* Items such as tampons, peripads, or razors are not considered medical waste and should be disposed of as you would any dressing.
- *Sharp objects, needles, blades:* Handle these items carefully to prevent cutting yourself. These objects should be placed in a puncture-resistant container and disposed of according to local rules (call your local health department or deparment of public works). Do not bend needles or try to recap them.
- *Dressing:* Wrap these items in a plastic bag and dispose of them according to local law (call your local health department or department of public works). You may have to double-bag them if you are transporting them as medical waste.
- *Plates, glasses, dishes:* Use separate utensils, disposable if possible. Clean reusable utensils in hot water and detergent. Use hot water, a sponge, and dry. Using the dishwasher for washing dishes is

preferable. In the chapter-opening scenario, Mrs. Day may be susceptible to infection due to the lack of infection control in the home (i.e., dishes not being washed properly). For infection control, if a dishwasher is not available, air dry the dishes rather than drying them with a dish towel.

- *Laundry:* Unsoiled laundry needs no special attention but should be washed or dry-cleaned normally. Soiled linen should be separated and handled with disposable gloves. Keep soiled linen in a double plastic bag lined with a cloth bag or pillowcase. Empty the contents of the plastic bag into the washing machine without touching the items, then throw away the plastic bag. Wash soiled linen each day with one of the following methods:

Machine washing (colorfast)	1 cup of household bleach in hot water and laundry detergent
Handwashing (colorfast)	2 tablespoons of household bleach in 1 gallon of warm water and laundry detergent; soak for 10 minutes and rinse
Machine washing (noncolorfast)	1 cup of Lysol in warm water and laundry detergent; wash again with water only to remove Lysol
Handwashing (noncolorfast)	2 tablespoons of Lysol in 1 gallon of warm water and laundry detergent; rinse at least three times to remove Lysol

Isolation Techniques (Transmission-Based Precautions)

Beyond standard precautions, additional precautions may be necessary when you care for a person with a highly contagious disease. These additional precautions can help decrease the chance of spreading the disease to others. Also, when an individual is highly susceptible to diseases, caregivers may have to protect the patient until his body is able to fight an infection. The physician will determine the type of isolation precaution to use. Transmission-based precautions include contact precautions, droplet precautions, and airborne precautions (see Guideline 7.4).

The use of gown, gloves, and mask should be determined with consultation of the physician. Wearing a gown protects you and the patient (see Guideline 7.5). Wearing a mask decreases the spread of airborne pathogens. Mask material filters the air the wearer breathes. A mask is sometimes worn to protect the patient, too. There are different types of masks, but they all filter the air. All should be applied the same way and changed after every patient encounter.

Basic handwashing is necessary even though gloves are worn. Wash your hands before and after every patient contact. The patient may have additional restrictions placed on her activity and the washing of her linen. Disposable dishes may need to be used.

GUIDELINE 7.4

Basic Isolation—Five Areas of Concern

- *Dressings:* Always dispose of dressings in plastic bags and according to local regulations. If the dressings are heavily soiled, double-bag them.
- *Urine/feces:* Flush urine and feces down the toilet immediately. Clean urinal, bedpan, or commode thoroughly with disinfectant.
- *Dishes:* Use disposable dishes and cups, if available. Wash dishes separately in hot water and soap. Do not let dishes soak or remain in the sink.
- *Linen:* Transport linen to the laundry area in separate plastic bags. If the linen is heavily soiled, double-bag it. Wash separately in hot water. Dry immediately.
- *Cleaning equipment:* Use a disinfectant. Dispose of cleaning water down the toilet. Dispose of cleaning rags in plastic bags.

Remember, standard precautions require that you protect yourself against contact with blood and body fluids. The use of isolation status may mean additional activities, but basic standard precautions must always be used. Double-bagging is a technique of placing contaminated articles in a plastic bag in an isolation room and then placing the closed bag into another plastic bag as it is placed in the trash or medical waste bin.

REGULATED MEDICAL WASTE

Regulated medical waste is defined as blood, blood products, sharp medical instruments such as needles, and dressings contaminated with body fluids. Many communities have regulations that specify how the residents may dispose of regulated medical waste. It is important that you know this information so that you can assist the patient and his family with proper disposal. Some towns have pickups, and some require residents to bring the waste to a central point. To find out the regulations in your area, contact the local health department or department of public works. These regulations protect local residents, the people who process the trash and waste, and the environment.

- *Human waste products:* Human waste products should be flushed down the toilet immediately and not discarded in the street, backyard, or street sewers.
- *Blood and body fluids:* Blood and body fluids should be cleaned up immediately. If the liquid can be flushed down the toilet, that is the best disposal method. Contaminated clothes should be washed separately in hot water and dried. Dressings and cleaning rags should be double-bagged in plastic and disposed of according to local regulations.

GUIDELINE 7.5

Using a Gown and Mask

• Gowns should be long enough to cover your clothing. The outside is considered contaminated. A wet gown is considered contaminated. Do not touch the outside of the gown when you remove it. Wear a clean gown for each patient contact. For instructions on putting on and taking off a gown, see Figure 7.7.

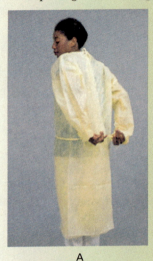
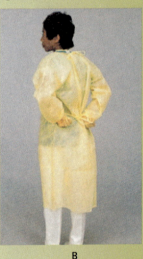

A   B

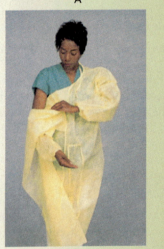
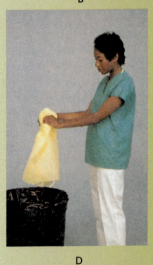

C   D

FIGURE 7.7 **A.** Tie the neck piece of the gown and overlap the back flaps. **B.** Tie the gown securely. Put on gloves now if you need them. **C.** To take off a gown, take off your gloves if you are wearing them. Untie neck and waist. Grasp shoulders. Turn gown inside out as you take it off. **D.** Fold up the town and discard. Do not reuse a gown. Wash your hands.

- Aprons should be worn to cover clothing during routine patient care.
- Masks should fit snugly over the nose and mouth. A wet mask is considered contaminated, as is the front of the mask. Do not wear a mask around your neck. A clean mask should be worn for each patient contact (see Figure 7.8). There are several different types of masks. Discuss with the physician which type is appropriate for your patient's condition.

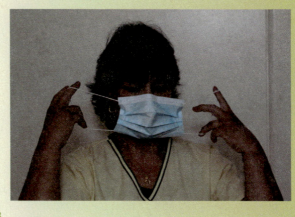

FIGURE 7.8

- *Needles (sharps):* Needles should be kept in a sharps container. A sharps container can be obtained by contacting the local health department. When the sharps container is full, secure the top and dispose of according to the local health department recommendations.
- *Medical supplies:* If supplies become contaminated (i.e., saturated wound dressings, rags used to clean up blood or vomit), they should be emptied (if necessary) and the equipment double-bagged and disposed of according to local regulation. This double-bagging procedure is most important when someone has an infectious disease such as AIDS or MRSA.

Summary

Infection control is a necessary part of safety while caring for someone in the home. It is especially important when the patient has an infection or a blood-borne disease. Make sure you understand how your patient's condition(s) are transmitted to others. This information will help ensure that you are taking the proper precautions to prevent the spread of the infection or disease. Being in contact with the local health department and department of public works will provide you with essential information about the use and disposal of contaminated medical supplies and equipment. Knowledge and practice of standard precautions keep you, the patient, and family members safe.

Chapter 8

Care of a Person's Environment

SCENARIO

Mr. Phom lives with his sister and her two adult children and their families in a small apartment above a bar. The children have all been in this country for ten years, but only the school-age children speak English. They act as interpreters whenever they are in the house. The extended family shops in Asian stores, watches Vietnamese television, and reads Vietnamese newspapers. The adults have never attempted to learn English. Mr. Phom is home from the hospital after an abdominal operation. His sister continues to be his primary caretaker, but she has to go to work each day and he is alone. An independent and private man, Mr. Phom does not accept assistance easily, and the language barrier presents a challenge. You assist him with his meals, which are left by the family. You have not been able to develop a way of finding out what Mr. Phom does when you are not in the house. Mr. Phom is in pain and self-medicates with native medication he buys over the counter in the local Asian store. The house is dark and the rugs are worn. You have offered to help with the laundry, but Mr. Phom's sister has refused this assistance.

HOMEMAKING TASKS

When agreeing to care for someone in her or his home, make sure to include the housekeeping tasks you will be expected to do. Be sure you know the answers to the following questions:

- Is the task related to the personal and therapeutic care of the patient?
- Can anyone else in the home or family do this task?
- Who will do this task when you are not in the home?

Remember, it is often difficult for families to realize what is important in keeping a house clean and that the caregiver is not there to perform all the housekeeping tasks. Clean environments keep harmful bacteria under control. By cleaning bathrooms regularly, the chances for the spread of communicable diseases are decreased. Foods stored in specific places are easy to find and can be used more often with less time and energy being spent to look for them. Accidents are less likely in areas kept orderly. It is especially important to keep clutter away from stairways and areas where people walk frequently.

Clean environments also tend to make us feel better. When things are looking their best, we are more often relaxed and comfortable. It also gives us a feeling of pride when others visit. A patient will tend to be healthier and happier in an environment that is clean and comfortable.

Cleaning a Person's Home

"Clean" usually refers to an area free of pathogens and clutter. To some people, a dust-free home is the only clean home. Others care little about dust. Such differences in values are important to recognize. Try to meet the patient's values. If your values and the patient's needs are different, you need to focus on the patient's values.

Cleaning equipment available to you in a house may differ from equipment in your house. Do not use any equipment unless you are sure how it works. If the equipment is not in good condition, do not use it. Encourage the family to check all equipment regularly and maintain it in perfect working order. This prevents accidents and assists with maintaining a clean and healthful environment. Use equipment only for the purpose for which it is intended.

Discuss all housekeeping tasks in the home with all people concerned. You might hold a meeting with the family members to decide what jobs need to be done to keep the household functioning. This discussion can be informal. After the group has made a list of jobs, discuss who will complete each task (see Table 8.1). Encourage all family members to make suggestions and offer help. Remember, the family is in a crisis situation, and people who may not usually participate in housekeeping tasks may be willing to help at this difficult time. A spirit of cooperation and flexibility should be encouraged. Children are important parts of families. Do not overlook them.

TABLE 8.1 Sample Work Plan

Day	Task	Who Will Do It
Monday		
Tuesday		
Wednesday		
Thursday		
Friday		
Saturday		
Sunday		

If someone is willing to help but does not know how, a "teacher" (either you or a family member) should be found. When teaching, remember the following:

- Make the explanation of the job as simple as possible.
- Help the individual, but do not do it for the person.
- Let the person do it his or her way if it gets the same results.

How to Keep a House Clean

Make a list of what you need to keep the house clean. Remember to use products already in the home. Do not insist that the individual purchase your brand of cleaning products. Your list might look like this:

Necessary Supplies	Nice to Have
Hot water	Dustpan
Soap or detergent	Vacuum cleaner
Broom	Scouring pads
Vinegar	Mop
Scrub pad, scrub brush	Wastebaskets
Baking soda, baking powder	
Bucket	
Trash container	

Be sure you know how to use the appliances in the house. If you are not sure, ask. When using any cleaning product, use the following care guidelines (see Table 8.2):

- Read the instructions on the label. Follow the directions in the order they are given and use the amount suggested (see Table 8.3).
- Do not mix cleaning products unless you have been instructed to do so. Mixed products may cause a chemical reaction that will hurt you and/or the surface you are cleaning.

TABLE 8.2   Basic Kinds of Cleaning Products

Products	Form	Uses	Cautions
Soaps and detergents	Liquid, powder, and solid.	All types of cleaning; personal cleaning.	Read label; protect eyes.
All-purpose cleaner	Liquid, powder, and solid.	All types of cleaning.	Read label; protect eyes.
Abrasives/bleach	Liquid, powder.	Surface soil; kills certain pathogens.	Read label; protect eyes and skin.
Specialty cleaners	Foam, liquid, powder, spray.	Specific jobs: metal, windows, etc.	Read label.

TABLE 8.3	Common Uses of Cleaning Products	
Task	**Product**	**Use**
Bathtub stains	White vinegar or paste of hydrogen peroxide and baking powder	Rub stain with rag dipped in vinegar, leave paste on stain overnight, and rinse.
Tile cleaner	Baking soda	Sprinkle on, rub with damp rag or sponge; rinse immediately because solution makes tile slippery.
Windows and painted surfaces	Mix carefully: 5 cups waters, 1 teaspoon detergent, 1 pint rubbing alcohol, ½ cup sudsy ammonia.	Wash area carefully, rinse well, dry.
Mattress stain solution	½ cup water and ½ cup white vinegar.	Dab solution on stain and let dry. Then rub the area with water and detergent; leave on for 10 minutes. Blot dry, rinse, and let mattress dry.

- Do not leave cleaners on a surface for a long time. Use care in how much you scrub a surface.
- Change the cleaning water when it is moderately dirty, and rinse if needed to avoid streaking or filming.
- Store all cleaning products safely away from children and pets, away from heat sources, and in their original containers. Store cleaning tools and supplies safely and as close as possible to where you will use them.
- Line garbage pails with plastic or paper bags. Do not put wet objects directly into paper bags. Wrap them first.

When using equipment, keep in mind the following safety points:

- Keep electrical equipment away from water. Never soak electrical equipment unless the manufacturer says that you can.
- Use equipment only as indicated by the manufacturer.
- Do not put sharp objects such as hairpins, knives, or screwdrivers into electrical equipment.
- Before repairing an electrical object, unplug it!
- Be sure all equipment is in good condition and does not have frayed cords.

Specific Housekeeping Tasks

DUSTING Dusting is done to prevent the spread of bacteria. In homes where people are particularly sensitive to dust, you may have to dust often. Dampen the rag with a light spray of water or a commercial spray to keep the dust from spreading. Dust with motions that will gather the dust into the rag and away from you. Dust from top to bottom. Dust pictures on walls, then objects on tables, and finally tables and cabinets. If the rag becomes soiled, change it.

WASHING DISHES   Dishes should be washed properly soon after meals. If a dishwasher is used or dishes are to be washed at a later time, scrape the food off the dish (a rubber spatula is a good tool to use for this job). Then rinse or soak the dishes in a basin of water.

- Place dishes on the counter to the left of the soapy dish water in the order in which they are to be washed: least dirty first (glasses, silverware, plates, cups, and saucers), most dirty last (pots and roasting pans).
- Wash dishes in the hot, soapy water and rinse in clear water in the pan to your right. Wash dishes in water hot enough to clean the grease from them and destroy as many microorganisms as possible.
- Drain dishes on a drain board placed to the right of the rinse water.
- Dry dishes with a clean cloth. If no clean cloths are available, allow dishes to air dry.

    Note: If you are left-handed, reverse the placement of the soapy water pan, clear water pan, and the place where the dishes are stacked and drained.

Keeping a kitchen clean is important. Just as food keeps us alive, it also feeds bacteria. Cleaning spills and taking proper care of leftover food is important. Trash should be disposed of regularly (before it falls out of the container). If the trash is wet, put it into a plastic bag first and then into the garbage can. Keep the garbage can clean. Wash it often!

- The stove should be wiped up regularly with soapy water to avoid spills becoming "cooked on."
- The refrigerator (or the place where food is kept cold) should be wiped out on a regular basis. If the refrigerator needs defrosting, discuss this with the family. Do not use sharp objects to poke at ice clumps when defrosting the refrigerator. If the refrigerator is self-defrosting, clean up spills promptly. Food tends to dry out faster in these models.
- Small appliances can be wiped down with soap and water or an all-purpose cleaner *after* they have been disconnected.
- Countertops should be free of food spills and grease. Counters are easier to wipe off if they are kept uncluttered. Areas around drawer handles and door pulls should be kept clean by wiping with a cloth (or sponge) and warm soapy water.

CLEANING BATHROOMS   Constant moisture in the air keeps bathrooms in need of regular cleaning to keep them free of bacteria and odors. If bathroom floors are ceramic tile, any water spilled on them can make them slippery and dangerous. Keep the floors dry.

Safety in bathrooms should always be on your mind. Before a patient uses a bathroom, check it for the following:

- Are there nonskid mats in the tub?
- Are there nonskid rugs on the tile floor?
- Are there grab bars in the shower or tub?
- Is there good lighting?
- Is there ventilation?

Cleaning shower walls and bathtubs can be minimal if everyone wipes the area out after each use. Encourage others to wipe out the area by keeping a cloth or sponge for this purpose near the bathtub.

Sinks and other bathroom fixtures should be cleaned regularly with cleanser and a rag. Do not destroy the surface of enamel fixtures by using cleaners that will scratch them.

To clean the toilet bowl, you need soap or detergent, a toilet bowl brush, and a rag or sponge. *Note:* Do not wipe anything else with this rag or sponge. Wash it after this task.

- Lift up the seat and put soap or detergent into the bowl.
- Scrub the inside of the bowl with a toilet bowl brush. Clean under the rim of the bowl.
- Let the suds stay in the bowl while you wash the outside.
- To avoid a possible chemical reaction, do not mix toilet bowl cleaner with any other cleanser (see Clinical Alert 8.1).
- Use clean hot water to rinse off all parts of the toilet with the sponge or rag.
- If there are water stains such as rust in the bowl, shake in ¼ cup of toilet bowl cleaner. Let stand about thirty minutes, then scrub and flush.

LAUNDRY Clean clothes are important for good health. They also make us look good and feel better about ourselves. Before washing any clothes, repair all tears, loose buttons, and jammed zippers. If you cannot do this, put the clothes aside and either repair them later or tell your patient about the need for the repairs. Such precautions will prevent the repair job from becoming a much larger task. Before washing, sort clothes by:

- *Color:* Dark colors should be washed separately from light colors.
- *Fabric:* Delicate fabrics cannot take as much scrubbing as can heavy-duty fabrics.

CLINICAL ALERT 8.1

Dangerous Household Cleaners

Any cleaners with ammonia, chlorine bleach, or formaldehyde should not be used in a home with young children, elders, or people who suffer from a respiratory condition. These chemicals can emit toxic fumes that can cause difficult breathing, coughing, or asthma attacks.

- *Degree of dirt:* Heavily soiled items should not be washed with lightly soiled ones.

As with any appliances that you use, either ask the patient how to operate the washer correctly or read the instructions in the owner's manual from the appliance manufacturer.

After sorting clothes, load the machine, being careful not to overload it. Put in the recommended amount of detergent and select the water temperature and amount of agitation. Starting the water and allowing the soap to dissipate prior to adding the clothes will prevent the soap from harming the clothing. Add fabric softener (if needed) after the water has soaked all the clothes.

Clothes dried out of doors conserve energy and have a fresh, clean smell. Take dry clothes immediately from a dryer because they will then need less ironing and you will save energy and time. If there is no washer in the home, find the closest Laundromat to take the clothes for washing. Ensure the patient is safe when you leave to do laundry or run other errands.

CARE OF RUGS AND CARPETING Ask your patient how to care for the carpets and rugs. Frequent vacuuming or sweeping will preserve the rugs and decrease lint and dust. If the patient has a vacuum cleaner, remember the following:

- Treat it as you would any electrical appliance.
- Ask how to change the dirt collection bag inside.
- Use the vacuum cleaner at a convenient time for the patient and family, when it will not disturb them.

When you find stains on a carpet or rug, you may treat them as follows:

- Ask the family if the stain is new and if they would like you to attempt to remove the stain. If it is an old stain, you will probably not be able to get it out.
- You may use commercial stain removers.
- You may mix water and baking soda into a solution and rub it into the stain. After it dries, vacuum.
- If the spot is sticky, sprinkle baking soda on it, then vacuum.

CARE OF FLOORS Keeping floors clean is important to the general well-being of the patient and her family. Clean floors decrease the spread of bacteria and provide a safe path in which people can walk.

- Sweep floors frequently, especially before washing them.
- Ask family members how they usually clean the floors. Wood floors often require special cleaners and are not cleaned with water.
- Use the detergent or cleanser according to the directions on the package. Do not let water remain on the floor.
- Most households have a mop for cleaning floors. If you do not find one, discuss this with the family or appropriate health care team member.
- Let the floor dry before walking on it or putting furniture back in place.

PEST AND BUG PREVENTION Pests and bugs may carry diseases and may annoy you and your patient. They may bite, cause skin irritations, or even frighten people. The best way to keep an area free of bugs, rodents, and other pests is to keep it clean and free of clutter.

- Put food away in closed containers; tin and glass are best.
- Clean up spills and crumbs.
- Take out garbage and trash.
- Keep garbage and trash in covered containers.
- Roaches and mice can pass through small cracks in walls and near pipes such as those under the kitchen sink. Talk to the patient or family about having someone caulk such holes.
- Do not let water stand inside or outside.

If you or any family member wish to use a commercial product to get rid of bugs or rodents, check with the physician to be sure that it is safe to use given the patient's condition.

BED MAKING You may have a patient who spends part of the day in bed. Other patients, though, cannot or must not leave bed at all. As a result, many patients are fed and bathed in bed and use a bedpan in bed.

Caregivers should make beds with no wrinkles in the sheets. Wrinkles are not only uncomfortable, they can restrict the patient's circulation and cause painful decubitus ulcers (pressure sores). When these wounds open, they often slow the patient's recovery. Decubiti can form quickly and are difficult to heal.

You may care for a patient in his own bed. Your patient may decide to sleep on a couch or a hospital bed in his home. Your patient may have a positioning device on his bed. These positioning devices assist him as he moves in the bed by providing him with something to grab for support. If the patient is at risk for falling out of bed, the mattress can be put on the floor or a specialty low bed can be used with a fall mat on the floor to prevent injury from falling.

- Keep the bed dry and clean—change linen when necessary.
- Keep the linen wrinkle free.
- Make the bed to suit your particular patient.
- Keep the bed free of food particles and crumbs.

See Guideline 8.1 for more information about bed making.

MAKING A BED THAT IS OCCUPIED The occupied bed is made when the patient cannot or must not leave the bed. The most important part of making an occupied bed is to get the sheet smooth and tight under the patient so no wrinkles rub against the skin. When making the bottom of this bed, your job will be easier if you divide the bed in two parts: the side the patient is lying on and the side you are making. By doing this, the weight of the patient is never on the side where you are working. Usually, the occupied bed is made

GUIDELINE 8.1

Bed Making

- Use linens that the patient has available.
- Try to make the bed according to the custom of the house. If you must change the custom of the house, explain your reasons to the patient and her family.
- Do not use a torn piece of linen. It may tear even more and could be dangerous.
- Never use a safety pin on any item of linen.
- Do not shake the bed linen. Shaking spreads harmful microorganisms to everything and everyone in the room, including you.
- Never allow any linen to touch your clothes.
- Dirty, used linen should never touch the floor.
- Put dirty linen in the place agreed upon by you and the patient's family.
- Some individuals prefer to use fitted bottom sheets. Others use flat sheets. The caregiver can make mitered corners with flat sheets. The mitered corners keep the sheets firm and smooth, and make the bed neat and attractive. See Figure 8.1 for instructions on mitering the corner of a bed.
- The bottom sheet must be firm, smooth, and wrinkle-free. This is important for the patient's comfort.

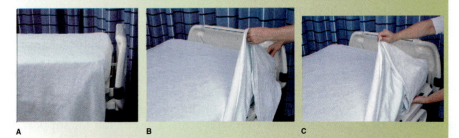

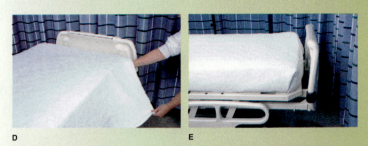

FIGURE 8.1 Mitering the corner of a bed: **A.** Tuck in the bedcover firmly under the mattress at the bottom or top of the bed. **B.** Lift the bedcover at a point so that it forms a triangle with the side edge of the bed and the edge of the bedcover is parallel to the end of the bed. **C.** Tuck the part of the corner that hangs between the matteress under the matrtress while holding he cover against the side of the bed mattress. **D.** Bring the point down toward the floor while the other hand holds the fold of the cover against the side of the mattress. **E.** Remove the hand and tuck the remainder of the cover under the mattress, if appropriate.

- By fan-folding the top of the bed (turning both the top sheet and the blanket down together), you make it easy for the patient to get in and out of bed.
- The draw sheet is about half the size of a regular sheet. When draw sheets are not available, a large sheet can be folded in half widthwise (with small and large hems together). The fold must always be placed toward the head of the bed and the hems toward the foot of the bed. You can also use a tablecloth. If you must protect the bed, a plastic tablecloth makes an excellent protective sheet. Never use plastic from a garment bag or garbage bag.
- The plastic draw sheet and disposable bed protectors protect the mattress. Plastics should never touch a patient's skin. When using a plastic draw sheet, be sure to cover it entirely with a cloth draw sheet.
- Some individuals do not use a draw sheet. Instead, small disposable bed protectors are placed on the bed under the client as necessary. These protectors are often expensive. Check with your patient and with his or her family before suggesting use of this product.
- To save linen and washing, a used clean top sheet may be used as a draw sheet or bottom sheet.
- A person who does not use his bed a great deal may not need the linen changed every day. Evaluate linen, home, patient, and the entire situation before you change the bed.
- Always use good body mechanics, no matter what kind of bed your patient is using.
- *Bottom of the bed* refers to the mattress pad (if used), the bottom sheet, and the draw sheets.
- *Top of the bed* refers to the top sheet, the blanket (if used), and the bedspread.
- You save time and energy by first making as much of the bed as possible on one side before going to the other side.

after giving the patient a bed bath. The patient should be covered with the bath blanket while you are making the bed. The sheets must be placed on the bed so the rough seam edges are kept facing the mattress and away from the patient's skin.

Some patients prefer the pillow to be moved with them from side to side as the bed is being made. Some patients will ask you to remove the pillow while making the bed. Either way is acceptable unless there is a medical contraindication (reason for not doing something). The physician will tell you if a particular bed position must be maintained.

Remember to talk to your patient while you make the bed. Continually notice his condition during the procedure (see Procedure 8.1).

SAFETY IN THE HOME

Safety is everyone's responsibility. The rules that govern safety in a home must become part of every procedure and every decision you make while caring for your patient. It is also important for you to remember that, by your actions, you are teaching family members. As they observe you practicing safety, they will be made aware of its importance.

PROCEDURE 8.1

Making an Occupied Bed

Rationale

Clean linen promotes cleanliness, good skin care, and comfort for bed-bound patients. Clean linen also helps prevent the spread of bacteria.

1. Assemble your equipment near the bed, in the order in which you will use them: A chair is useful for this purpose; two large sheets; one plastic draw sheet, if used; one cotton draw sheet, if used; disposable bed protectors, if used; one bath blanket, if available; pillowcase(s); one blanket; one bedspread; and a container for dirty laundry.
2. Wash your hands.
3. Ask any visitors to step out of the room, if appropriate.
4. Tell the patient you are going to make the bed.
5. If you are working on a hospital bed, lower the backrest and knee rest until the bed is flat, if that is allowed. Raise the bed to its highest horizontal position and lock in place.
6. Loosen all the sheets around the entire bed.
7. Take the bedspread and blanket off the bed, and fold them over the back of the chair. Leave the patient covered only with the top sheet.
8. If using a bath blanket, cover the patient with it by placing it over the top sheet. Ask the patient to hold the bath blanket. If he is unable to do this, tuck the top edges of the bath blanket under the patient's shoulders. Without exposing him, remove the top sheet from under the bath blanket. Fold the top sheet and place it over the back of a chair.
9. If the mattress has slipped out of place, move it to its proper position touching the headboard. Remember to use proper body mechanics. If you cannot move the mattress, ask for assistance.
10. Ask the patient to turn onto his side toward the opposite side from where you are standing. Help the patient to turn if necessary. If the patient cannot turn, have him stay on his back but move as far as possible toward the side. Be careful how the patient's hands are placed. Adjust the pillow to suit the patient's needs. Check it for items such as dentures and eyeglasses.
11. Fold the cotton draw sheet toward the patient and tuck it against his back. Protect him from any soiled matter on the bedding (see Figure 8.2).
12. Roll the bottom sheet toward the patient and tuck it against his back. This strips your side of the bed down to the mattress.
13. Take the large clean sheet and fold it in half lengthwise. Do not permit the sheet to touch the floor or your clothing.
14. If using a flat sheet for the bottom sheet, place it on the bed, still folded, with the fold running along the middle of the mattress. The small hem end of the sheet should be even with the foot edge of the mattress. Fold the top half of the sheet toward the patient. This is for the other side of the bed. Tuck the folds against his back, below the plastic draw sheet.
15. Tuck the sheet around the head of the mattress by gently raising the mattress with the hand closest to the foot of the bed and tucking with the other hand.

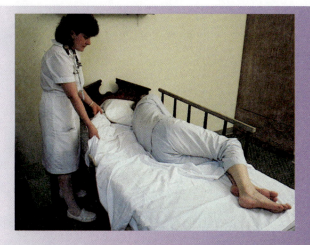

FIGURE 8.2

16. Miter the corner at the head of the mattress. Tuck in the clean bottom sheet on your side from head to foot of the mattress.
17. Pull the plastic draw sheet toward you, over the clean bottom sheet, and tuck it in.
18. Place the clean cotton draw sheet over the plastic sheet, folded in half. Keep the fold near the patient. Fold the top half toward the patient, tucking the folds under his back, as you did with the bottom sheet. Tuck the free edge of the draw sheet under the mattress (see Figure 8.3).
19. Ask the patient, or help him, to roll over the "hump" onto the clean sheets toward you.
20. Remove the old bottom sheet and cotton draw sheet from the bed. Put them into the container for soiled linen. Pull the fresh bottom sheet toward the edge of the bed. Tuck it under the mattress at the head of the bed and make a

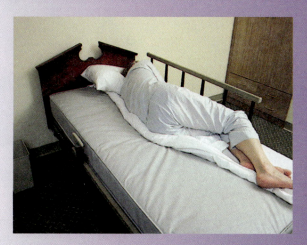

FIGURE 8.3

(continued)

mitered corner. Then pull the bottom sheet under the mattress from the head to the foot. Do this by rolling the sheet up in your hand toward the mattress and pull it as you tuck it under.

21. One at a time, pull and tuck each draw sheet under the mattress.
22. Have the patient turn on his back.
23. Change the pillowcase, and place the pillow under the patient's head. If necessary, assist the patient with placing the pillow under his head.
24. To put the pillowcase on a pillow:
    a. Hold the pillowcase at the center of the end seam.
    b. With your hand outside the case, turn the case back over your hand.
    c. Grasp the pillow through the case at the center of the end of the pillow.
    d. Bring the case down over the pillow.
    e. Fit the corner of the pillow into the seamless corner of the case.
    f. Fold the extra material from the side seam under the pillow.
    g. Place the pillow on the bed with the open end away from the door.
25. Spread the clean top sheet over the bath blanket with the wide hem at the top. The middle of the sheet should run along the middle of the bed. The wide hem should be even with the head edge of the mattress. Ask the patient to hold the hem of the clean sheet, if he can, while you remove the bath blanket, moving toward the foot of the bed. Do not expose the patient.
26. Tuck the clean top sheet under the mattress at the foot of the bed. Make sure you leave enough room for the patient to move his feet freely. Miter the corner of the sheet if the patient likes this.
27. Spread the blanket over the top sheet. Be sure the middle of the blanket runs along the middle of the bed. The blanket should be high enough to cover the patient's shoulders.
28. Tuck the blanket in at the foot of the bed if the patient likes this. Make a mitered corner with the blanket.
29. Place the spread on the bed as the patient prefers.
30. Go to the other side of the bed, turn the top covers back and miter the top sheet, then miter the blanket. Be sure the top covers are loose enough that the patient can move his feet.
31. To make the cuff:
    a. Fold the top hem edge of the spread over and under the top hem of the blanket.
    b. Fold the top hem of the top sheet back over the edge of the spread and blanket to form a cuff. The rough edge of the hem of the sheet must be turned down so the patient does not come in contact with it.
32. Raise the backrest and knee rest to suit the patient, if this is allowed.
33. Lower the entire bed to its lowest horizontal position.
34. Make sure the patient is comfortable.
35. Put all used linen in the proper place.
36. Wash your hands.

It is your responsibility to protect your patient and be continually aware of her safety. Make yourself aware of potential hazardous situations and their remedies in each home where you work. It is also your responsibility to protect yourself. Be careful! Be aware! Be alert!

General Safety Rules

This section is designed to make you aware of the most common safety hazards in a home. More accidents occur in the home than in any other place, for several reasons:

- People are careless.
- People do not have the same safety inspections in homes as are required in commercial buildings.
- People are not aware of the potential hazards that exist in homes.

GENERAL SAFETY RULES YOU SHOULD FOLLOW

- Discuss emergency communication with the patient and his or her family members. If no telephone is available, determine the best method of communicating.
- Arrange for any unsafe conditions to be fixed.
- When you see something on the floor that does not belong there, pick it up. If you see spilled liquid, wipe it up.
- Avoid slippery floors.
- If slippery floors cannot be avoided, walk on them carefully.
- Remove scatter rugs. If you cannot remove them, tack them down.
- Be sure to set the brakes on the wheelchair when a patient is getting in or out.
- Do not work in poor light.
- Do not use any piece of equipment unless you are sure you know how it works.
- Keep the telephone numbers of the police, rescue squad, fire department, and poison control center near each telephone.
- Read labels. If a container does not have one, do not use the contents.
- Know how to leave the house in case of fire.
- Be aware of what accidents are most prevalent at different ages.
- Do not attempt a task if you have any doubt that you can do it safely.
- Do not reach into a garbage can or trash basket. You may hurt yourself on sharp objects.

SAFETY PRECAUTIONS FOR CHILDREN

- Small children should never be left unattended when they are awake.
- Every child in a protective device should be checked frequently.
- Articles used in the child's care should be kept out of reach of a toddler when they are not being used. Watch especially for needles, water, safety pins, medications, matches, electrical equipment, syringes, and thermometers.
- Toys should never be left carelessly on the floor. Be especially alert to pick them up because they could cause someone to fall. Also, remember to clean up spills and messes such as food, urine, and feces.
- The sides of a child's crib should be up at all times except when someone is giving direct care to the child.

- Keep doors to stairways and the kitchen closed and locked.
- Keep venetian blind cords out of the reach of children.
- Be sure no small toys or objects that could be swallowed are in children's beds or cribs.
- Be sure no large objects on which the child could stand are in the bed or crib. The child might fall out of bed as a result.
- Keep all poisonous substances in a high place behind locked doors.

SAFETY PRECAUTIONS FOR THE ELDERLY Abilities change as we age. Unfortunately, few people realize this fact. Therefore, they attempt tasks that they can no longer do safely. As a caregiver, be aware of the capabilities of the individual you are caring for. Also keep in mind these general rules:

- Ensure adequate lighting for every task.
- Be alert to sensory changes (for example, sight, hearing, and smell).
- Protect your patient from falling. Recovery from falls takes a long time.
- Protect your patient from burns. Temperature sensation becomes less accurate as we age. Run cold water through a faucet after you run hot water so your patient will not burn himself if he touches the faucet. Test bath water yourself.
- If a confused patient tells you she is going to do something that you know to be harmful, take her seriously and protect her.

ELECTRICITY Electricity is a great help in our lives. If we misuse it, however, it can cause a great deal of damage (see Figure 8.4). Follow these precautions:

- Make sure all electrical equipment you use is in good condition.
- Be sure the cords are not frayed and that you are using the proper tool for the job.
- Do not put electrical cords under rugs. They may fray and go unnoticed under a rug. This is a perfect place for a fire to start.
- Be sure your hands are dry before you use any electrical equipment.
- Do not change fuses or touch circuit breakers unless you are sure you know what you are doing.
- Do not run all household appliances at the same time in an effort to save time.

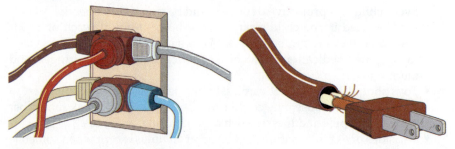

FIGURE 8.4 Examples of unsafe electrical plugs.

CLINICAL ALERT 8.2

Smoking Safety

If your patient smokes and wears oxygen, it is imperative that the oxygen tank and tubing are removed from the patient when they go outside to smoke. Oxygen will remain in the tubing and is flammable when smoking. Lighting materials within twenty feet of someone wearing oxygen can start a fire. If your patient has burn holes in his clothing, use a nonflammable smoking apron to prevent burns. These aprons can be purchased at medical supply stores. If your patient is at risk of burning his fingers due to smoking, use cigarette extenders to prevent finger burns. Extenders can be purchased at any convenience store.

SMOKING   Some patients and some of their visitors may smoke. If a patient permits smoking in his or her home, you may have to tolerate it unless smoking is not allowed for medical reasons or because oxygen is present. Keep in mind the following rules if people smoke in the house (see Clinical Alert 8.2):

- Be sure ashtrays are provided and used.
- Never empty warm ashtrays into plastic bags, plastic wastebaskets, or containers. When you empty ashtrays, be sure the contents are cool. Wet the ashes if you are in doubt.
- An individual who has been given a sedative should not smoke.
- A confused person should not smoke.
- A patient in bed should not smoke unattended.
- Check chairs, upholstery, and blankets for ashes or cigarettes if your patient is smoking.
- If an individual has hand tremors, light her cigarette and assist her as she smokes.

SAFETY IN THE KITCHEN   Some people cook in a hurry and think about many other things while they work. This leads to various types of accidents common to the kitchen area. Keep in mind the following basic safety rules when you are in the kitchen:

- Keep a fire extinguisher in the kitchen.
- Do not leave grease on the stove. Clean it up.
- If you have a grease fire, do not put water on it. Use a chemical-type fire extinguisher or baking soda to smother it. If the fire occurs in a pot or pan with a lid, use the lid to smother it.
- Do not leave cooking pots unattended.
- Have good lighting in the kitchen.
- Be alert when carrying hot liquid.
- Keep paper towels, napkins, and potholders away from the burner.
- Keep the kitchen floor clean and free of clutter and spills.
- Store knives so that blades are protected.

- Electric cooking does not produce a visible flame, so be sure to check that the dial is at the setting you want or at OFF.
- If you or the patient has a pacemaker, stay out of the kitchen when a microwave oven is working.

SAFETY IN THE BATHROOM   Many accidents occur in the bathroom. Young and old alike have these accidents. You must be alert to potential hazards that exist due to conditions in the room and your patient's abilities.

- Is the toilet secure to the floor? Is the seat secure to the toilet?
- Can your patient get up and down safely? Can he sit without additional support?
- Are the hot and cold water faucets marked correctly?
- Is the tub deep, and can the individual climb in and out safely?
- Does the person feel weak while bathing?
- Is there ventilation in the bathroom?
- Are the floor tiles slippery when wet? Is there a secure bathmat on the floor?
- If there are grab bars, are they secure in the wall? Towel bars were not designed to support weight. Special bars may be necessary. Contact the occupational therapist if you believe these bars are needed.
- If you must use electrical equipment such as hair dryers or shavers, be sure your hands, body, and feet are dry.

PROPER STORAGE   Dispose of articles in well-ventilated containers. Do not keep used rags in closed containers. They can catch fire by a process called spontaneous combustion, which means they will burn as a result of their own heat. Dispose of these rags before this happens.

Do not store flammable liquids near any source of heat. Flammable liquids are those that can burn. Keep them in the garage but away from cars. Use flammable liquids in a well-ventilated area to reduce the risk of fire and the risk of illness due to the fumes.

Do not keep piles and piles of newspapers. Make arrangements for them to be given to a recycling plant or recycle them regularly with the local department of public works.

FIRE PREVENTION

Fire safety means following three rules:

1. Preventing fires
2. Doing the right things if fire should occur
3. Protecting your patient and yourself

Fires start because of three ingredients: heat, fuel, and oxygen. The following are common causes of fire:

- Smoking and lighting materials
- Misuse of electricity
- Defects in heating systems

- Spontaneous combustion
- Improper rubbish disposal
- Improper cooking techniques
- Improper ventilation

Making a Fire Plan

If you don't already know the layout of the home, take time to learn the layout and ask yourself the following questions:

- Where are the exits from this house in case of fire?
- How would I remove the patient from this house in case of fire?
- If the patient is bed-bound, how would I remove him from the fire scene?
- Are there fire extinguishers in this house, one for grease fires and one for other types of fires?
- Are there smoke detectors in this house? Do they work?
- Does the family have a fire evacuation plan?
- What special precautions, indicated by the town fire department, should be taken so that fire personnel are aware of small children, bed-bound residents, or people dependent on oxygen or ventilators?

What to Do in Case of Fire

Seal off the fire! If the fire is behind a closed door, do not open it! (See Figure 8.5.) Take another route out of the building to safety. If you must go through a smoke-filled room, put a cloth (a wet one if possible) over your mouth and nose and one over your patient's nose. Crawl along the floor to safety or keep your patient as low to the ground as possible (see Figure 8.6). Keeping in mind the word *RACE* will help you remember the steps to take in case of a fire (see Figure 8.7):

- **Remove** your patient from the house.
- **Activate** the fire department by calling from a neighbor's house or a cell phone.

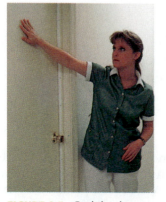

FIGURE 8.5 Feel the door.

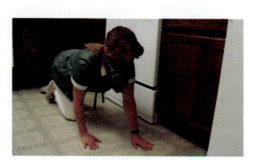

FIGURE 8.6 Crawl on the floor.

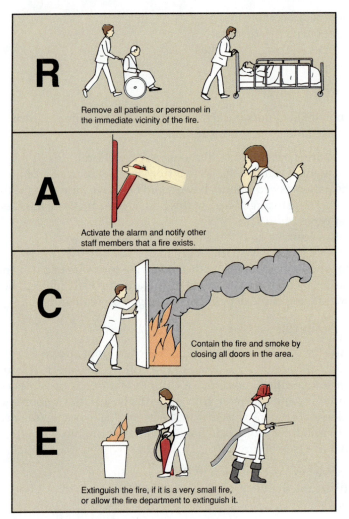

R Remove all patients or personnel in the immediate vicinity of the fire.

A Activate the alarm and notify other staff members that a fire exists.

C Contain the fire and smoke by closing all doors in the area.

E Extinguish the fire, if it is a very small fire, or allow the fire department to extinguish it.

FIGURE 8.7 In case of a fire, remember the word RACE.

- **Contain** the fire and smoke by closing all doors in the area.
- **Extinguish** the fire, if it is a very small fire, or allow the fire department to extinguish it.

POISONS

Children frequently swallow objects not meant to be swallowed. This is considered poisoning. Some people often forget that they took their medication and take additional doses of it. A confused person may take one medication when she really wanted another one. All of these situations are considered instances of poisoning. Prevention is the best treatment for poisoning.

- Keep all poisons and medications locked away from children and confused patients.
- Never keep food products near poisons or cleaning products.
- Make it a habit to read labels each time you pick up any container.
- Call the poison control center for assistance if you have any suspicion that someone has swallowed a poisonous substance or has taken an overdose of medication.
- Instructions for antidotes appear on the bottles of many potentially dangerous substances; unfortunately, these antidotes are not always correct. Do not use them. Call the poison control center and follow the instructions that the attendant relays to you.

OXYGEN SAFETY

Patients may have oxygen prescribed to them for many different reasons. They may be instructed to use the oxygen in different ways, but the safety rules are always the same:

- Never permit smoking in the room where the oxygen tank is kept. This is true if the tank is open or shut.
- Do not use electrical appliances such as heating pads, hair dryers, or electric shavers near oxygen. Keep the plugs out of the wall while the oxygen is running. If a plug is pulled from the outlet while the oxygen is running, a spark could cause an explosion.
- Remove cigarettes, lighting materials, and ashtrays from the room.
- Do not use candles or open flames in the room.
- Do not rub oil, alcohol, or talcum powder on the patient while the oxygen is running.
- Avoid combing a person's hair while she or he is receiving oxygen. A spark of static electricity from the comb or the hair can set off an explosion.
- Wool blankets, nylon, and certain synthetic fabrics can cause static electricity, an electric spark sent into the air. Remove items made from these materials from the individual's room. Use cotton items when possible.
- Check the equipment regularly for leaks and improper functioning.
- Ask for careful instructions about which valves you may touch and which valves should not be moved by contacting the company that delivered the oxygen; the contact information should be on the tank.

RESTRAINTS VERSUS POSITIONING DEVICES

A positioning device is different from a restraint. Restraints should only be used in a hospital setting under twenty-four-hour supervision and a physician's care. Every patient has the right to a safe environment and to

CLINICAL ALERT 8.3

Restraints

Restraints are the least desirable way to provide a safe environment for a patient. They often frighten the patient and her or his family members. Explore with the family and the physician other methods of controlling and keeping the patient safe. Try familiar music, a soft radio station playing in the background, family members taking turns staying with the patient, and talking to the patient in her or his native language.

have his dignity and his rights as a person maintained. Tying a human being to a chair or bed does not support these rights. Restraint devices, while appearing to protect an individual, may actually violate his rights and could be identified as a form of abuse. See Clinical Alert 8.3 for more information.

At a medical facility, the physician should make sure all of the following questions have been answered before considering a restraint:

- Can someone sit with the patient to provide comfort, distraction, and direction during times the patient is most likely to wander?
- Has the medication regime been reviewed to be sure that the mediations are not contributing to the confusion?
- Can activities such as music, television, reading, and visitors be used as diversions?
- Can positioning devices (such as a saddle cushion or self-releasing seat belt displayed in Figure 8.8) be used as reminders to patients instead of actual restraints?

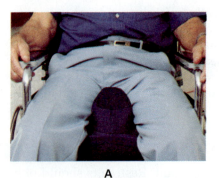

A **B**

FIGURE 8.8 Restraint alternatives; (A) saddle cushion, which prevents sliding forward; (B) self-releasing safety belt.

A positioning device is anything added to a chair or bed that aids the patient in posture, safety, and/or comfort. These devices should be used only when prescribed by a physician. Here are examples of positioning devices:

- A wedge or several pillows can be to prop a person so she can sit up at an angle in bed.
- A saddle cushion helps the patient stay in the wheelchair versus slipping out of the chair.
- A tray can be connected to a wheelchair for the patient to rest a casted arm in an elevated position.
- A self-releasing seat belt can help the patient by securing him in a wheelchair when he is seated, but he can release it himself when he would like to stand.

Summary

Keeping a home clean and comfortable can aid in a patient's recovery and/or sustain her or his quality of life. Use the tools in this chapter to identify supply or equipment needs. Be sure to make a schedule for regular cleaning and eliminate any safety concerns. Care of the environment is important; however, you must always ensure that your patient is safe before you take time to clean. The patient is always the priority.

Chapter 9

Planning, Purchasing, and Serving Food

SCENARIO

Mr. Patel has lived in the United States since he was a little boy. He is fluent in English and his native language. Although he lives in a primarily homogeneous neighborhood, he works in a big factory many miles away. Mr. Patel has developed a heart condition and has been placed on a salt- and calorie-restricted diet. He has been used to eating out each day or dining with friends at their houses. He cooks only simple dishes and uses mostly canned food. He is sure that his condition will improve because he has no symptoms and takes his medications every day that he works. He is not receptive to suggestions about meal planning or taking his lunch to work (see Figure 9.1)

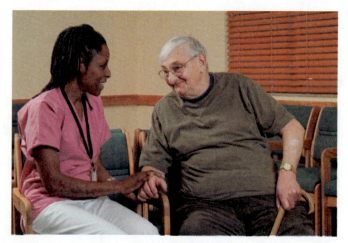

FIGURE 9.1

BASIC NUTRITION

Eating properly is important for all people. Good nutrition is especially important for a person whose body is in a weakened condition. Food gives us energy to carry out the day's activities and is necessary to rebuild body tissue. Eating is also a social activity. In some homes, it is the only time when all family members come together. Many family and personal preferences and practices are associated with food. Do not assume that each family is the same.

Nutrients are substances that our bodies need to repair cells, maintain cells, and grow new ones. Each nutrient comes from many sources. It does not matter from which sources you get the nutrient as long as you get it in sufficient supply. A person unable to get the proper amount of a nutrient from food takes supplements. It is necessary for proper bodily function that a balance be kept among all nutrients—not too much of one or the other.

Dietary requirements differ at different stages of life. Children need more protein and calories than older persons need, but older persons need more of other nutrients depending on their condition.

All foods have been divided into five main food groups: dairy, grains, proteins, fruits, and vegetables. In an effort to help consumers make better food choices, the US Department of Agriculture (USDA) has developed a communications inititiave called MyPlate, which is based on *2010 Dietary Guidelines for Americans*. MyPlate illustrates the five food groups using a familiar mealtime visual: a dinner table place setting.

Although diet will often be as important to the health of your patient as medication or exercise, the patient and his family may not understand this fact. Refer to Chapter 2 for ideas on how to teach the family the importance of food and the proper diet while incorporating family and cultural preferences. If you do not understand certain practices, you may discuss them with the patient or a family member in a respectful and nonjudgmental manner.

Personal Preferences

We all know foods we like and dislike or will not eat. Sometimes, a patient will not eat a food for a cultural reason, a religious reason, or an unexplainable reason. You must respect these preferences and plan meals and diets taking these personal wishes into consideration. Discuss these situations with the physician or a dietician so that you will be able to include all the nutrients in the patient's meals and still adhere to her or his wishes. Your goal is to understand the patient's and family's habits so that you can honor them when planning menus. Observe what foods your patient eats and when she or he eats them.

Standards for a Healthy Diet

Various daily food guides have been developed to help healthy people meet the daily requirements of essential nutrients and to facilitate meal planning. Food group plans emphasize the general types or groups of foods

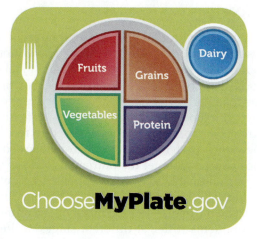

FIGURE 9.2   MyPlate

rather than the specific foods because related foods are similar in composition and often have similar nutrient values. For example, all grains, whether wheat or oats, are significant sources of carbohydrates, iron, and the B vitamin thiamine.

The new USDA MyPlate (see Figure 9.2) has changed considerably from earlier versions of the food guide pyramid developed by the US Department of Agriculture in 1992. Released in 2011, MyPlate reflects guidelines based on updated nutritional knowledge gained from research and data. Consult the US Department of Agriculture MyPlate website (www.choosemyplate.gov) for more information.

PLANNING, SHOPPING FOR, AND SERVING A MEAL

Planning

Mealtime is important. It should be a pleasant change in a patient's day. The atmosphere, the place, and the way the food is served are important in stimulating an appetite. Try to serve a patient in a room free from unpleasant odors and where the patient can be comfortable. Keep the room at a comfortable temperature and as noise-free as possible. It is often helpful to let the patient decide what foods he wishes to eat and when he prefers to eat. Mealtime is more pleasant when a preferred food is served when the patient is hungry.

Menu Planning

As the caregiver, you may find it necessary to purchase food for the patient. First, develop a menu of foods to prepare. Be sure the menu planning is based on the patient's diet and preferences. It is important to keep in mind the patient's ability to chew and swallow as you prepare food.

Consider the recommended servings from MyPlate. Check the ingredients the patient has on hand, and then make a shopping list. A list will help avoid unnecessary trips to the store for forgotten ingredients. It will also prevent buying foods already on hand and, if grouped by types of food, avoid extra steps in the market. When planning a meal, remember the following tips:

- *Variety:* A well-balanced diet consists of nutrients from many different kinds of food. No one food is perfect.
- *Texture:* Combining crispy foods with smooth, soft foods makes each texture seem more interesting. Unless the patient is on a special diet and food texture is controlled, choose different types of texture within each meal served.
- *Flavors:* If all foods in the meal have a strong distinctive taste, they will compete with one another and overwhelm the patient's taste buds. Keep the strong-flavored foods as the spotlight and milder-tasting foods as the background in a meal. Season food as the patient prefers and her diet permits.
- *Temperature:* Cook food at the correct temperature. Ask the patient at what temperature he prefers his food served. Not everyone enjoys their food hot or cold. Some people like ice. Some do not.
- *Taste:* Cook meals to the patient's taste. Discuss with the patient and his or her family members which spices they like and how they usually season their food.
- *Shape:* Prepare food with familiar shapes. Some families always slice their tomatoes, some cut them into chunks. Ask how food is prepared in this household.
- *Color:* Give each meal eye appeal by keeping colors compatible. A sprig of parsley, radish roses, olives, or carrot curls may make an interesting dash of color to an otherwise drab-looking meal.
- *Cost:* Few patients are free to spend an unlimited amount of money on their food. Plan meals within their budgets and do not cause waste.

Include all food eaten during a day in your planning. Food may be eaten at three traditional meals or as snacks throughout the day. Plan meals as close to the patient's usual eating habits as possible.

When a patient's diet is changed, special care should be taken to try to keep this new diet as close to the diet of the other family members as possible. For example, although food for a patient on a salt-free diet should be separated from other family members' food before salt is added, the food may be the same.

Food habits can also be influenced by the patient's religious beliefs or ethnic background. Jewish households may keep a kosher kitchen, which means that utensils and equipment used for meat products are kept separate from those used for dairy products. Meat and dairy products may or may not be eaten at the same meal. The degree to which a patient keeps a kosher home should be discussed with the family. The impact of this upon the prescribed diet should be discussed with the physician or dietician.

Other ethnic groups may not eat pork, shellfish, or beef. Vegetarians eat no animal meat or by-products. These foods or foods made from them should not be ingredients in any prepared foods that you may purchase for a vegetarian household.

People with strong bonds to their ethnic backgrounds may choose foods unfamiliar to you. Patients often ignore a prescribed diet to eat foods more familiar to them. Encourage patients to stay on their therapeutic diet and adapt your menus as much as possible within the therapeutic diet recommendations.

Most of the time, your patient's therapeutic diet can be adapted to meet her ethnic preferences. If you are unfamiliar with her dietary habits, talk with the patient, family members, and/or dietician so that you will learn and be able to help your patient keep within her ethnic tradition.

Food Allergies

Patients may have food allergies that cause mild skin irritations or even severely affect their ability to breathe. Be alert to all of a patient's allergies. Do not take it upon yourself to introduce any new food, even in small amounts. Sometimes children have food restrictions if one of their parents is highly allergic to a substance.

PURCHASING FOOD WISELY   When purchasing packaged foods, *read the labels.* The ingredients lists on labels are critical to a person on a special diet. People on a low-sodium or salt-free diet should read the product label and see if salt was used in preparing the food item. The sodium listed on the labels of all foods for that day should not exceed 1500 mg. Foods such as canned soup, cottage cheese, and hot dogs can exceed the daily limit in one serving. Patients whose diet restricts sugar can tell by reading the label if sugar has been used in the product. People sensitive to certain types of foods or chemicals will find the label's list of ingredients helpful in planning what to eat (see Figure 9.3).

Labels also provide information on the amount in the container. Some labels list the number and amount of servings. Often, labels contain the calories per serving of the product. This information might be important to a patient whose caloric intake is being monitored. The label may also list nutrients in the food and their amounts.

Products that contain more than one ingredient, such as spaghetti in meat sauce, must list all ingredients used in making the product. The ingredient found in the greatest amount is listed first. In comparing two different brands of spaghetti in meat sauce, you can see that a can that listed meat first and flour last would have more meat than one that listed flour first and meat last.

Grocery Shopping

Before you go shopping for your patient, be sure that family members or other emergency contacts know that you are leaving the home. Usually, patients and their families will be encouraged to assume responsibility for shopping

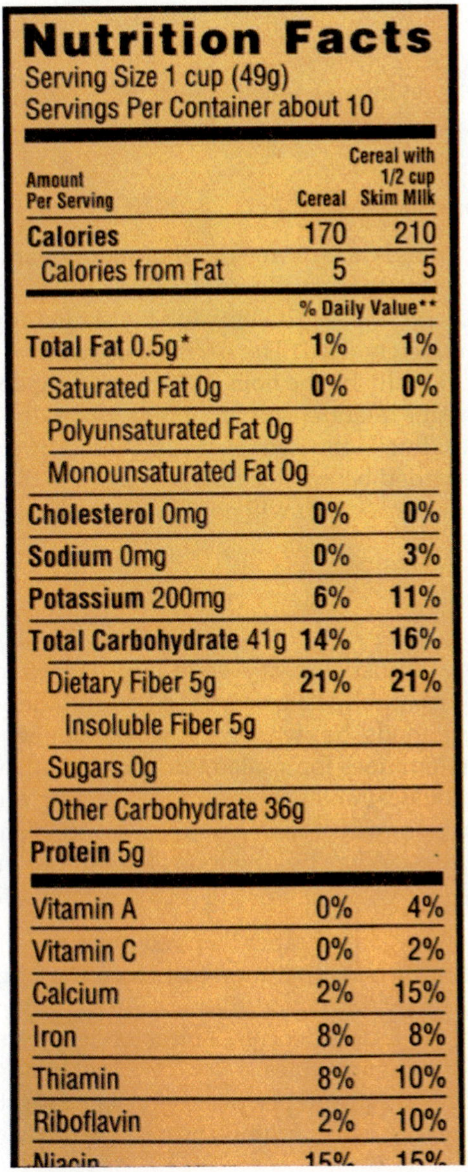

Nutrition Facts

Serving Size 1 cup (49g)
Servings Per Container about 10

Amount Per Serving	Cereal	Cereal with 1/2 cup Skim Milk
Calories	170	210
Calories from Fat	5	5
	% Daily Value**	
Total Fat 0.5g*	1%	1%
Saturated Fat 0g	0%	0%
Polyunsaturated Fat 0g		
Monounsaturated Fat 0g		
Cholesterol 0mg	0%	0%
Sodium 0mg	0%	3%
Potassium 200mg	6%	11%
Total Carbohydrate 41g	14%	16%
Dietary Fiber 5g	21%	21%
Insoluble Fiber 5g		
Sugars 0g		
Other Carbohydrate 36g		
Protein 5g		
Vitamin A	0%	4%
Vitamin C	0%	2%
Calcium	2%	15%
Iron	8%	8%
Thiamin	8%	10%
Riboflavin	2%	10%
Niacin	15%	15%

FIGURE 9.3   Nutritional label

for themselves and managing their own budgets. Sometimes, however, you will be asked to help with shopping for a patient within the family's budget. Before you go shopping:

- Prepare a list and discuss it with the patient.
- Discuss the size of the purchase, money available, likes and dislikes, and favorite stores.
- Be sure your patient will be safe while you are out shopping.

After you shop:

- Save all receipts.
- Carefully write down how much money you were given, how much you spent, and how much change you brought back.

Convenience Foods

Convenience foods (foods with some or all of the preparation already done) generally cost more than those made from scratch. But if only one or two people are eating the food, the ingredients for the scratch process might spoil before they are completely used. The decision about which is most practical must be made individually by the household (including you).

Purchasing larger quantities of an item is generally cheaper than buying small quantities. But, if the item is rarely used or if storage is limited, it may have to be discarded before it is finished. Discuss this with your patient before you go to the store so you will not have to make this decision while at the supermarket.

Good Buys

Foods in season are almost always a good buy. Menus should be planned with seasonal foods in mind. The cost will be less and the selection greater.

When selecting foods, be aware that the best quality is not always necessary. In choosing tomatoes for a salad, the most attractive and usually the most costly would be desirable. However, in selecting tomatoes for tomato sauce, a less expensive product with perhaps a blemish on the skin might be considered a better buy. When buying foods high in protein, you can reduce the cost by:

- using poultry when it is cheaper than red meat
- considering cuts of meat that may cost more per pound but give more servings per person
- learning to prepare less-tender cuts of meat for casseroles or crock pot meals
- serving eggs or egg substitutes
- substituting dried bean and pea dishes for higher-cost meats
- using fillers such as bread crumbs or pasta to make a meat dish serve more people

Storing Food

After shopping for food economically, it is essential that you store it properly. Proper storage prevents loss of nutrients and possible food poisoning. If your patient does not have good storage facilities, limit the amount of food purchased to what space is available to store the food appropriately. Some people do not have sole use of a refrigerator or stove. Work with your patient so that food can be stored safely.

GENERAL STORAGE HINTS

- Do not buy more food than you can safely store.
- Keep refrigerators operating properly by defrosting them when needed.
- Check the expiration date on food before purchasing it. Choose the food with the longest time before expiration.
- Rotate food at home by using the most recently purchased food last.
- Dry ingredients such as flour, sugar, cereal, and pasta products should be stored in tightly covered containers.

TIPS FOR SPECIFIC FOODS

- *Meats:* Refrigerate all meats. Ground meat and variety meats spoil more quickly than others, so use them soon after purchase.
- *Fruits and vegetables:* Keep most fresh fruits and vegetables in the refrigerator in plastic bags, tightly covered containers, or the crisper.
- *Bread:* If wrapped properly, bread can be frozen to keep it unable for a long time.
- *Milk:* Instant nonfat dry milk can be used in many of the same ways as whole milk and can be stored for much longer periods without refrigeration.
- *Canned foods:* Store in a cool, dry place.
- *Frozen foods:* Keep in the freezer at a temperature of 0°C.

Preparing a Meal

Encourage the participation of the patient and family members if at all possible to make the meal preparation process fun for everyone. Prior to cooking a meal, have everyone wash their hands. Wash any fresh fruits or vegetables you are using to prevent the spread of germs. If you are cutting vegetables or fruit, do not use the same knife or cutting surface that you have used or will be using to cut meat products. Wash your hands after any contact with meat products. When preparing foods, be aware of the amount of energy you use. By doing this, you will save time and money, and indicate your concern for the patient's resources. Keep the following hints in mind:

- Use the oven to prepare more than one food at a time. For example, if you are going to bake a cake, do it at the same time the casserole is heating up in the oven.
- Do not preheat the oven longer than necessary.
- Put the pot or pan on the correct-size burner. The burner should be as close to the size of the pot or pan as possible. Too big a burner wastes fuel.
- Cover pots while food in them is cooking.
- Make one-dish meals.
- Make enough food for more than one meal and reheat the remaining servings.

- If you are using an electric range, turn off the heat a few minutes before the food is ready.
- Use the correct appliance for the job. Use a small toaster oven for small jobs and the big oven for big jobs.

METHODS OF COOKING

- *Bake or roast:* Cook with dry heat in a confined space, such as an oven.
- *Boil:* Cook in a liquid hot enough for bubbles to break on the surface.
- *Braise:* A long, slow cooking method that uses moist heat in a tightly covered vessel at a temperature just below boiling. The cooking liquid should just barely cover the food to be braised. Braising is a good way to cook tough meats and vegetables because the long cooking breaks down their fibers.
- *Broil:* Cook directly under or above a source of heat.
- *Fry:* Cook food in fat or oil. When only a small amount of fat is used, the process is called pan frying or sautéing. When larger amounts of fat are used—enough to cover the food—the process is called deep frying or deep fat frying.
- *Poach:* A method of cooking used to preserve the delicate texture of foods and to prevent toughening foods. The food is covered by water or another liquid. Depending on the type of food being cooked, the liquid may be either boiling or close to the boiling point.
- *Steam:* A method of cooking in which the food is exposed to the steam of boiling water. The food must be above the liquid, never in it. The container is kept closed during cooking to let the steam accumulate. Steaming keeps a high proportion of the original flavor and texture of the foods because the nutrients are not dissolved in the cooking liquid, as is the case with boiling or poaching. Steaming is a more time-consuming way of cooking, however.
- *Stew:* A process of long, slow cooking of the food in a liquid in a covered pot with seasoning. It is good for tenderizing tougher cuts of meat.

GETTING A PATIENT READY FOR A MEAL

Before serving a meal to a patient, wash the patient's hands and clean the eating area. Serve the patient in an orderly and friendly fashion. Prepare small portions, especially if the patient has a poor appetite. A great deal of food will only make him uncomfortable. Serve the meal as the patient wants it. Some people want their soup first; some want their salad first. Accommodate the patient unless there is a health reason why you may not. The place where people eat is important. If a patient enjoys eating in the living room, serve him there. If he would rather eat in his bedroom and you know of no reason not to, serve him there.

An important part of serving a meal to a patient is your observations about the patient at mealtime:

- How is the person's appetite?
- Does she eat foods on her diet?
- What foods does she avoid?
- Is there any discomfort associated with eating?
- Does the patient drink fluids?
- Does the patient eat several big meals, or does she eat all day long?
- Who serves the patient when you are not there?

Serving a Meal

A poor appetite does not mean that the body's need for food is lowered. The sick person's body is in a weakened condition. The patient needs as much food as ever—if not more—to return to health. The surroundings and the food served should be as cheerful, attractive, and appetizing as possible. The sight and aroma of food often make a person hungry. You can increase a patient's appetite by showing him what he will be eating. Also, people have a better appetite for foods they especially like. Therefore, if a patient asks for a particular food (and if he is permitted to have it), serve it to him.

Mealtime is often one of the highlights of the day for a convalescent patient or a patient who is not extremely sick. Mealtime is a break in an often boring routine. It gives the person something to look forward to.

- Tell the individual you will be serving her a meal.
- Most people enjoy company during mealtime. Visitors and family members should be encouraged to remain with the patient and even eat with the patient if that is appropriate.

Keep the following tasks separate from the patient's mealtime:

- Before or after the meal, offer the patient the bedpan or urinal.
- After the meal, offer the patient oral hygiene.

THE THERAPEUTIC DIET

The appropriate type of diet will be determined by the doctor. The dietitian will help the patient plan her diet and work with you. The therapeutic diet will be planned to incorporate the patient's likes and dislikes, her ethnic background, and her budget (see Tables 9.1, 9.2, 9.3. and 9.4).

It is your responsibility to follow the diet plan when preparing the patient's meals and to offer feedback to the dietician. Assist the patient and family members with incorporating the therapeutic diet into the family's usual eating habits. If there are any questions about the diet or its preparation, call the dietitian. If the patient is not eating the food on the diet, the dietitian should be notified.

TABLE 9.1 Types of Patient Diets

Type of Diet	Description	Common Purpose	Foods Often Recommended	Foods to Avoid
Normal, regular	Provides all essentials of good nourishment in normal forms.	For people who do not need special diets.	Not applicable	Not applicable
Soft (mechanical)	Same foods as on a normal diet, but chopped or strained.	For people who have difficulty chewing or swallowing.		
Bland	Foods mild in flavor and easy to digest; omits spicy foods.	For people who need to avoid irritation of the digestive tract, as with ulcer and colitis.	Puddings, creamed dishes, milk, eggs, plain potatoes.	Fried foods, raw vegetables or fruit, whole-grain products.
Low-residue	Foods low in bulk; omits foods difficult to digest.	Spares the lower digestive tract; for people with rectal diseases.		Whole-grain products, uncooked fruits and vegetables.
High-calorie	Foods high in protein, minerals, and vitamins.	For underweight or malnourished people.	Eggnog, ice cream, frequent snacks, peanut butter, milk.	Not applicable
Low-calorie	Foods low in fats and complex carbohydrate, cereals, low-fat desserts.	For people who want to lose weight.	Skim milk, fresh fruit and vegetables, lean meat, fish.	Fried foods, sauces, gravies, rich desserts.
Low-fat	Limited amounts of butter, cream, fats, and eggs.	For patients who have difficulty digesting fats and may have gall bladder, cardiovascular, and/or liver disturbances.	Veal, poultry, fish, skim milk, fresh fruits and vegetables.	Bacon, butter, cheese, fried foods, liver, whole milk, ice cream, chocolate.

Diet	Description	Purpose	Foods allowed	Foods to avoid
Low-cholesterol*	Low in eggs, whole milk, cheese, and meats.	Helps regulate the amount of cholesterol in the blood.	Fruits, vegetables, cereals, grains, nuts, vegetable oil.	Organ meats (for example, liver)
Diabetic*	Balance of carbohydrates, protein, and fats; devised according to the needs of individual person.	For a diabetic patient: match food intake with insulin and nutritional requirements.	Fresh fruits and vegetables, low-sugar products.	High-sugar foods, alcohol, carbonated beverages.
High-protein	Meals with high-protein foods, such as meat, fish, cheese, milk, and eggs.	Assists in the growth and repair of tissues wasted by disease; assists in wound healing.	Milk, meat, eggs, cheese, fish	Not applicable
Low-sodium (low-salt)	Limited amount of foods containing sodium; no salt allowed at the table.	For people whose circulation would be impaired by fluid retention, who have hypertension, or who have certain heart or kidney conditions.	Puffed wheat and rice or shredded wheat, fruits, fruit juices.	Canned vegetables, ham, luncheon meats, frankfurters, most cheeses.
Salt-free*	No salt	Not applicable	Most fresh or frozen vegetables.	Not applicable

*See additional charts provided in this chapter.

TABLE 9.2	Foods High in Cholesterol
Milk	Whole milk, cream, soft cheeses, high-fat cheeses, ice cream, sour cream.
Breads/cereals	Pastry, sweet rolls, snack crackers, doughnuts, egg noodles.
Meat	Prime meat, organ meat, animal fat, lard, sausage, bacon, luncheon meat.
Eggs	Egg yolks.
Fats/oils	Butter, lard, coconut oil, palm oil, margarines high in saturated fats, dressings made with egg yolks.
Desserts	Ice cream, pies, cakes, milkshakes.

TABLE 9.3	Foods High in Potassium	
Apricots		Low-sodium baking soda
Avocados		Molasses
Bamboo shoots		Nuts
Bananas		Nectarines
Beet greens		Oranges
Bran		Potato with skin
Chocolate		Spinach
Coffee		Sweet potato
Low-sodium baking powder		Wheat germ

Figure 9.10 is a recipe for a main dish that is versatile, nutritious, easy to prepare, and economical. For more information on topics related to nutrition, see the Resource Page at the end of this book.

FEEDING OR ASSISTING A PATIENT

Some patients cannot feed themselves and therefore need to be fed. Here are some example situations that require you to assist a patient with eating a meal:

- The individual cannot use her hands.
- The doctor wants the patient to save her strength and to be on complete bed rest.
- The person may be too weak to feed herself.
- The patient is too confused to sit and eat a meal on his own.

Usually, it is hard for an adult to accept the idea of being unable to feed herself. Patients who cannot feed themselves may feel resentful and depressed. Be friendly and natural. Talk pleasantly but not too much. Encourage each patient to do as much as he can.

TABLE 9.4   Foods High in Salt

A-1 Sauce	Anchovies	Bacon	Barbecue sauce
Bologna	Bouillon cubes or powders (regular)	Buttermilk	Canned gravies or sauces
Canned ravioli or spaghetti	Canned soups	Canned stews	Canned vegetables
Catsup (ketchup)	Caviar	Celery salt	Cheese doodles
Chili sauce	Corned beef	Cheese—regular, processed, and spreads	Chinese food, canned or restaurant
Frozen, breaded meats and fish	Frozen TV dinners	Ham—smoked or cured	Hamburger Helper mix
Herring	Horseradish	Hot dogs/frankfurters	Kitchen Bouquet
Knockwurst	Kosher meats	Liverwurst	Lox
Luncheon meats	Malted milk	Meat tenderizers	Monosodium glutamate (Accent)
Mustard	Nuts—salted	Olives	Onion salt
Party spread and dips	Pastrami	Pickled pigs' feet	Pickles
Popcorn—salted	Relishes	Salami	Salted snack foods— pretzels, potato chips, corn chips
Sardines	Sauerkraut	Sausage	Scrapple
Sea salt	Seasoned salt	Smoked salmon	Smoked tongue
Soy sauce	Tomato juice—regular	Worcestershire sauce	

Tips for Feeding a Patient

- Allow patients to feed themselves as much as possible; give assistance only as needed.
- Do not rush the feeding; sit if possible.
- Be gentle with forks and spoons; straws may help in feeding liquids (if straws are approved by the speech therapist).
- If your patient is confused, try serving or feeding one bowl of food at a time. Alternatively, you can feed a patient several times throughout the day.
- If the patient won't sit for a meal (if she keeps pacing or leaving the table), try giving her finger foods so she can feed herself as she walks around the home.
- Keep the conversation pleasant and make the meal a highlight of the day.
- Feed foods separate rather than mixed together (unless it is the patient's preference to have them mixed).

- When offering a glass, cup, or utensil, first touch it to the patient's lips.
- Record the intake and output of food and any liquid (if requested by the health care team).
- If anything out of the ordinary occurs while you are feeding a patient, record these observations.

Safety Factors

Be sure a patient can swallow before you put food in his mouth. Some patients will be able to swallow one food and not another. Pay special attention to the food temperature. If a food is hot, tell the patient and then offer him a small amount. If the food is cold, do the same. Keep food on a table away from the patient's bed so that the patient can change position without spilling the food. If a patient is blind, name each mouthful (each type of food and liquid) before you offer it to him.

EFFECTS OF CHEMOTHERAPY AND RADIATION ON A PATIENT'S DIET

Many people who receive chemotherapy and radiation therapy change their eating habits due to periods of nausea, vomiting, appetite loss, and/or constipation. It is helpful to consult with the dietitian so that the best possible diet, taking nutrients from the five food groups and the minerals and vitamins, can be planned. Here are several helpful hints for these patients:

- Decrease intake of red meats; many people prefer fish, chicken, turkey, and other nonmeat foods high in protein.
- Use plastic utensils; some people complain of a bitter taste from metal utensils.
- Maintain adequate fluid intake of cool, clear liquids.
- Eat small, frequent meals; chew food well; eat warm, not hot, food.
- Decrease intake of sweets and fried or fatty foods; this change decreases nausea and decreases intake of empty calories.
- Remain in a sitting position for two hours after meals.
- Eat non-gas-producing foods.

YOUR ROLE AS A CAREGIVER

In addition to the points already listed for the patient, follow these guidelines:

- Discuss the patient's fiber intake with your supervisor.
- Provide a pleasant, quiet atmosphere for meals.
- Vary the diet.
- If the patient has difficulty eating by himself or being neat as he eats, protect his clothes with a large napkin (use of clothing protectors that look like an infant's bib can be demeaning).

Summary

For many of us, food is the highlight of the day. We plan our activities around mealtimes and use food as the purpose of a party or get-together. When the ability to plan, prepare, and serve meals diminishes, it can affect our desire to eat. Illness or medications can make food unappealing, or a prescribed diet may not fit our usual eating habits. At these times, a caregiver can provide variety and socialization for meals. Don't be afraid to be creative! Try new ways of setting the table or different background music, or invite various people to join the patient for a meal. Figuring out ways to make mealtimes more appealing will help the patient respond more positively to eating foods that are needed for health.

Chapter 10

Basic Body Movement and Positions

SCENARIO

Mrs. Mahamoud suffered a broken hip from a fall in her kitchen. She was trying to retrieve a dish from a high shelf and slipped off a stool. Her sons are young adults and are in college and working. Prior to her fall, Mrs. Mahamoud was active in her neighborhood religious activities, but she is unable to drive now. Her husband works six days a week and spends his free time with his elderly father living nearby with his also elderly aunt. Mrs. Mahamoud exercises when she is reminded and when someone is there to assist her, but she does not initiate the exercises. She remains in bed until everyone has left the house in the morning and then gets up using her own procedures. Her husband communicates with the doctor and the therapists via telephone. Mrs. Mahamoud manages to keep the house tidy and cook simple meals. She seldom eats with the family, preferring to eat after everyone is finished at the table. Shopping for food poses a serious problem because Mrs. Mahamoud cannot go herself and does not want to ask her family for help.

BODY MECHANICS

The term *body mechanics* refers to the way of standing and moving one's body to prevent injury, avoid fatigue, and make the best use of strength. If you understand the rules of good body mechanics and apply them to your work and everyday life, you will be less tired and will feel better at the end of the day. Once you understand how to control and balance your body, you will understand how to control and balance your patient's body. Body mechanics is a major safety factor for both of you. Remember, low-back problems are a leading cause of employee sick time. It is most important that you learn good body mechanics to protect your back and your ability to care for your patient.

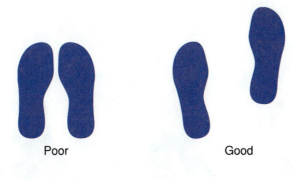

Poor   Good

FIGURE 10.1

Base of Support

The base of support determines how stable your balance will be. Try standing with both feet together. How far can you reach forward? Sideways? You probably lost your balance quickly. Now stand with your feet separated about six to eight inches, with one foot a half-step ahead of the other. Repeat reaching forward and sideways. You can reach farther this time before losing your balance because, by separating your feet, you made your base of support larger and your balance more stable (see Figure 10.1).

Center of Gravity

The center of gravity of any object you hold is the point at which you have the greatest control over the object with the least amount of effort. A person's center of gravity is located around the pelvic area (see Figure 10.2). When moving or assisting a patient, support him through his center of gravity. By holding a person close to his center of gravity and your center of gravity, you will have the greatest amount of control with the least amount of effort. The individual will also feel that you have control and will be more likely to trust you and follow your directions.

Balancing

When you must lift heavy objects, spread your feet apart and bend your knees. This position will lower your center of gravity, increase stability, and broaden your base of support. To balance yourself, your center of gravity must remain within your base of support. Getting up from a sitting position is one example: Some people have difficulty getting up from a sitting position because they are afraid to lean forward far enough. Their center of gravity is not balanced over their base of support. If you help them move their buttocks out over their feet (properly positioned), they will usually balance quite well and learn to lose their fear (see Guideline 10.1).

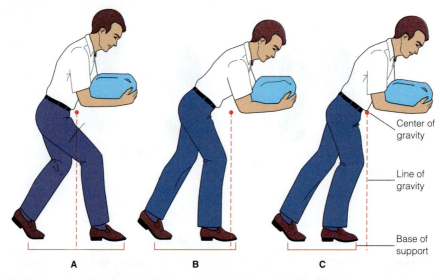

FIGURE 10.2 A. Balance is maintained when the line of gravity falls close to the base of support. B. Balance is precarious when the line of gravity falls at the edge of the base of support. C. Balance cannot be maintained when the line of gravity falls outside the base of support.

GUIDELINE 10.1

Good Body Mechanics

- When an action requires physical effort, use as many groups of muscles as possible. For example, use both hands rather than one hand to pick up a heavy piece of equipment.
- Use good posture. Keep your body properly aligned. Keep your back straight. Have your knees bent. Keep your weight evenly balanced on both feet.
- Check your feet when you lift something. They should be at least twelve inches apart. This position will give you a broad base of support and good balance (see Figure 10.3).
- If you think you may not be able to lift the load, or if it seems too large or heavy, find help.
- Lift smoothly to avoid strain. Always count one, two, three with both the patient and with other helpers.
- If you must move or lift a heavy object or person, use a lumbar support. A support can be obtained from the agency medical supply store or a pharmacy. When you want to change the direction of movement:
  - Pivot (turn) with your feet.
  - Turn with short steps.
  - Turn your whole body without twisting your neck and back.
- Get close to the load being lifted.
- When you move a heavy object, it is better to push, pull, or roll it rather than lift and carry it.

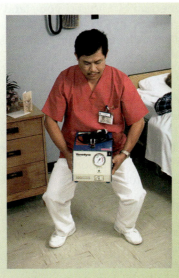

FIGURE 10.3

- Use your arms to support the object. The muscles of your legs, not the muscles of your back, actually do the job of lifting. The muscles that bend your elbow are stronger than the ones that straighten it out; your greatest lift power is in pulling.
- When you do work such as giving a backrub, making a corner on a bed, or exercising a patient, work with the direction of your efforts, not against them.
- When working with a patient in a hospital bed (bathing, dressing, exercising, etc.), raise the bed to a comfortable position for you. Also, move the patient close to the side of the bed where you are working.
- When working with a patient in a bed that cannot be raised up and if you must stand, put one foot up on a footstool to relieve the pressure on your lower back. Remember the same rules of a broad base of support: Use the strongest muscles for the work and keep your center of gravity close to your work.
- Avoid twisting your body (or your patient's body).

Strongest Muscles

Generally, muscles that flex (bend) joints are the strongest. In your arms, you have the greatest power and control when you lift with your palms facing up. In your legs, your hip flexors and your knee flexors are strongest, which explains why you should bend your hips and knees slightly when using good body mechanics. This position puts the muscles in the best position to do heavy work. Your strongest muscles are not in your back, so do not expect your back to do heavy work. Keep the following points in mind:

- Knowing how your body balances means you will know how your patient's body balances.
- Use proper body mechanics to protect your back; it is the only one you have.

- Use proper body mechanics *whenever* you stand or move. It cannot be a behavior you use only on the job.
- An injured back is painful, inconvenient, and costly.

DAILY ABILITY LEVEL

Each person is different. Depending on many factors, such as age, disability, weather, and family pressures, a patient may be totally or partially dependent on you, or she may be fully independent. Activities performed one day may be impossible the next. It is your responsibility to check the daily ability level of the individual you are caring for before you ask her to perform an activity. Observe the patient's activity tolerance each day (see Guideline 10.2).

Checklist to Assess Daily Ability Level

- Can the patient hear and understand you?
- Can the patient follow directions?
- How much can the patient do alone?
- How does the patient look?
- What are her vital signs?
- Will pain be a factor in this activity?
- Are joint motions limited?
- Does the patient tire easily?

GUIDELINE 10.2

Assisting Patients

- Expect the patient to do as much as possible.
- Help only when needed.
- Work at the patient's level and speed.
- Direct activity instead of asking for it. For example, say, "It is time to stand, Mrs. N" instead of "Do you want to stand up, Mrs. N?" (If Mrs. N says, "No!" what do you do then?)
- Plan ahead. Gather all equipment and put it in place before you begin the activity.
- Know your own capabilities.
- Give the patient short, simple directions.
- Praise the patient for following directions. If he does something incorrectly, stop the activity and redirect him until the correct activity is done. That way, the patient will get used to doing the activity the correct way only.
- Your body language (your tone of voice, facial expression, the way you touch, etc.) will be more strongly received than the meaning of the words you use. Make sure your nonverbal messages fit the words you use.
- Touch is the most important of the senses. You will be touching your patient during care. If you are comfortable with this, your patient will be, too.
- Always use smooth, steady motions with patients. Avoid sudden, jerking movements.

Your role is to help the patient complete the activity, not to do it for her. Because you may not be in the house all the time, the patient and her family must know how to give care when you are not there. By setting a good example, you will teach and you will assist the patient and her family in accepting whatever limitations remain.

BODY SUPPORT AND ALIGNMENT

Many of your tasks require lifting and moving patients. Some patients will be able to help you. Some will not. A bedridden person must have his position changed at least once every two hours. Proper support and alignment of the patient's body are important.

The individual's body should be straight and properly supported; otherwise, his safety and comfort might be affected. The correct positioning of the person's body is referred to as body alignment or bed positioning. Arrangement or adjustment of the patient's body is made so that all parts of the body are in their proper positions in relation to each other. Proper body alignment can be seen in proper standing posture. When people lie in bed, it is often necessary to use pillows and rolled-up towels to keep this alignment. Some conditions and injuries, as well as special patient care treatments, make it difficult or even dangerous for an individual to be in a certain position. The patient's physician will tell you about any special positions that your patient requires.

A person unable to move needs to have her position changed every two hours to:

- minimize the possibility of muscle tightness (contractures)
- reduce the chance of skin breakdown
- maintain proper body alignment
- make the patient comfortable
- avoid delaying rehabilitation

A patient improperly positioned during the first part of her illness can develop problems that must be taken care of before rehabilitation can begin. This additional step often prevents or delays exercises and activities that would allow a patient to function more fully. For example, if a patient who is not properly positioned in bed develops a decubitus, or bed sore, this must heal before she can start exercises.

COMMONLY USED POSITIONS

A patient can be positioned on the back, stomach, either side, or in a position halfway between side lying and stomach lying. The person's diagnosis, condition, and comfort determine which position to use. Remember, just because an individual cannot move without help when asked does not mean that he will stay for two hours in the correct position. Keep checking your patient for proper positioning (see Procedures 10.1 and 10.2).

PROCEDURE 10.1

Rolling the Patient (Log Rolling)

1. Wash your hands.
2. Tell the person you are going to roll him to his side as if he were a log.
3. Lock any wheels on the bed.
4. Raise the whole bed to the best height for you.
5. Remove the pillow from under the patient's head, if allowed.
6. Move the person to your side of the bed on his back (see Figure 10.4).

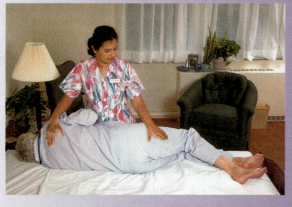

FIGURE 10.4

7. While holding the patient at his hip and shoulder, roll the patient toward you onto his side. Turn him gently (see Figure 10.5).

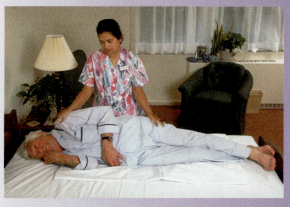

FIGURE 10.5

8. Place the patient in a good bed position, and remake the top covers of the bed.
9. Wash your hands.

PROCEDURE 10.2

Raising the Head and Shoulders

Rationale

Keeping good body alignment helps prevent decubiti, respiratory problems, and general discomfort. Some people require assistance to sit up. Sitting up comfortably and safely prevents poor body alignment. Using correct procedures prevents injury to you and the person for whom you are caring.

1. Never pull on an arm to lift a patient up. If assistance is required, slide your arm under the shoulder blade to lift. Or raise the head of the bed, if possible.
2. If the patient has some strength in one or both arms, "plant" your feet in the proper position, hold your arm out steady, and let her pull up on you; that way, you remain stationary while she does the work. You then have one hand free to adjust the pillow or blankets as desired.
3. Remember, good body mechanics are important to success (see Figure 10.6).

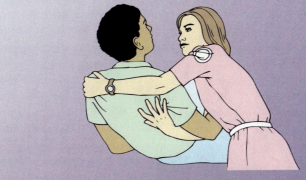

FIGURE 10.6 The patients hand should be under your armpit and placed on your shoulder or across his waist.

MOVING PATIENTS IN BED

For good positioning, the patient must be up at the head of the bed. If your patient can stand, even briefly, have her sit over the edge of the bed. Help her to stand and move her buttocks up toward the head of the bed. Repeat the process until she is in a good position to lie back down with her head at the top of the bed. In this way, you not only have your patient back where you want her, but she will have exercised her muscles, heart, balance system, and coordination system all at the same time. You have taught her a valuable activity that she can use in the future when she is stronger (see Procedure 10.3).

When an individual needs help to move, a pull sheet can help you move the patient in bed. A regular extra sheet folded over many times and placed under the person serves as a pull sheet. The cotton draw sheet can also be used as a pull sheet. When moving the patient, roll up the pull sheet tightly

PROCEDURE 10.3

Moving a Patient Up in Bed with the Patient's Help

Rationale

Keeping a person in good body alignment helps prevent decubiti, respiratory problems, and general discomfort. Working with the patient prevents injury to both patient and caretakers, and allows the patient to be an active participant in his care.

1. Wash your hands.
2. Tell the patient you are going to help him move up in the bed.
3. Lock wheels on the bed, if possible.
4. Raise the whole bed to a height best for you.
5. Remove the pillow from under the patient's head and place it at the head of the bed to prevent the patient from hitting his head on the headboard when you move him up.
6. Put one hand under the patient's shoulder. Put your other hand under the patient's buttocks (see Figure 10.7).

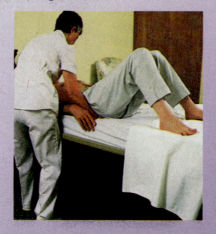

FIGURE 10.7

7. Tell the patient to bend his knees and brace his feet firmly on the mattress.
8. Tell him to put his hands on the mattress to help push.
9. Have your feet twelve inches apart. The foot closest to the head of the bed should be pointed toward the head of the bed.
10. Bend your knees. Keep your back straight.
11. Face the patient and turn slightly toward the head of the bed; bend your body from your hips.
12. On the count of three, have the patient pull with his hands toward the head of the bed and push with his feet against the mattress.
13. At the same time, help him to move toward the head of the bed by sliding him with your hands and arms.
14. Put the pillow back in place. Reposition the patient correctly.
15. Make him comfortable. Lower the bed to the lowest horizontal position, if possible.
16. Wash your hands.

on each side next to the patient's body. Grip the rolled portion underhand to slide the patient into the desired position. By using the pull sheet, you avoid friction and irritation to the individual's skin that touches the bedding. If there is another person available to help, have that person stand on one side of the bed while you stand on the other. At the same time, use the sheet to pull the patient to the top of the bed (see Procedure 10.4).

PROCEDURE 10.4

Moving a Patient Up in the Bed Alone

Rationale
Keeping a person in good body alignment helps prevent decubiti, respiratory problems, and general discomfort. Using aids to assist you will help prevent injury to both you and your patient.

1. Wash your hands.
2. Tell the patient you are going to move her up in bed. Say this even if she appears unconscious.
3. Ask the visitors to leave, if appropriate.
4. Remove the pillow from the bed. Place it on a chair or any other convenient location.
5. Lock wheels on the bed, if possible.
6. Raise the whole bed, if possible, to a height that is comfortable for you.
7. Stand at the head of the bed. One foot should be as close as possible to the bed, the other slightly behind.
8. Reach over the top of the draw sheet. Roll the edge and grab it.
9. On a count of three, lock your arms and back into one unbendable unit and shift your weight to your back leg. The patient will slide easily to the top of the bed with the sheet. Make sure you do this slowly and use good body mechanics (see Figure 10.8).

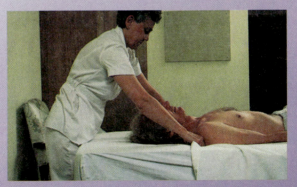

FIGURE 10.8 Use the sheet and good body mechanics to move the patient.

10. Replace the pillow. Position the patient correctly. Return the bed to its original horizontal position.
11. Wash your hands.

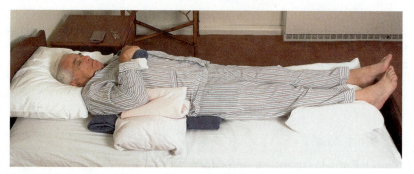

FIGURE 10.9 Support the patient in bed with pillows and towels to their comfort level.

General Positioning Rules

- A rolled-up washcloth makes an excellent support for the hand.
- If an arm or leg is swollen, try to keep the part higher than the heart. Gravity will help the extra fluid drain from the limb.
- Any open skin will heal more quickly if pressure is reduced and air is allowed to circulate around it.
- Position and support only nonfunctional parts of the body. The rest should be left to freely move, which will help the blood to circulate.

Proper positioning can help a patient maintain or recover his or her best possible state of health.

Tips for Positioning a Patient on His or Her Back

- Place a small comfortable pillow under the individual's head.
- Use a small hand towel folded under the shoulder blade of the weak side.
- Place a bath towel folded under the hip on the weak side.
- Use a washcloth rolled up in the hand on the weak side.
- Place a weak arm and elbow on a pillow higher than the heart.
- Put a small pillow under the calf of the weak leg, with the heel hanging off the mattress edge (see Figure 10.9).
- Loosen the top sheet so pressure is removed from the toes (see Procedure 10.5).

USING THE CORRECT TERMS

Patients who need physical therapy or any other types of assistance usually have some type of disability. They may have a weakness or an injury on one side. Do not refer to this side as the bad side. There is nothing bad about it. Instead, refer to it as the involved side because it is involved in the treatment. Refer to the other side as the uninvolved side. Calling

PROCEDURE 10.5

Moving a Patient to One Side of the Bed on the Patient's Back

Rationale

Keeping a patient in good body alignment helps prevent decubiti, respiratory problems, and general discomfort. When assistance is unavailable, use the correct procedure, even if it takes time. The correct procedure will prevent injury to both you and your patient.

1. Wash your hands.
2. Tell the patient you are going to move him to one side of the bed on his back without turning him. Explain that this is a safety measure so that, when he is turned to his side, he will be in the center of the bed.
3. Lock any wheels on the bed.
4. Raise the whole bed to the highest position best for you.
5. Lower the backrest and footrest, if this is allowed.
6. Loosen the top sheets, but do not expose the patient.
7. Place your feet in good position: one close to the bed and one back. Slide both your arms under the patient's back to his far shoulder, then slide his shoulders toward you by rocking your weight to your back foot (see Figure 10.10).

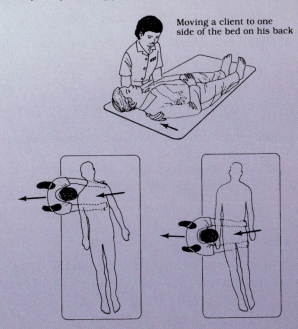

Moving a client to one
side of the bed on his back

FIGURE 10.10

8. Keep your knees bent and your back straight as you slide the patient.
9. Slide both your arms as far as you can under the patient's buttocks, and slide his buttocks toward you the same way. Use a pull (turning) sheet whenever possible for helpless patients.

10. Place both your arms under the patient's feet and slide them toward you.
11. Replace and adjust the pillow, if necessary.
12. Remake the top of the bed.
13. Make the patient comfortable. Lower the bed to its lowest horizontal position.
14. Wash your hands.

your patient's weak side the bad side will only discourage him or her from using it.

If your patient understands the concept of right and left, refer to her limbs in those terms. At times, you will have to touch the arm or leg you want her to move. You may also have to demonstrate the activity first.

You will hear the words *functional* and *nonfunctional*. *Functional* describes the usefulness of something. It may be an activity or a body part. An activity such as folding clothes, making salad, or combing one's hair is a functional activity because it produces a desired result. Nonfunctional body parts will not perform a useful activity.

You can see that words are important: They describe the way you feel and the way you see the patient and his or her disability.

Positioning a Patient on the Uninvolved Side

- Place a small pillow under the head. Keep the head in alignment with the spine.
- Roll a large pillow lengthwise, and tuck it in at the patient's back to prevent him from rolling and to give him support.
- Place a pillow in front to keep the arm the same height as the shoulder joint.
- Use a medium pillow between the patient's knees (the top knee may be slightly bent or both may be bent).
- Place a small pillow between the ankles and feet.
- Use a large pillow at the stomach area (if the patient wishes) for the patient to roll onto (see Figure 10.11).

Positioning a Patient on the Involved Side

The same principles of positioning for the uninvolved side are used for positioning the involved side. But keep the following additional points in mind:

- The patient's comfort will be the key to how and where support should be used.
- Change the patient's position more frequently than when he is positioned on the uninvolved side.
- Disability can come with lessened sense of pain and recognition of pressure. Check the involved side for signs of pressure and skin irritation.

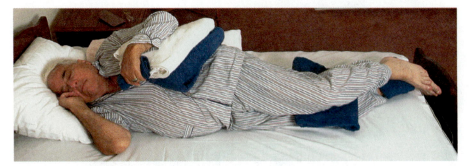

FIGURE 10.11   If laying on their side, find the center of gravity through positioning.

ELASTIC SUPPORT STOCKINGS (TED HOSE)

Once you have positioned a patient in bed successfully, it is important to make sure the patient is comfortable. In addition, elastic support hose may have been prescribed by the physician. Support hose are used to improve the patient's circulation and blood return to the heart because they exert pressure on the leg veins. Stockings may be ordered postoperatively or at any time during the patient's care.

Support hose, also called elastic stockings, come in various sizes and models. Some are up to the knee, and some may be up to the groin area. The model is prescribed by the physician and usually sized by the company or a technician who can come to the home. Using the correct size is important to prevent pressure areas from forming where the stocking ends. Stockings may also vary in weight and color and may be made to order. For applying the stockings, see Procedure 10.6. To remove stockings, roll them down and carefully pull away from the patient's toes. Never pull stocking toes while the whole stocking is still on the foot. Be sure to inspect the foot and the leg when you remove the stockings. Report any red, tender, or puffy areas immediately to the physician.

PROCEDURE 10.6

Applying Support Stockings

Rationale

Correctly applied support stockings increase circulation and provide comfort and support to the patient.

1. Assemble equipment: clean and dry support stockings.
2. Wash your hands.
3. Have the patient assume a supine position in the bed with her legs exposed.
4. Gather the stocking in your hands from the top until you reach the toe.
5. Insert the patient's toe into the toe of the stocking.

6. Pull the stocking up the leg. Be sure it is smooth and not twisted.
7. Repeat the procedure on the second leg.
8. Assist the patient into a safe, comfortable position.
9. Wash your hands.

Summary

Moving items or a person takes a great deal of physical energy, especially if the person is unable to provide assistance. As a caregiver, you need to conserve your energy and maintain your strength to continue to care for your patient. To accomplish this task, ensure that you have appropriate equipment to move yourself, others, and equipment comfortably. Regular exercise and listening to pain in your body will allow you to stay strong and healthy and thus continue in your valuable role. If you experience weakness or pain when repositioning or moving a patient, be sure to visit your doctor to prevent further injury.

Chapter 11

Skin Care

SCENARIO

Mr. Flannery has always been active in sports. He is now in a full leg cast following his recent skiing accident. He lives alone and talks on the phone most of the day. His social life, which centered on his sports life, decreased, and he seldom has visitors. His work friends call during the day but do not visit him. He is confident that he will return to his job as a supervisor at a local tree service. Mr. Flannery has no regular eating schedule. He drinks about six cans of soda a day and says that he does not like water. He also believes that limiting his fluid intake will limit his need to get up and go to the bathroom. Mr. Flannery reports that his cast itches, and he has red areas on his back near his shoulders.

BASIC SKIN CARE

Providing an Environment for Good Skin Care

Good skin care is one of the prime responsibilities of the caregiver. It is much easier to prevent skin deterioration than to heal a problem with the skin. The skin must be inspected daily for changes, reddened areas, tender places, sore areas, cuts, bruises, and areas of breakdown (see Figure 11.1). It is important to recognize patients who are at risk of skin breakdown and protect them from the danger of skin issues. Besides being observant of your patient's skin condition, you must provide a safe environment for your patient. By protecting your patient from cuts, bruises, and excessive pressure, you prevent injury to the skin.

General Factors Affecting Skin

Many conditions working together affect the health of your patient and the condition of your patient's skin:

- Disease process (i.e., diabetes, circulatory disorders, neuropathy)
- Medication (i.e., steroids, anti-inflammatory medications)

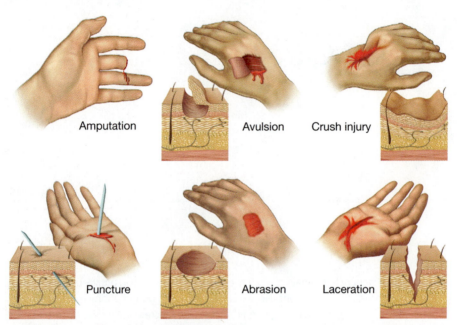

FIGURE 11.1   There are many ways to injure the skin. Here are examples of open injuries.

- Nutrition (i.e., low protein, calcium, albumin)
- Assistance or lack of assistance in her home when you are not with her
- Exercise, positioning, and mobility
- Health habits (i.e., smoking, alcohol use, being overweight)
- Financial resources

High Risk Factors

The primary cause of skin breakdown is pressure on body parts, especially the bony prominences. Bony prominences are places where the bones are close to the skin (see Figure 11.2). Pressure on these areas decreases circulation, leading to decubitus ulcer formation. These areas are the shoulder blades, elbows, knees, heels, ankles, and backbone (see Figure 11.3). Because these areas are covered by thin layers of skin that receive a smaller blood supply than other areas, they are at high risk of break down. Friction is another way that skin issues develop. For example, an obese patient may develop skin issues where skin surfaces rub together, causing friction in areas such as under the breasts, between the folds of the buttocks, and between the thighs. In addition, these areas may not get enough air, which can cause yeast to grow. Left untreated, this condition can also cause skin ulcers to develop.

Shearing is another force that can cause skin breakdown. Shearing occurs when the skin moves one way and the bone and tissue under the skin moves another. This can happen when a patient is transferring from one

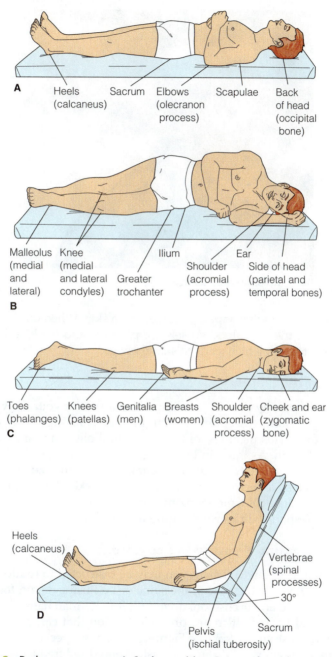

FIGURE 11.2 Body pressure areas: A. Supine position; B. Lateral position; C. Prone position; D. Fowler's position.

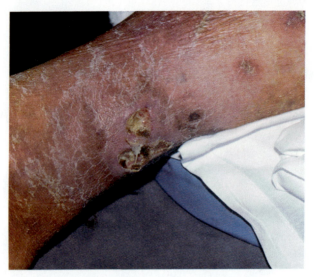

FIGURE 11.3 Decubitus or pressure ulcer.

surface to another or when tape is removed from skin. When this happens, the skin is pinched, the tiny blood vessels are pinched, and the blood supply to the skin is decreased, which leads to skin damage.

Skin Care of the Elderly

Skin care of the elderly patient is an important aspect of your daily care. The elderly are especially susceptible to skin problems. Aging brings a gradual loss of skin tone. This includes loss of the natural oils, leading to dry, itchy, scaly, or rough skin. As the skin loses its underlayer of fat, the skin becomes thin, fragile, and unable to sense or maintain temperature adequately. With aging, there is also a decrease in circulation to the skin. Protecting a patient from extreme heat or cold, moisturizing the skin, and relieving pressure areas become your responsibilities when caring for the elderly.

Ways of Decreasing Pressure to Body Areas

When a patient is in a wheelchair, you may be instructed to reduce the pressure to the back under the base of the spine or legs using an air, foam, or gel cushion. If you use an air cushion, do not fill it more than half-full. For areas like elbows and heels (which are prone to friction that can cause pressure sores), you may use sheepskin (see Figure 11.4). These special pads should be placed against the skin and should be washed and dried frequently. For pressure relief while in bed, an egg-crate mattress placed on the mattress under the sheet decreases pressure on the back and permits air to circulate. Often a physician or physical therapist will prescribe a specialty mattress for prevention of pressure areas or for healing of pressure ulcers. Specialty mattresses are usually air mattresses that have a pump attached to alternate the air in

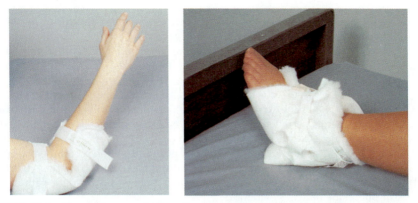

FIGURE 11.4   Sheepskin or professionally made boot can be used for elbows and/or heels.

the mattress, or they are mattresses that move slightly to relieve pressure on pressure areas. If a specialty mattress is used, do not use a fitted sheet or add layers to the mattress because this practice will decrease the effectiveness of the specialty mattress. Health care professionals may also recommend a heel floating device, which can be as simple as a foam-constructed wedge that keeps the heels off the bed. In any case, it is important to ask for a demonstration on use of the equipment. Misuse of the equipment can lead to further skin deterioration.

GENERAL OBSERVATIONS

Observe the condition of the patient's skin each time you visit (see Guideline 11.1). Be sure to note temperature, cleanliness, and dryness. Any difference between two extremities (i.e., one leg being larger than the other, one arm being warm and the other cold) is important and should be reported to the physician immediately. Watch for bruises and scratches. A bruise could indicate a reaction to a medication, a change in diet, a change in the patient's ability to complete certain tasks, a safety issue, or abuse. Try to determine when the bruise appeared, note how big it is, the color, how long it lasts, and if it becomes worse or improves.

GUIDELINE 11.1

Basic Skin Care

- Observe the patient's skin each day as you provide care, especially when bathing or caring for incontinence. Report any changes, including bruising, to the health care team.
- Care for the skin gently. A simple act, such as accidentally scratching the skin, can introduce bacteria and lead to infection. Accidentally stubbing a toe can

cause many weeks of discomfort. Protect your patient and his or her skin from all injuries.

- Protect your patient from exposure to the sun, wind, cold, and rain. If your patient insists on sitting in the sun, encourage the use of a protective lotion with sunscreen.
- Keep the patient's body as clean and dry as possible. A patient need not bathe daily unless he or she exercises heavily or perspires heavily. It is important to keep a patient's perineum clean and dry, but a complete bath on a daily basis is often unnecessary. Use a mild soap to wash the patient, and be sure to dry each body area thoroughly. Do not use perfumes, bubble bath crystals, or bath salts because they tend to dry the skin and make the tub slippery. If itchy skin is a problem, discuss with the nurse what can be added to the bathwater or put on the patient's skin for relief.
- If the patient is incontinent, keep her clean and dry no matter how often you must wash her and change the bed. Do not put the patient in rubber pants because they are irritating to the skin. To protect the bed and to make cleaning the patient easier, use a disposable bed protector. A bed protector allows the soiled area to be cleaned easily and often (especially if the bed isn't a specialty mattress). These pads protect the linen on which the patient lies. Change the bed linen immediately when it becomes wet, and be sure that the plastic side of the protector never touches the patient's skin.
- Many new types of disposable products support a patient who is incontinent. Before you request that your patient purchase any product, discuss with him which product would be most appropriate and fit within the family budget.
- Use lotion on the skin to prevent contact with any bodily discharges or drainage from a wound. Use powder and cornstarch sparingly, and be sure to wash it all off when you bathe the patient. Both tend to cake in body creases creating a breading ground for bacteria.
- Turn the patient often. You should change the patient's position at least every two hours. The family should follow this schedule when you are not there. Move the patient slowly to avoid causing sheet burns or shearing.
- Be careful when using bedpans. Pressure from sitting on the rim causes friction when getting on and off the pan, and friction can worsen the skin condition. Never leave your patient on the bedpan longer than necessary. Use care when removing the bedpan. Avoid spilling urine on the skin because urine can irritate and cause skin damage. Padding the rim of the bedpan can reduce some pressure. Powdering the rim will also minimize friction.
- Keep linen wrinkle-free and dry at all times.
- Remove crumbs, hairpins, and any other hard objects from the bed promptly.
- Do not let the patient lie on catheters or any type of tubing because it can cause pressure areas.
- Be alert to the effects of medications on the skin.
- Do not rub the skin in a harsh manner. Always rub the skin with lotion and in a circular motion. Rubbing stimulates the circulation of blood to the skin, but hard rubbing can damage fragile skin.
- Keep walkways clear of furniture so the patient will not bump his or her toes or legs.
- Encourage good eating habits and adequate intake of fluids.

DECUBITUS ULCERS

Decubitus ulcers, or pressure sores, occur where the skin has broken because of pressure. Both external and internal factors affect the skin's breakdown. External factors may be abrasions, scratches, burns, or chemicals. Internal factors may be swelling, abscesses, or allergic reactions. Disease may also cause skin breakdown. An elderly or ill patient may have poor circulation as part of the disease process, which leads easily to decubitus formation. The pressure can also come from the weight of the body lying in one position too long or from splints, casts, or bandages. In the chapter-opening scenario, Mr. Flannery is likely developing pressure areas on his back as evidenced by the red areas. Even wrinkles in the bed linen or lying on a catheter tube can cause a decubitus ulcer. Decubiti are often made worse by continued pressure, heat, moisture, and lack of cleanliness. Irritating substances on the skin, such as perspiration, urine, feces, wound drainage, or even soap, tend to make decubiti worse. If a decubitus ulcer is not treated, it will quickly become larger, very painful, and even infected. Some decubitus ulcers that are untreated can tunnel to the bone, where an infection can occur in the bone. Such an infection often requires surgery to remove the infection or amputation of the affected limb(s).

A decubitus ulcer is the responsibility of the entire health team. Therefore, as the caregiver, you must know how to recognize decubiti when they occur. Report the first sign of decubiti to the nurse on the health care team so that steps can be taken to prevent further damage. Initial detection and consistent care prescribed by the physician can prevent the red area from worsening.

Signs of a Decubitus Ulcer

The signs of a decubitus ulcer are a warm area of skin, redness, tenderness, discomfort, and a feeling of burning (see Clinical Alert 11.1). After this, the skin often becomes gray in color, which means that the blood supply to the area is greatly decreased. If the condition is allowed to continue, a blister will form. Finally the skin will actually break and a wound will appear (see Figure 11.5). If you notice any one of these signs, notify the nurse or physician and relieve the pressure to the area. By doing this, you may well prevent further skin breakdown. When the skin is broken, a decubitus ulcer has formed.

CLINICAL ALERT 11.1

Red Areas of Skin

It is important to report persistent redness on skin to the nurse or physician. Pain does not always accompany a red area on the skin due to lack of circulation to the area, but if such an area on the skin is left untreated, further skin damage can occur. While waiting to see the nurse or physician, reposition the patient frequently to relieve the pressure on the reddened area and massage around the area to stimulate circulation. The nurse may recommend using a barrier cream (similar to diaper cream used on infants) if the area (for example, the buttocks) is likely to get wet or soiled.

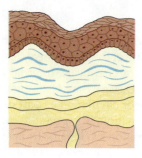

Inflammation or redness of the skin that does not return to normal after 15 minutes of removal of pressure. Edema is present and involves the epidermis. Skin may or may not be broken.

(a)

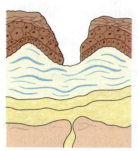

Skin blister or shallow skin ulcer. Involves the epidermis and dermis. Looks like a shallow crater. Area is red and warm and may or may not have drainage.

(b)

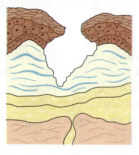

Full thickness skin loss exposing subcutaneous tissue; may extend into next layer. Edema, inflammation, and necrosis present. Drainage present that may or may not have an odor.

(c)

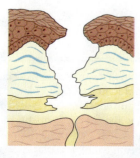

Full thickness ulcer. Muscle and/or bone can be seen. Infection and necrosis present. Drainage present that may or may not have an odor.

(d)

FIGURE 11.5 Stages of skin breakdown.

Care of a Decubitis Ulcer

Specific treatment for a decubitus ulcer is prescribed by a doctor; however, the wound must be kept clean and the rules of asepsis followed. The patient must be positioned so that pressure is removed from the decubitus. If care is a simple, nonsterile dressing, you may be assigned to clean the area and cover it. Be sure you understand the procedure. Ask the nurse to advise you of the way to fasten the dressing. If tape is used, alternate the site where the tape is applied so the tape doesn't cause irritation. Be gentle when removing the tape.

If the patient is incontinent and urine and/or feces continue to drain into the wound, discuss alternatives with the nurse. The patient's care plan may have to be changed so that the decubitus remains dry and can heal (for example, a temporary catheter may be needed to keep the wound dry).

Encourage all the practices of good basic skin care to prevent further skin deterioration and improve the healing climate. Often, even with good practices, patients suffer from skin breakdown. It is important for you to feel that you have done all you could to prevent this. But do not feel guilty if the patient, despite your efforts, forms a pressure ulcer. Sometimes, other contributing factors occur over which you have no control.

Once in a while, a decubitus ulcer does not heal with conservative care and the patient must be placed on medication or hospitalized. It is the goal of your good care to prevent this from happening.

Family Care of the Patient's Decubitus Ulcer

A decubitus ulcer must be cared for twenty-four hours each day. You, as the caregiver, will perform the care while you are in the house. The patient's family members will assume the care the rest of the time. It is important to the healing of the decubitus ulcer that the care be done regularly. If the care is not carried out throughout the day, healing will either be delayed or not take place at all.

You may notice that no healing is occurring. If you believe the patient's family is unable to care for the wound in your absence, or you find out the family is definitely not caring for the decubitus ulcer, report this to the physician. Skin care is a twenty-four-hour concern and must be shared by all caregivers. For more information on wounds, see the Resource Page at the end of the book.

BASIC FOOT CARE

Feet are often the site of many problems because of decreased circulation, infection, poor nutrition, and poor care. Although you will not be able to help your patient reverse all conditions, you will be able to help prevent further deterioration.

Many chronic diseases predispose people to foot problems. Diseases such as diabetes, arthritis, chronic obstructive pulmonary disease COPD, and hypertension often cause foot problems because of lack of circulation, poor nutrition, and decreased physical ability to care for the feet.

Patients may not notice changes in their feet. You will have to observe and report changes on the following conditions to the doctor:

- Pain either while resting or during exercise
- Changes in sensation on skin or in the feet, usually tingling, "pins and needles," or numbness
- Change in color, such as to blue or dark red
- Decreased temperature sensation—sensitivity to cold
- Increased fluid—edema or swelling (see Figure 11.6)
- Dry, cracked skin
- Presence of open areas, such as ulcers or blisters
- Toenails that are thick and curling into the toes
- Absence of toenails

If you notice any changes in your patient's feet, report these changes to your supervisor, who will help you establish a foot care regime for your patient. Remember, do not cut your patient's toenails or apply any over-the-counter medication to open areas! The basic guidelines for foot care are the following:

1. Inspect the feet each day for changes before you wash them.
2. Wash and dry feet daily. Feet should be washed with mild soap in warm water and dried well, especially between toes. Soaking is not desirable or needed. If the skin is dry, a lubricant or cream can be applied. Check to see if this is permitted. Use of heavily scented soaps or lotions may cause skin irritation.
3. Do not cut nails, corns, or bunions. Observe these and report changes or pain. A podiatrist or the nurse should cut nails and perform any removal of excess skin.
4. Help your patient choose proper shoes. They should fit well and give support. They should be proper for the time of year and the activity he or she will be doing. Going barefoot is not advised because lack of shoes decreases support and permits injuries to toes and feet. Socks or

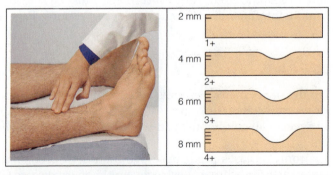

FIGURE 11.6   Assess edema by pressing your finger firmly against the patient's skin for several seconds (especially in the ankle area). After removing your finger, observe for lasting impression or indentation.

stockings should be worn. Certain socks are the best because they allow air to circulate and absorb perspiration. Socks and stockings should be the proper size: Socks that are too big cause irritation; socks that are too small constrict circulation. Do not use garters or rubber bands to hold up socks or stockings. If your patient has been prescribed ted hose (elastic stockings), see Chapter 10 for instructions about their use.

5. Check the temperature of bathwater. If a patient has decreased temperature sensation, she may not notice that the water is too hot. The patient should not use heating pads to keep warm; instead, she should wear cotton socks and down slippers indoors and insulated boots outdoors. Walk in well-lit and clear areas. Do not try to walk in areas with trash or other debris. In warm weather, keep your patient's feet protected from hot sand, boardwalks, objects on the beach, and the sun.

6. Encourage your patient to wear the correct shoes for each activity.

7. Diet is important for the health of the entire body. A patient should consult a nutritionist for specific foods that will affect feet. For example, if circulation is a problem, discuss decreasing the use of caffeine.

If you notice the following problems, immediately call the appropriate member of the health care team:

Problem	Immediate Action
Swollen legs and feet	Elevate the legs and feet on a chair or couch and report this condition.
Pain	Stop exercise or activity, rest, and call your supervisor.
Open skin areas	Do not put on socks or bandage with tape. Cover with clean dressing and call your supervisor.
Temperature variations: hot and cold skin	Cover lightly with blanket and report either condition. Do not use a hot water bottle or ice.

RADIATION THERAPY AND THE SKIN

Radiation therapy uses a specialized type of energy ray to stop the growth of cancer cells by destroying the cells' ability to grow and reproduce. Radiation is used at various times in the treatment of cancer.

During the first visit to the radiation center, lines are drawn on the skin to indicate the target for the radiation. It is important not to wash off these marks. The skin within these marks may appear red or burned. Should the skin break, contact the physician immediately. Care for the skin gently with cool water. Do not wash the area with soaps nor apply lotions. Protect the radiation site from sunlight. Cover it with loose-fitting clothing that will not scratch or irritate the area.

Should the patient need to shave in the radiation site, use only electric razors. Check with the physician about the type of shaving cream to be used, and make sure it is specific for electric razors. Do not use hair-removal chemicals or lotions.

CHEMOTHERAPY AND THE SKIN

Chemotherapy is a general term used to describe the use of drugs to treat cancer. There are many differences in the way drugs are given, how often they are given, and how each person responds. Be sure to follow the plan of care for your patient; do not change it without consulting the health care team.

Chemotherapy works by destroying cancer cells' ability to reproduce. Unfortunately, normal cells also pick up some chemicals, which can cause side effects.

- Sometimes, a dry mouth and throat is a problem. The patient can eat moist foods and drink fluids. Also, eating cold, soft foods is easier. Bland foods help avoid further irritation.
- Mouth care is important. Gently use a soft-bristle toothbrush followed by a nonirritating mouthwash without salt or alcohol. Keep lips moist and lubricated.
- If you think professional dental care is necessary, tell the patient's physician.
- Hair follicles frequently are affected by drugs, and hair falls out. Often the hair grows back when the patient stops taking the drugs. It is important to help your patient feel as attractive as possible at this time. Wigs are often used. Men often wear hairpieces. Some women wear turbans or hats. It is important to keep the scalp clean and free of irritations.
- Skin rashes often occur generally over the body or in specific areas. A nonirritating lotion or cornstarch-based powder can be used. Contact the nurse if itching becomes severe or if the skin is broken.

Individuals receiving radiation and/or chemotherapy are under a great deal of stress. Their skin condition is important because it is a visible sign to them and their family that they are ill and experiencing side effects from the treatments. Your role as a caregiver is to assist patients in maintaining a clean body and one that minimizes the side effects to the skin from cancer treatments.

Summary

Optimal skin care can prevent your patient from skin breakdown. Skin breakdown, whether a cut, bruise, or pressure area, can be very painful. These deteriorations of the skin can easily become infected and cause further problems in the body. Therefore, remember the importance of offering fluids frequently, moisturizing the skin, serving nutritious meals, and moving the body at least every two hours to prevent the patient's skin from breaking down. As always, report any unusual findings in your patient's skin to the physician as soon as possible.

Chapter 12

Personal Care

Mr. Ricci lives with his wife, tends his garden, and makes his own wine in the basement each year. He takes medication, but his wife is unable to say what it is. "He takes care of himself," she says. Mr. Ricci is a retired steel worker and is very independent. He continues to care for his personal needs, although his wife says that he is often unable to wash himself thoroughly. The family, which is large and lives nearby, visits each weekend, and Mrs. Ricci takes great pride in the fact that she cooks for all thirteen of them. She says the children stop by during the week on their way home from work. "They think we do not know they are checking up on us," Mrs. Ricci says, "but at least they come."

ORAL HYGIENE

People who are ill need frequent oral hygiene. They may have a bad taste in their mouth. The tongue may become coated, or they may have sore gums. A clean, fresh-feeling mouth improves appetite, communication, general appearance, and dental health. It gives a feeling of well-being and decreases mouth odor.

Oral hygiene includes the cleansing of the mouth, gums, and teeth or dentures. This procedure should be done twice a day and after meals whenever possible.

Oral hygiene is part of every patient's care, whether he is conscious or unconscious, eating or not eating, self-sufficient or partially dependent. Unconscious patients cannot respond to you or tell you they need oral hygiene. It is your responsibility to see that each patient receives oral hygiene. If the patient can be responsible for cleaning his teeth and mouth, encourage him to continue doing so. If he is unable, however, you as the caregiver must do it for him (see Procedure 12.1).

PROCEDURE 12.1

Oral Hygiene

Rationale

A clean mouth and clean teeth help prevent oral problems and promote fresh breath and a general feeling of well-being. *Be sure that your patient can spit out water before you allow him to take it.*

1. Assemble your equipment: fresh water, cup, straw (if necessary), toothbrush and toothpaste, emesis basin (or sink) or small basin, face towel, disposable gloves, floss, mouthwash (optional).
2. Wash your hands.
3. Ask visitors to step out of the room, if appropriate.
4. Explain the procedure to the patient.
5. Have the patient sit up or assist her to the sink.
6. Spread the towel across the chest to protect her. Put on gloves.
7. Offer her water to rinse the mouth.
8. Hold the emesis basin under the chin so she can spit out the water.
9. Put toothpaste on the wet toothbrush.
10. Offer the toothbrush to the individual if she can brush her own teeth. If she is unable to do so, you must do it. Use a gentle motion, starting above the gum line and going down the teeth. Repeat this until you have brushed all the teeth (see Figure 12.1).

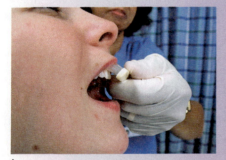
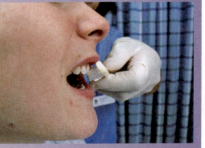

A

B

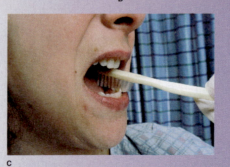

C

FIGURE 12.1 Sometimes the home health aide will be required to brush a patient's teeth. These pictures demonstrate the technique used to brush the surfaces of the teeth.

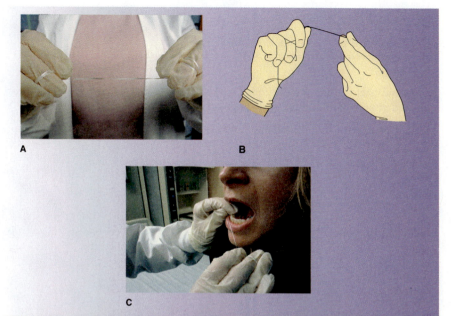

FIGURE 12.2   A. Stretch the floss between your third finger of each hand. B. Floss the upper teeth by using the thumbs and index fingers to stretch the floss. C. Floss the lower teeth by using the index finger to stretch the floss.

11. Offer water to rinse her mouth.
12. If the patient is able to floss on her own, provide her with floss to achieve this task. If the patient is not able to perform this task, then you must do so (see Figure 12.2).
13. Offer mouthwash if she likes it.
14. Prior to putting away equipment, make the patient comfortable.
15. Clean and put away the equipment. Remove your gloves.
16. Wash your hands.

Cleaning Dentures

Patients who wear dentures (false teeth) also require oral hygiene. Pieces of food must be removed from gums and the tongue. The gums must also be stimulated to ensure good circulation. Gums should be stimulated with a soft toothbrush whenever dentures are removed. Dentures need not be cleaned each time they are removed if the patient removes them several times a day. They can, however, be soaked in a cleansing solution each time. They should be brushed thoroughly at least once every 12 hours (see Procedure 12.2).

Be careful while you are handling dentures. They are expensive and difficult to replace. Always put them in a carefully marked denture cup. Do not wrap them up in tissue, put them under a pillow, or leave them on a night table. They could be thrown out by accident.

PROCEDURE 12.2

Oral Hygiene for Patients Who Wear Dentures

Rationale

Food and bacteria that collect under dentures cause discomfort and mouth odor. Clean dentures promote general well-being and help prevent oral problems.

1. Assemble your equipment: tissues, denture cup, small basin or emesis basin, toothbrush or denture brush, denture-soaking solution, towel, disposable gloves, denture toothpaste.
2. Wash your hands.
3. Ask visitors to step out of the room, if appropriate.
4. Tell the individual you wish to clean his dentures.
5. Spread the towel across the chest to protect his bedclothes. Put on gloves.
6. Ask the patient to remove his dentures. Have tissue in the emesis basin ready to receive the dentures. Help if the patient cannot remove the dentures herself (see Figure 12.3).

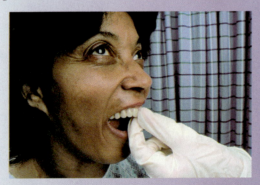

FIGURE 12.3 Remove the top dentures by first breaking the suction.

7. Take the dentures to the sink in the basin. Hold them securely.
8. Line the sink with a paper towel or washcloth so that if the dentures slip out of your hand, they will be cushioned as they fall. Fill the sink with water.
9. Apply toothpaste or denture cleanser to the dentures. With the dentures in the palm of your hand, brush them until they are clean. *Do not use kitchen cleanser or abrasive cleansers.*
10. Rinse the dentures thoroughly under cool water.
11. Fill the denture cup with denture soaking solution, cool water, or mouthwash and water. Place the dentures in the cup, and cover it.
12. Help the patient rinse his mouth with water and/or mouthwash.
13. Have the patient replace the dentures in his mouth if that is what he wants. Be sure the dentures are moist before replacing them. Ask the patient if he uses denture adhesive and assist in applying the adhesive if necessary. Insert the dentures if the patient is unable to do so and desires the dentures to be inserted (see Figure 12.4).
14. Leave the labeled denture cup with clean solution where the patient can easily place the dentures if he takes them out between cleanings.

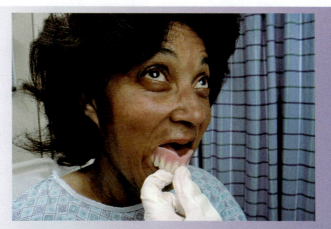

FIGURE 12.4   When inserting the denture. Be sure to do so at a slight angle.

15. Clean your equipment and replace it in the proper place.
16. Remove gloves and wash your hands.

ORAL HYGIENE FOR THE UNCONSCIOUS PERSON   Be careful not to overlook mouth care of a person who is unconscious. A responsible caregiver always remembers to give frequent and thorough oral hygiene to an unconscious patient. Proper oral hygiene prevents oral tissues from cracking and bleeding. If you share the care of a patient with family members, be sure they observe you giving oral hygiene so they will learn, by your example, the necessity of this procedure (see Procedure 12.3).

PROCEDURE 12.3

Oral Hygiene for the Unconscious Patient

Rationale

Unconscious patients often breathe through their mouths, which dries lips and mucous membranes. Careful, frequent care and observation are necessary to prevent oral problems. *Do not put water into the patient's mouth.*

1. Assemble your equipment: towel, disposable gloves, small basin or emesis basin, special disposable mouth care kit (if such a kit is not available, you will need a tongue depressor padded with several gauze squares; make sure the gauze squares are fastened securely to the tongue depressor), lubricant (such as glycerine or a solution of glycerine and lemon juice).

(continued)

2. Wash your hands.
3. Ask visitors to step out of the room, if appropriate.
4. Tell the patient what you are going to do. Even though the patient seems unconscious, she may hear you.
5. Stand at the bedside and turn the patient's face toward you. Put on gloves.
6. Support the patient's face on a pillow covered by a towel.
7. Put a small basin on the towel under the patient's chin.
8. Place the mouth care equipment near you so you do not have to move.
9. Wipe the patient's entire mouth (roof, tongue, and inside the lips and cheeks) with the swab or the tongue depressor dipped in solution. *Do not put your fingers in the patient's mouth. She may close her mouth and injure you.*
10. Put used swabs in the basin. The swabs will leave a coating of glycerine solution on the entire mouth and tongue. This will protect and lubricate the oral tissues.
11. Dry the patient's face with a towel.
12. Using a clean applicator, put a small amount of lubricant on the patient's lips.
13. Make the patient safe and comfortable.
14. Clean your equipment and put it in the proper place.
15. Remove your gloves and wash your hands.

ASSISTING A PATIENT WITH DRESSING AND UNDRESSING

Allow a patient to choose her own clothes if she wishes to do so. If the individual is in her bed most of the day, bedclothes are preferred (be sure they are not wrinkled). If a patient spends most of the day out of bed, encourage her to dress in street clothes.

If a patient has a method of dressing herself that suits her and is safe, allow her to continue using her personal method. For example, some patients may not zip up their dresses all the way or always leave the top button on a shirt unbuttoned. Individualization is always necessary. Remember not to expose the person unnecessarily as you assist her. In this way, you will avoid chilling and/or embarrassing her.

Remember: An injured or inflexible (rigid) arm or leg is first into the garment and last out (see Procedure 12.4).

PROCEDURE 12.4

Assisting a Patient with Dressing and Undressing

Rationale

Dressing in familiar street clothes gives the patient a feeling of well-being, normalcy, and inclusion in the family. Assisting rather than dressing the person reinforces independence and control.

1. Assemble your equipment: the patient's clean clothes.
2. Wash your hands.
3. Ask visitors to leave the room, if appropriate.

4. If the patient can sit on the edge of the bed, assist him into this position. Avoid exposing him. If he must remain in bed, assist him into a flat position on his back.

5. Put on underwear and trousers or pajamas. If a leg is injured, place it into the underwear or pajamas first, followed by the other leg.

6. Ask the person to stand up, if possible, and pull the pants to his waist. If he is in bed, have him lift his buttocks as you pull up his pants.

7. To put on an over-the-head shirt (or other garment), place an injured arm into the shirt first. Then put the neck of the shirt over the patient's head. Finally, guide the other arm into the shirt.

8. To put on a button shirt, place the sleeve over an injured arm first. Bring the shirt to the back of the patient and guide the other arm into the sleeve.

9. Assist the patient with socks or stockings. Do not use round garters because they decrease circulation.

10. Assist with shoes. Be sure they fit well and give support. Look for any blisters or red areas on the feet.

11. Make the individual comfortable.

12. Wash your hands.

ASSISTING A PATIENT WITH BATHING

There are several important reasons for bathing an individual:

- Bathing takes waste products off the skin.
- Bathing cools and refreshes the person.
- Bathing stimulates the skin and improves circulation.
- Bathing requires movement of the muscles.
- Bathing provides a good opportunity for the caregiver to observe the patient.
- Bathing provides an opportunity to talk with the patient.

Individuals receiving care at home may not need to have a complete bath each day. They may prefer to have a partial bath at times. Most people are used to bathing themselves privately. Some individuals are embarrassed by having another person do this for them. Demonstrate your understanding of the patient's feelings by keeping him covered and not exposing him, and by bathing him in a professional and reassuring manner. Patients who tire easily may prefer to have a different part of the body bathed each day. The frequency of your patient's baths will depend on climate, need, skin condition, and the patient's diagnosis. Discuss your patient's preferences with the nurse, and try to meet the patient's preferences (see Guideline 12.1).

The physician or nurse will indicate which type of bath to give your patient. Do not change the type of bath unless you check with the physician or nurse and discuss the change. There are four types of baths:

1. *The complete bath:* This is usually given in bed. If the patient is weak or unable to bathe himself, it is your responsibility to bathe him. When you are giving the bath, the patient will usually give you little or no assistance (see Procedure 12.5).

GUIDELINE 12.1

Bathing

- Usually, the complete bath is given as part of morning care. However, if your patient enjoys his bath at another time of day, try to follow his request.
- Take everything to the bedside *before* you start the bath.
- Always cover the person with a bath blanket before giving the complete bath. If you do not have a bath blanket, use a thin blanket, big towel, or terry cloth bathrobe.
- Use good body mechanics. Keep your feet separated, stand firmly, bend your knees, and keep your back straight.
- When you use soap, keep it in the soap dish, *not* in the basin of water.
- Observe safety rules.
- Use lotions and creams the individual normally uses. Deodorant is used only if the patient requests it and after the entire bath is completed.
- Check the pockets of the bedclothes for personal items before putting them in the laundry.
- Talk to the person as you bathe him.
- Keep the individual's body in proper alignment.
- Change the water as often as you need to so that you have warm, clean water at all times.
- Continually observe the person for distress. If he appears tired or uncomfortable, stop the bath.

PROCEDURE 12.5

The Complete Bed Bath

Rationale

Giving a bed bath improves circulation, provides a general feeling of well-being, and provides an opportunity to examine the patient's skin and body. This is an opportune time as well to interact.

1. Assemble your equipment: soap in a soap dish, washcloth, disposable gloves, several bath towels, washbasin, powder, deodorant, clean gown or pajamas, bath blanket or large towel, orange stick for nail care if used by your agency, lotion for backrub, comb, hairbrush.
2. Wash your hands.
3. Ask visitors to step out of the room, if appropriate.
4. Tell the patient you are going to give him a complete bed bath.
5. Offer the bedpan or urinal.
6. Assist the patient with oral hygiene.
7. Take the bedspread and regular blanket off the bed. Fold them loosely over the back of a chair, leaving the patient covered with the top sheet.
8. Place the bath blanket over the top sheet. Ask the patient to hold the blanket in place.

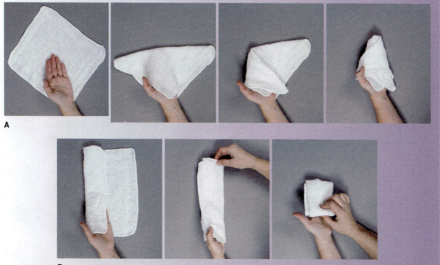

FIGURE 12.5   Making a bath mitt: A. Triangular method; B. Rectangular method.

9. Remove the top sheet from underneath without uncovering (exposing) the patient. Fold the sheet loosely over the back of the chair if it is to be used again; if it is not, put it in the laundry bag.

10. Lower the headrest and knee rest of the bed, if possible and if permitted. The patient should be in a flat position, as flat as is comfortable for him.

11. Raise the bed to its highest horizontal position, if possible.

12. Remove the patient's nightclothes and jewelry. Keep the patient covered with the bath blanket. Place the nightclothes in the laundry bag, and put the jewelry in a safe place.

13. Fill the washbasin two-thirds full of water. Ask your patient how he likes the water—hot, warm, or cool. Test it with your whole hand. Then let him test it with the inside of his hand.

14. Help the patient to move to the side of the bed closest to you. Use good body mechanics. Put on gloves.

15. Put a towel across the patient's chest and make a mitten with the washcloth (see Figure 12.5). Wash the patient's eyes from the nose to the outside of the face. Be careful not to get soap in his eyes. Rinse and dry by patting gently with the bath towel.

16. Put a towel lengthwise under the patient's arm farthest from you. This will keep the bed from getting wet. Support the arm with the palm of your hand under his elbow. Then wash his shoulder, armpit (axilla), and arm. Use long, firm strokes. Rinse and dry the area well.

17. Place the basin of water on the towel. Put the patient's hand into the water and let it soak. Be sure to support the arm and the basin. Wash, rinse, and dry the hand well. Place it under the bath blanket.

18. Wash, rinse, and dry the arm, hand, axilla, and shoulder closest to you in the same way.

19. Clean the patient's fingernails with an orange stick.

(continued)

20. Place a towel across the patient's chest. Fold the bath blanket down to the patient's abdomen. Wash and rinse the patient's ears, neck, and chest (Note the condition of the skin under a female patient's breasts). Dry the area thoroughly.

21. Cover the patient's entire chest with the towel. Fold the bath blanket down to the pubic area. Wash the patient's abdomen. Be sure to wash the umbilicus (navel) and in any creases of the skin. Dry the patient's abdomen. Then pull the bath blanket up over the abdomen and chest and remove the towels.

22. Empty the dirty water. Rinse the basin and refill it.

23. Fold the bath blanket back from the patient's leg farthest from you.

24. Put a towel lengthwise under that leg and foot.

25. Bend the knee and wash, rinse, and dry the leg and foot. Support the leg if the patient is unable to do so. Take hold of the heel for more support when flexing the knee.

26. If the patient can easily bend his knee, put the washbasin on the towel. Then put the patient's foot directly into the basin to wash it. Support his leg and the basin. Protect the ankle area from too much pressure on the basin.

27. Observe the toenails and the skin between the toes for general appearance and condition. Look especially for redness and cracking of the skin. Take away the basin. Dry the patient's leg and foot and between the toes. Cover the leg and foot with the bath blanket and remove the towel.

28. Repeat the entire procedure for the leg and foot closest to you. Empty the basin, and rinse and refill it with clean water.

29. Ask the patient to turn on his side with his back toward you. If he needs help in turning, assist him.

30. Put the towel lengthwise on the bottom sheet near the patient's back. Wash, rinse, and dry the back of the neck, back, and buttocks with long, firm, circular strokes. Give the patient a back rub with warm lotion. The patient's back should be rubbed for at least a minute and a half. Give special attention to bony areas for example, shoulder blades, hips, and elbows. Look for red areas. Dry the patient's back, remove the towel, and turn him on his back.

31. Offer the patient a soapy washcloth to wash his genital area. Give him a clean, wet washcloth to rinse himself well. Give him a dry towel for drying himself. If he is unable to do this for himself, it is your responsibility to wash the patient's genital area. Provide for privacy at all times.

32. Put a clean gown or pajamas on the patient. *Note:* Usually, the patient's hair is combed and the bed is changed; however, this depends on the needs of *your* patient.

33. Arrange the bed so that your patient is comfortable and safe.

34. Clean your equipment and put it in its proper place.

35. Remove gloves and wash your hands.

2. *The partial bath:* A patient may take care of some of her own bathing requirements. When this is the case, you will be responsible for bathing only the areas that are hard for her to reach (back, feet, and/or genitalia).

3. *The tub bath:* This bath is given in a tub. Sometimes, you will be asked to help the patient with a tub bath into which he puts medication. Be sure that the patient or his family can assume responsibility for the medication when you are not there (see Procedure 12.6).

PROCEDURE 12.6

The Tub Bath

Rationale

Tub bathing provides a relaxing atmosphere for the patient and an opportunity for you to observe the patient's skin.

1. Assemble your equipment: bath towels, nonskid bathmat on the bathroom floor, washcloths, disposable gloves, soap, nonskid bathmat to be used in the tub, chair for the patient to sit on (or use the commode), clean gown or pajamas, equipment to wash the tub before and after your patient's bath.
2. Check the tub. Wash it if necessary.
3. Wash your hands.
4. Ask visitors to leave the room, if appropriate.
5. Tell the patient that you would like to assist her with her tub bath.
6. Assist the patient to the bathroom.
7. For safety, remove all electric appliances from the bathroom. Check the grab bars for stability. Check to see that there is proper ventilation.
8. Fill the bathtub half full with water. Ask your patient how she likes the bath water—warm, hot, or cool. Run cold water through the faucet last so it will be cool if the patient should touch it. Test the water for temperature. Have the patient test the water.
9. Assist the patient in undressing and getting into the bathtub.
10. Let the patient stay in the bathtub as long as permitted, according to your instructions. Give her privacy as is safely appropriate.
11. Help the patient wash herself as needed. Wear gloves.
12. Empty the tub. It is easier to exit an empty tub than a full one.
13. Put one towel across the chair or the commode. Have the patient sit on this.
14. Allow the patient to dry as much of her body as she can. Assist her with putting on clean bedclothes or street clothes.
15. Assist the patient out of the bathroom to her bed or chair. Make her comfortable.
16. Return to the bathroom. Clean the tub and bathroom as necessary.
17. Remove all used linen and put them in the proper place.
18. Wash your hands.

4. *The shower:* The patient is bathed under running water with a stand-by assist from the caregiver.

The Partial Bath

Your patients should be encouraged to take as active a part in their care as their medical condition allows. It may be easier, faster, and more efficient for *you* to bathe your patient, but do not let the patient know how you feel. Remember, as a caregiver, you will have to leave the patient after a period of time. It is your responsibility to help her gain her independence so she can function when you are gone. She will gain this independence and self-confidence only if you encourage her to take an active part in her care. A partial bath routine must be individualized to suit the needs of your patient. However, always keep in mind certain rules involving safety and patient ability:

- Assist the patient with establishing a bathing routine to save her energy.
- Allow the patient to bathe as much of her body as she can safely reach.
- Bring a basin to her bed, or assist the patient to the bathroom.
- Take a chair into the bathroom or have the patient sit on the toilet covered by a towel.
- Be observant of safety while the patient is bathing.
- Give the patient privacy as she bathes.

The Tub Bath and Shower

Your patient may want a tub bath. Some houses do not have showers. Some patients are used to taking baths rather than showers. Some baths are prescribed for therapeutic reasons. For safety, you must be sure that you can carry out tub bath.

Handheld Showers

Some patients may have a handheld shower in their bathroom. A handheld shower is attached to the tub or shower (see Procedure 12.7) and allows the user to direct the water to a single place on the body or head. Apply the same safety precautions you would use for a regular shower, but keep the following additional considerations in mind:

- Remember to keep the patient covered and warm when using this appliance so that his privacy is protected and his body temperature is maintained.
- Test the water temperature away from the patient.
- Be extra careful when changing water-flow direction so neither you nor the bathroom gets an unexpected shower.
- Remember to turn off the water after you are finished using the appliance.

PROCEDURE 12.7

Assisting a Patient with a Shower with or Without a Shower Chair

Rationale

A shower provides a relaxing atmosphere for the patient and an opportunity for you to observe the patient's skin.

1. Assemble your equipment: bath towels, nonskid bathmat on the bathroom floor, soap, shower cap (optional), washcloth, gloves, nonskid bathmat in the shower, clean pajamas or street clothes, equipment to clean the shower before and after your patient's shower, a shower chair (optional).

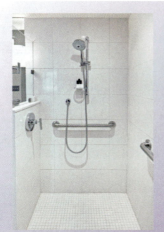

FIGURE 12.6

2. Check the shower. Wash it if necessary.
3. Wash your hands.
4. Ask visitors to leave the room, if appropriate.
5. Tell the patient that you would like to assist him with his shower.
6. Assist the patient to the bathroom.
7. For safety, remove all electrical appliances from the bathroom. Check to make sure the grab bars are secure (see Figure 12.6). Check ventilation.
8. Position the shower chair in the shower or tub.
9. Turn on the shower and adjust the water temperature. Ask your patient how he likes the water—hot, warm, or cool.
10. Assist the patient into the shower.
11. Give the patient as much privacy as is safely appropriate.
12. When the patient is finished washing, turn off the water and assist the patient out of the shower. Assist the patient with washing and drying those body areas he finds difficult to reach. Wear gloves when washing or drying the patient.
13. Help the patient with dressing as needed. Assist the patient out of the bathroom to his bed or a chair. Make him comfortable.
14. Return to the bathroom. Clean the shower and bathroom as necessary.
15. Remove all used linen and put in the proper place.
16. Wash your hands.

GIVING YOUR PATIENT A BACKRUB

Rubbing a patient's back refreshes her, relaxes her muscles, and stimulates circulation. Because of pressure from the bedclothes and lack of movement to stimulate circulation, the skin of a patient who spends a great deal of time in bed needs special attention (see Procedure 12.8).

PROCEDURE 12.8

Giving a Patient a Backrub

Rationale

Giving a backrub promotes circulation and provides an opportunity to help the patient relax and to check his back and arms for any skin changes (see Figure 12.7).

1. Assemble your equipment: towels, disposable gloves, lotion of the patient's choice, and a basin of warm water (optional).
2. Wash your hands.
3. Ask visitors to leave the room, if appropriate.

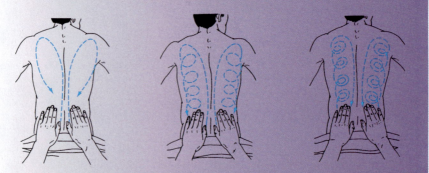

FIGURE 12.7

4. Tell the patient you are going to give him a backrub.
5. Raise the bed to its highest horizontal position, if possible. Ask the patient to turn on his side or abdomen so that you can reach his back easily. Have him positioned as close as possible to the side of the bed where you are working.
6. Warm the lotion by placing the container in a basin of warm water. Put on gloves.
7. Expose the patient's back and buttocks. Do not overexpose him.
8. Pour a small amount of lotion into the palm of your hand.
9. Rub your hands together, using friction to warm the lotion.
10. Apply lotion to the entire back with the palms of your hands. Use firm long strokes from the buttocks to the shoulders and the back of the neck and shoulders.
11. Use proper body mechanics. Keep your knees slightly bent and your back straight.
12. Exert firm pressure as you stroke upward from the buttocks toward the shoulders. Use gentle pressure as you move your hands down the back. Do not lift up your hands as you massage.
13. Use a circular motion on each bony area. Continue this rhythmic rubbing motion one to three minutes.
14. Dry the patient's back by patting it with a towel.
15. Assist the patient in putting on a gown or pajamas.
16. Reposition the patient. Make him comfortable.

17. Arrange the top sheet of the bed neatly.
18. Arrange the bed so that your patient is safe and comfortable.
19. Put your equipment back in its proper place.
20. Remove gloves and wash your hands.

Backrubs are usually given as part of morning care after the patient's bath. They are also given in the evening before a patient goes to sleep and during the day whenever a patient changes position or requires this procedure.

Sometimes, a patient does not enjoy having his back rubbed. Respect his wishes. Do not take it personally if a patient refuses a backrub. He just may not enjoy this particular activity.

HAIR CARE

It is important to keep your patient's hair neat and clean. This prevents scalp and hair breakdown, improves the individual's appearance, improves circulation to the scalp, and improves the person's general feeling about him- or herself.

There are various methods of washing a person's hair (see Guideline 12.2):

- Bed shampoo (see Procedure 12.9)
- Shampoo at the sink
- Shampoo in the shower (usually done by the patient)
- Dry shampoo

Before you wash a person's hair, consider two important points:

- Can the individual safely remain in the required position during the procedure?
- Are there any instructions from health care professionals *not* to wash the patient's hair?

GUIDELINE 12.2

Hair Care

- Keep the individual free of drafts.
- Never cut, color, or do a chemical treatment on someone's hair unless you are trained to do so.
- Never use a hot comb or curling iron on a patient's hair unless you know how to use the device safely.
- Style the patient's hair as he or she is accustomed to having it styled.

PROCEDURE 12.9

Giving a Shampoo in Bed

Rationale

Clean hair promotes general health and well-being. Being well groomed promotes self-esteem.

1. Assemble your equipment: patient's comb and brush, patient's shampoo, conditioner (optional), several containers of warm to hot water (as patient prefers), chair, pitcher, large basin or pail to collect dirty water, bed protectors, several large bath towels, washcloth, disposable gloves, water trough (or 1½ yards of 60-inch-wide plastic to make one), cotton balls (optional), bath blanket, waterproof pillow (optional), electric blow dryer (optional), curlers (optional).
2. Wash your hands.
3. Ask visitors to leave the room, if appropriate.
4. Tell the patient that you are going to shampoo her hair in bed.
5. Raise the bed to the highest horizontal position, if possible. Lower the headrest if possible. Ask the patient what water temperature she prefers.
6. Place a chair at the side of the bed near the patient's head. The chair should be lower than the mattress. Put on gloves.
7. Inspect the patient's hair for knots and lice. If the patient has knots, carefully comb them out. If the patient has lice, stop the procedure and report this to the nurse. Lice are tiny black insects that live on hair and scalp and can spread quickly to others. Place a shower cap on the patient's head until treatment can be done.
8. Place a towel on the chair. Place the large basin or pail on the towel.
9. This step is optional. Remove the pillow from under the patient's head. Cover the pillow with a waterproof case. Have the pillow under the small of the patient's back so that when she lies on it, her head is tilted backward.
10. Put the bath blanket on the patient. Fan-fold the top sheets to the foot of the bed without exposing the patient.
11. Ask the patient to move across the bed so that her head is close to where you are standing.
12. Place the bed protectors on the mattress under the patient's head (see Figure 12.8).
13. Put small amounts of cotton in the patient's ears for protection.
14. Place the shampoo trough under the patient's head. A trough can be made by rolling up the sides of the plastic sheet to make a channel for the water to run into the pail. Three sides must be rolled to make the channel. The top edge should be rolled around a rolled bath towel. Place the edge with the rolled towel in it under the patient's neck and head. Have the open edge hanging into the pail on the chair.
15. Loosen the pajamas so the patient is comfortable and no clothing is in the trough.
16. Ask the patient to hold the washcloth over her eyes.
17. Pour some water over the patient's hair. Use a pitcher or a cup. Repeat until the hair is completely wet.
18. Apply shampoo and, using both hands, wash the hair and massage the scalp with your fingertips. Avoid using your fingernails because they could scratch the patient's scalp.

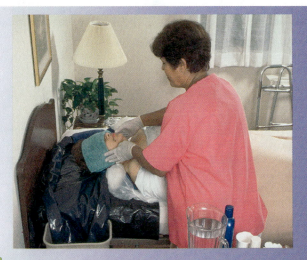

FIGURE 12.8

19. Rinse the shampoo off by pouring water over the hair. Have the patient turn her head from side to side. Repeat this until the hair is free of soap.
20. If the patient uses a conditioner, apply it after reading the directions.
21. Dry the patient's forehead and ears.
22. Remove the cotton from the patient's ears.
23. Raise the patient's head and wrap it in a bath towel.
24. Rub the patient's hair with a towel to dry it as much as possible.
25. Remove the equipment from the bedside. Be sure the patient is in a safe, comfortable position before you leave.
26. Comb the patient's hair as she is accustomed to having it done. You may leave a towel spread over the pillow under the patient's head as her hair dries or you may set the patient's hair. If an electric blow dryer is available, use it on low or cool.
27. Remove the bath blanket and, at the same time, bring up the top sheets to cover the patient.
28. If possible, lower the bed to its lowest horizontal position.
29. Make the patient comfortable.
30. Clean your equipment and put it in its proper place.
31. Remove gloves and wash your hands.

Shampooing at the Sink

If a patient can sit with her head over the sink, this procedure is preferable to a bed shampoo. It is faster and easier (see Procedure 12.10).

Combing a Person's Hair

As with other types of personal care, a patient may be unable to take care of his own hair. When this is the case, it is your responsibility to comb and brush his hair. This almost always makes him look better and feel better (see Procedure 12.11).

PROCEDURE 12.10

Shampooing a Patient's Hair at the Sink

Rationale

Clean hair promotes general health and well-being. Being well groomed promotes self-esteem.

1. Assemble your equipment: patient's comb and brush, patient's shampoo, pitcher for water (optional), chair that allows the patient to sit comfortably facing the sink, several towels, washcloth, disposable gloves, cotton balls (optional), electric blow dryer (optional), curlers or curling iron (optional).
2. Wash your hands.
3. Ask visitors to leave the room, if appropriate.
4. Assist the patient to the sink. Be sure a chair is available for her to sit on if she tires.
5. Place a towel around the patient's shoulders. Put on gloves.
6. Inspect a patient's hair for knots and lice. If the patient has knots, carefully comb them out. If the patient has lice, stop the procedure and report this to the nurse. Place a shower cap on the patient to prevent the lice from spreading to you.
7. Put a small amount of cotton in the patient's ears for protection.
8. Give the patient a washcloth to cover her eyes.
9. Ask the patient what temperature she prefers the water. Adjust it according to her preferences.
10. Ask the patient to lean forward (or backward if the sink is the barber-shop type) so that her head is over the sink.
11. Wet her head thoroughly.
12. Apply shampoo and, using both hands, wash the hair and massage the scalp with your fingertips. Avoid using your fingernails because they may scratch the patient's scalp.
13. Rinse the shampoo off by pouring water over the hair.
14. Dry the patient's forehead and ears. Have her assume a comfortable position. Raise the patient's head and wrap it in a towel.
15. Remove the cotton from the patient's ears.
16. Rub the patient's hair with a towel to dry it as much as possible.
17. Comb the patient's hair as she is accustomed to having it done. You may leave a towel around the patient's shoulders while her hair is drying. Leave a towel under the patient's head if she prefers to lie down as her hair dries. You may also set curlers in a patient's hair and use the electric blow dryer set on low or cool.
18. Make sure that the patient is comfortable and safe following this procedure.
19. Clean your equipment and the area you used.
20. Remove gloves and wash your hands.

PROCEDURE 12.11

Combing a Patient's Hair

Rationale

A patient's appearance plays a role in his self-image. Combing and styling hair is usually done according to patient's personal preference, which should be respected regardless of the patient's age or health status.

1. Assemble your equipment on the bedside table: towel, comb or brush, any hair product the patient uses, hand mirror (if available).
2. Wash your hands.
3. Ask visitors to leave the room, if appropriate.
4. Tell the patient you are going to brush or comb his hair.
5. If possible, comb the patient's hair after the bath and before you make the bed. Some patients prefer to have their hair combed while sitting in a chair.
6. Lay a towel across the pillow, under the patient's head. If the patient can sit up in bed, drape the towel around his shoulders.
7. If the patient wears glasses, ask him to take them off before you begin, unless this makes the patient uncomfortable. Be sure to put the glasses in a safe place.
8. Part the hair down the middle to make it easier to comb.
9. Brush or comb the patient's hair carefully, gently, and thoroughly in his usual style.
10. For the patient who cannot sit up, separate the hair into small sections. Then comb each section separately, using a downward motion. Comb the loose end first and work up, in smaller sections, toward the head, always combing in downward motions. Ask the patient to turn his head from side to side. Or turn it for him so that you can reach the entire head.
11. Arrange the patient's hair the way he wants it.
12. If the patient has long hair, suggest braiding it to keep it from tangling.
13. Be sure you brush the back of the head.
14. Remove the towel when you are finished.
15. Let the patient use the mirror.
16. Make the patient comfortable.
17. Wash your hands.

SHAVING A PERSON'S BEARD

A regular morning activity for most men is shaving the beard. A patient is often well enough to shave himself. In this case, you will give him any help necessary, such as setting up the equipment he needs. Sometimes, however, patients cannot shave themselves. In such cases, you will do it. Certain individuals may not be permitted to shave or be shaved; the physician or nurse will inform you if this is the case.

Shaving can be done only with an electric razor or a safety razor. Never use an electric razor if the patient is receiving oxygen (see Procedure 12.12).

PROCEDURE 12.12

Shaving a Patient's Beard

Rationale

A patient's appearance plays a role in his self-image. Shaving facial hair is a key part of daily grooming for many men.

1. Assemble your equipment at the bedside: basin of water (very warm to hot), shaving cream, safety razor or electric razor, face towel, disposable gloves, mirror, tissues, aftershave lotion (optional), face powder (optional), washcloth
2. Wash your hands.
3. Ask visitors to leave the room, if appropriate.
4. Tell the patient that you are going to shave his beard.
5. Adjust a light so that it shines on the patient's face but not in his eyes.
6. Raise the head of the bed if possible and if allowed. Put on gloves.
7. Spread the face towel under the patient's chin. If the patient has dentures, be sure they are in his mouth.
8. Put some warm water on the patient's face or use a damp warm washcloth to soften his beard.
9. If using a razor, apply shaving cream generously to the face.
10. With the fingers of one hand, hold the skin taut (tight) as you shave in the direction that the hair grows. Start under the sideburns and work downward over the cheeks. Continue carefully over the chin. Work upward on the neck under the chin. Use short firm strokes.
11. If using a razor, rinse it often in the basin of water.
12. Areas under the nose and around the lips are sensitive. Take special care in these areas.
13. If you nick the patient's skin, wash the area and put a small piece of tissue on the cut or a Band-Aid if necessary. If it is a significant cut or the bleeding will not stop, call the physician.
14. If you used a razor, wash off the remaining shaving cream when you have finished.
15. Apply aftershave lotion or powder as the patient prefers.
16. Make the patient comfortable.
17. Clean your equipment and put it in its proper place.
18. Remove gloves and wash your hands.

ASSISTING A PATIENT WITH TOILETING

Toileting is usually a private activity and one not openly discussed. The amount of assistance you give varies with the patient's physical condition. The patient may be embarrassed. You may be embarrassed. Your role is to assist the patient with this important and normal bodily function in a way that is both acceptable to her and safe to you. People often associate special words with elimination. Knowing these words may make the communication between you and your patient easier. Try to keep to the schedule and way the individual usually toilets because a routine will help when you are not there.

Body waste elimination is important if the body is to maintain its health and function. You will be asked to report any abnormalities in your patient's eliminations. Often, this information will provide an indication of your patient's health status. Report the following to the physician:

- Frequency changes in elimination (using the toilet more or less than normal)
- Color (if urine is dark brown, red, or completely clear; if stool is black or gray)
- Odor (foul, out-of-the-ordinary smell)
- Any pain with elimination
- Out-of-the-ordinary inability to control elimination
- Any foreign material, such as blood or mucous

Some patients cannot leave bed to use the bathroom. These patients require a urinal and a bedpan (see Figure 12.9). The urinal is a container into which the male patient urinates. The bedpan is a pan into which he defecates (moves his bowels). The female patient uses the bedpan for urination and defecation. There are times, however, when a female urinal must be used. You should always cover the bedpan and remove it from the patient's bedside to the bathroom as quickly as possible after use. At this time, you would collect a specimen, if required. You would also measure the urine, if necessary (see Procedure 12.13).

Some patients can climb out of bed but cannot walk to the bathroom. For these patients, your supervisor will arrange to have a portable commode brought to the house (see Procedure 12.14). Whenever the patient uses the portable commode, you are responsible for cleaning it just as if he had used the bedpan or urinal.

When a patient is told he may go to the bathroom, you are responsible for assisting him to the bathroom and observing all the rules of safety.

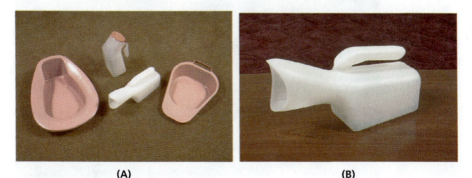

(A)   **(B)**

FIGURE 12.9   (A) Two different types of bedpans male and female urinals (B) Female urinal.

PROCEDURE 12.13

Offering the Bedpan

Rationale

Carefully and skillfully placing the bedpan prevents physical discomfort and decreases the patient's emotional discomfort with needing assistance for this intimate task.

1. Assemble your equipment: bedpan and cover (or fracture bedpan and cover), toilet tissue, washbasin with water or wet washcloth, soap, talcum powder or cornstarch, hand towel, disposable gloves.
2. Wash your hands.
3. Ask visitors to leave the room, if appropriate. You may, however, wish to demonstrate this procedure to the patient's family members.
4. Ask the patient if he would like to use the bedpan. Put on gloves.
5. Warm the bedpan by running warm water inside it and along the rim. Dry the outside of the bedpan with paper towels and put talcum powder or cornstarch on the part that will touch the patient. If the patient is going to move his bowels and a specimen is not needed, place several sheets of toilet tissue or a slight bit of water in the bedpan. This will make cleaning it easier.
6. Raise the bed to the highest horizontal position, if possible.
7. Fold back the top sheets so that they are out of the way.
8. Raise the patient's gown, but keep the lower part of his body covered with the top sheets.
9. Ask the patient to bend his knees and put his feet flat on the mattress. Then ask the patient to raise his hips. If necessary, help the patient to raise his buttocks by slipping your hand under the lower part of his back. Place the bedpan in position with the seat of the bedpan under the buttocks.
10. Sometimes a patient cannot lift his buttocks to get on or off the bedpan. In this case, turn the patient on his side with his back to you. Put the bedpan against the buttocks. Then turn the patient back onto the bedpan (see Figure 12.10).
11. Replace the covers over the patient.

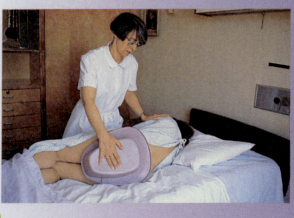

FIGURE 12.10

12. Raise the backrest and knee rest, if allowed, so the patient is in a sitting position.
13. Put toilet tissue where the patient can reach it easily.
14. Ask the patient to signal when he is finished.
15. Leave the room to give the patient privacy.
16. Remove gloves and wash your hands if you are going to do another task.
17. When the patient signals, return to the room.
18. Wash your hands and put on gloves.
19. Help the patient to raise his hips so you can remove the bedpan.
20. Help the patient if he cannot clean himself. Turn the patient on his side. Clean the anal area with toilet tissue.
21. Cover the bedpan immediately. You can use a disposable pad or a paper towel if no cover is available.
22. Take the bedpan to the patient's bathroom. Remove gloves and wash your hands.
23. Return to the patient. Offer the patient the opportunity to wash his hands in the basin of water.
24. Make the patient comfortable.
25. Put on gloves and note the excreta (feces or urine) if there is an odd amount, odor, or color.
26. If a specimen or sample is required, collect it at this time. Measure the urine, if necessary.
27. Empty the bedpan into the patient's toilet.
28. Clean the bedpan and put it in the proper place. Cold water is always used to clean the bedpan. You may also use a toilet brush, if one is available.
29. Remove gloves and wash your hands.

PROCEDURE 12.14

Offering the Urinal

Rationale

Carefully and skillfully placing the urinal prevents physical discomfort and decreases the patient's emotional discomfort with needing assistance for this intimate task.

1. Assemble your equipment: urinal and cover, basin of water or wet washcloth, soap, towels, disposable gloves.
2. Wash your hands.
3. Ask visitors to leave the room, if appropriate. You may, however, wish to demonstrate this procedure to the patient's family members.
4. Ask the patient if he wishes to use the urinal. Put on gloves.
5. Give the patient the urinal. If the patient is unable to put the urinal in place, put his penis into the opening as far as it goes. If the patient cannot hold it in place, you will do so. Raise the head of the bed if it is possible to do so and the patient prefers.
6. Ask the patient to signal when he is finished.
7. Leave the room to give the patient privacy. Remove gloves and wash your hands.

8. When the patient signals, return to the room. Wash your hands and put on gloves.
9. Take the urinal. Be careful not to spill it. Cover it and take it to the patient's bathroom. Remove gloves and wash your hands.
10. Return to the patient. Put on gloves. Help him wash his hands in the basin of water or with a wet washcloth. Remove gloves and wash your hands.
11. Make the patient comfortable.
12. Put on gloves. Check the urine for color, odor, and amount.
13. Measure the urine, if necessary. Collect a specimen or sample at this time, if necessary.
14. Empty the urinal into the toilet. Rinse the urinal with cold water.
15. Clean the urinal according to your agency's policy and return it to the proper place.
16. Remove gloves and wash your hands.

CARE OF THE PERINEAL AREA

Perineal care or peri-care is the gentle cleansing of the perineal area or perineum. This may be necessary following the birth of a child, following surgery, or when a female patient does not take a full bath but wishes to clean the genital area. This procedure promotes healing, helps prevent infection, and refreshes the patient. The use of a squeeze bottle—or peribottle—is encouraged, rather than cleansing the area with a washcloth. The bottle directs a stream of water so that it removes waste or drainage without damaging the skin. The use of the bottle also enables patients to clean themselves even if they cannot reach the area with their hands (see Procedures 12.15, 12.16, and 12.17).

PROCEDURE 12.15

Assisting a Patient with a Portable Commode

Rationale
Using a commode in a safe and private manner is more comfortable and familiar than using a bedpan or urinal.

1. Assemble your equipment: portable bedside commode, toilet tissue, basin of water or wet washcloth, soap, towel, gloves.
2. Wash your hands.
3. Ask visitors to leave the room, if appropriate. However, you may want to demonstrate the procedure to the patient's family members.
4. Tell the individual you are going to assist her onto the commode. Put on gloves.
5. Put the commode next to the bed in a position to which she can safely transfer.
6. Using proper body mechanics and transfer techniques, assist the patient onto the commode.
7. If you do not have to collect a specimen, leave a small amount of water in the bottom of the pail. This will make cleaning it easier.
8. If the patient is safe, leave the room to give her privacy.
9. Remove gloves and wash your hands if you are going to do another task.

10. When the patient signals you that she is finished, return and wash your hands. Put on gloves.
11. Offer the patient toilet tissue to clean herself. If he is unable to do so, it is your responsibility to clean her. After doing so, remove gloves and wash your hands.
12. Assist the patient back to bed.
13. Offer her the basin of water or wet washcloth to wash her hands.
14. Make the person comfortable. Put on gloves.
15. Remove the pail from the commode. Cover it and carry it to the bathroom.
16. Check the excreta (feces or urine) for odd color, amount, or odor.
17. Measure output if that is ordered. If a specimen or sample is required, collect it at this time.
18. Empty the pail into the toilet and clean it according to your agency's policy.
19. Put the pail back into the commode.
20. Remove gloves and wash your hands.

PROCEDURE 12.16

Care of the Perineal Area of a Mobile Patient

Rationale

Keeping the perineum clean and free of discharge and bacteria is an important part of personal care and contributes to general health and well-being.

1. Assemble your equipment: two peribottles or squeeze bottles, mild soap, clean dressings (or peripads) and undergarments, towels, gloves, garbage bag for soiled dressings, warm water (or periwipes as appropriate).
2. Wash your hands.
3. Ask visitors to leave the room, if appropriate.
4. Tell the patient what you are going to do and what you expect. Put on gloves.
5. Remove old peripads or dressings and discard in a paper or plastic bag. Note the drainage, color, amount, and odor.
6. Assist patient onto the commode or toilet.
7. If using the bottles and water:
   a. Fill one bottle with warm, soapy water and the other with warm, clean water.
   b. Place the bottle filled with soapy water parallel to the perineum. Let the water drain over the perineum. Move the bottle so that the whole perineal area is cleansed for at least two minutes. You may have to refill the bottle.
   c. Rinse the perineum with plain warm water.
8. If using periwipes, wipe the perineal area. Be careful to wipe in one direction only, from front to back. Several wipes should be used and then discarded in the trash bag.
9. Assist the patient to stand up.
10. Pat the area dry. This may not be necessary if periwipes are used.
11. Assist the patient with clean dressings and undergarments. Make the patient comfortable.
12. Clean the equipment and commode.
13. Remove gloves and wash your hands.

PROCEDURE 12.17

Care of the Perineal Area of a Bedridden Patient

Rationale

Keeping the perineum clean and free of discharge and bacteria is an important part of personal care and contributes to general health and well-being.

1. Assemble your equipment: two peribottles or squeeze bottles, mild soap, clean dressings (or peripads) and undergarments, towels, gloves, garbage bag for soiled dressings, warm water (or periwipes as appropriate).
2. Wash your hands.
3. Ask visitors to leave the room, if appropriate.
4. Tell the patient what you are going to do and what you expect. Put on gloves.
5. Assist the patient to lie down in the supine position.
6. Assist the patient in opening his or her legs and bending at the knees.
7. Drape the legs to allow dignity for the patient (see Figure 12.11).
8. Remove old peripads or dressings and discard in a paper or plastic bag. Note the drainage, color, amount, and odor.
9. Assist patient onto the bedpan (see Chapter 16 for directions).
10. If using the bottles and water:
    a. Fill one bottle with warm, soapy water and the other with warm, clean water.
    b. Place the bottle filled with soapy water parallel to the perineum. Let the water drain over the perineum. Move the bottle so that the whole perineal area is cleansed for at least two minutes. You may have to refill the bottle.
11. Rinse the perineum with plain warm water.
12. If using periwipes, wipe the perineal area. Be careful to wipe in one direction only, from front to back. Several wipes should be used and then discarded in the trash bag.
13. Assist the patient as you remove the bedpan.
14. Pat the area dry. This may not be necessary if periwipes are used.
15. Assist the patient with clean dressings and undergarments. Make the patient comfortable.
16. Clean the equipment and commode.
17. Remove gloves and wash your hands.

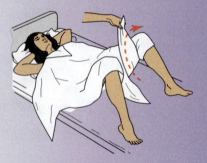

FIGURE 12.11

Summary

Providing personal care for someone at home involves supporting the patient while honoring the household culture at the same time. There are bound to be changes in one's lifestyle after an event or illness that requires home care. During these changes, it is important to respond to the emotional and physical needs of both the patient and family members, while at the same time always taking into account the family's culture. For instance, if the event is childbirth, reactions in the family may vary. With this event, you will mostly likely be asked to reinforce the family's culture and their customs in dealing with the new baby and the new mother. If you do not understand some of the actions, discuss the reasons behind the actions with the patient and/ or family member as appropriate. If you believe some actions are unsafe or are contrary to your agreed-upon role, discuss this with the patient and other family members. Whether it is a new child or a chronic illness that the patient and family have to adjust to, you may suggest changes in routine or actions that in your experience have worked. Do not be offended if the family chooses not to adopt your suggestions. There are many ways to accomplish the same goal, and each family must set up a system that is comfortable for the family members when you leave.

Chapter 13

Rehabilitation of the Individual Receiving Care at Home

SCENARIO

Mr. Robinson lives in a small basement apartment. He has lived all his life in this neighborhood and knows all the nearby families. Although he has never married and has no family of his own, he is included in many of his neighbors' activities. Prior to his retirement, Mr. Robinson worked as a railroad conductor. He now goes for walks and spends time in the playground watching the children. Recently, he fell in the street and broke his wrist, and it is still in a splint. Mr. Robinson usually remembers his physical therapy appointments, but he missed two recently, stating that he forgot them. The physical therapist has given Mr. Robinson daily exercises, but he admits he does not do them regularly. The neighbors are concerned; they think Mr. Robinson has not been as visible as usual, and when they do see him, he does not look as neat and clean as he has in the past. They are also sure he has lost weight.

REHABILITATION

Rehabilitation is the process of relearning how to function, in the best possible way, as an independent person despite a disability. Rehabilitation is not easy and not always pleasant but, with proper direction and encouragement, the individual can accomplish her goals. Sometimes, a person will use a brace or support for an injured body part. When providing home care, it is important to have a full understanding of the care and use of the equipment. The way in which you assist the patient will communicate to her if you really believe she will succeed or if you believe her attempts are useless. Be alert to your verbal and nonverbal communications.

Establishing a Routine

Before a therapist establishes a routine for the patient, he reviews the whole patient profile, including his environment. Your objective reporting during this assessment will help establish a useful individualized program for your patient. Factors considered during this assessment include the following:

- *Active motion:* The amount of active motion that the patient has
- *Passive motion:* The amount of passive motion that the patient has
- *Symptoms:* Symptoms of all medical diagnoses that may affect function
- *Sensory deficits:* Sensory deficits in vision, hearing, speech, touch, balance, or proprioception (knowledge of limb position in space with eyes covered)
- *Mental attitude:* How does the patient see his situation? His disability?
- *Attitude:* Is he depressed, euphoric, angry, cooperative, resentful, or frustrated? Is he motivated? In other words, does he want to try to do things for himself?
- *Ability:* What can the patient do for himself? What does he attempt to do?
- *Previous level of function:* Which limb is dominant (used for most activities)? What did the patient do before he became disabled? If a person did not want to do something before an illness, he may not be motivated to do it afterward.
- *Priorities:* A priority is something the patient wants to do. Often, the priority might not seem important, but achieving it makes the patient feel less handicapped. It could be a little thing like putting on make-up, setting hair, shaving, tying shoes, using the telephone, or signing checks.
- *Equipment:* What is the patient using now, and what does he need to help him function; for example, hospital bed, commode, crutches, catheter, walker, cane, brace, splints, or adaptive equipment such as built-up spoons or dressing sticks?
- *Environmental barriers:* Are there any objects and/or structures in the patient's home that make it difficult for him to care for himself? Some examples are a second-floor bathroom when a patient cannot climb stairs, throw rugs that can trip him, narrow doorways that prevent him from moving from room to room in a wheelchair, heavy furniture that he cannot pass in a walker or with crutches or a cane, or a bed without hand rails to help him sit up.
- *Support system:* Who is involved in the care of a patient? Besides the home health aide, will family members or friends help him regain functional independence?

PHYSICAL THERAPY

Muscles, Joints, and Movement

Joints are where two or more bones meet to form a movable area of the skeletal frame. Muscles move the bones. Unused muscles can shorten and tighten, which makes the joint motion painful and limited. Muscle shortening can happen in a short time. Therefore, it is important that patients are helped to use their muscles by encouraging them to do normal daily activities and their prescribed exercises. Figure 13.1 shows joint movements that are necessary to allow optimal movement.

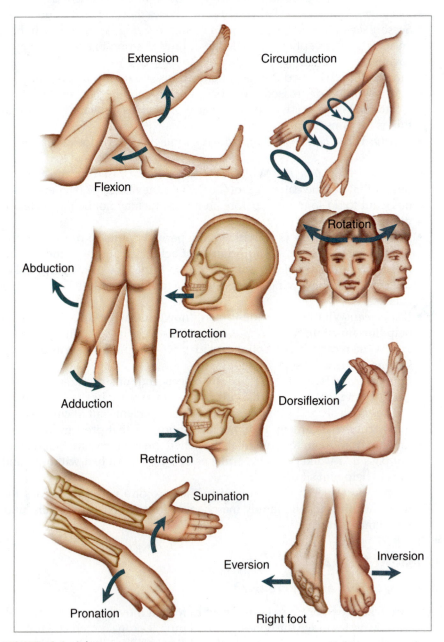

FIGURE 13.1   Joint movements.

GUIDELINE 13.1

Assisting with ROM Exercises

- Do not start ROM exercises until you have received specific instructions for your patient.
- Never take a patient beyond the point of pain. Pain is a warning sign and should be heeded. Report patient pain to the patient's therapist or physician.
- Report to the therapist if the patient does not do the exercises when you are not in the house.
- Report to the therapist if the patient is finding the exercises harder rather than easier to do.
- Use the flat part of your hand and fingers to hold the patient's body parts. Do not grip with your fingertips. Some people are sensitive to pressure. Some people are ticklish.
- If you forget what to do, think of your own body and how it works.
- Talk to the patient. Explain what is being done and why. Even if the person does not appear to understand, the tone of your voice and touch of your hands can help you communicate.
- Better communication greatly improves your chances for patient cooperation.
- Do each exercise three to five times or as you have been instructed.
- Follow a logical sequence during the exercises so that each joint and muscle is exercised. For example, start at the head and work down to the feet.
- Be gentle—never bend or straighten a body part farther than it will go normally.
- Slow, steady movement of a tight muscle will help the muscle relax and also increase the joint range.
- Include the family members or caregivers in the activity so they can learn and continue the exercises when you are not there.

Range-of-Motion Exercises

There are four types of range-of-motion (ROM) exercises (see Guideline 13.1); each is ordered for a specific purpose:

Type of ROM Exercise	Patient	Helper
Passive	Not applicable	Takes patient through ROM Patient does not help
Active/assist	Active motion	Helps make motion easier; moves part farther than patient can
Active	Done totally by patient	Not applicable
Resistive	Active motion	Makes exercise harder by providing resistance to motion but allows completion of motion (see Procedure 13.1)

PROCEDURE 13.1

Range of Motion

Rationale

Correct movement of joints and muscles assists the patient to remain independent, contracture-free, and mobile. It also contributes to increased strength and sense of well-being.

1. Wash your hands.
2. Explain to the patient that you are going to help him exercise his muscles and joints.
3. Ask visitors to leave, if appropriate.
4. Prior to doing range-of-motion exercises, offer the patient the bedpan or urinal.
5. Drape the patient for modesty.
6. Raise the bed to the highest horizontal position, if possible.
7. Move the patient close to you.
8. Proceed with the exercises as you have been instructed (see Figure 13.2).
9. Make the patient comfortable.
10. Wash your hands.

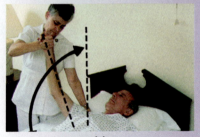

(a)

Shoulder flexion, with elbow straight, raise arm over head, then lower, keeping arm in front of you the whole time.

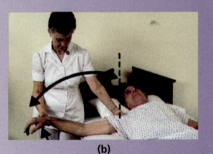

(b)

Shoulder abduction and adduction, with elbow straight, raise arm over head, then lower, keeping arm out to the side the whole time.

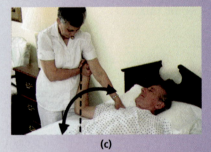

(c)

Shoulder internal and external rotation, bring arm out to the side. Do not bring elbow out to the shoulder level. Turn arm back and forth so forearm points down toward feet, then up toward head. With arm alongside body and elbow bent at 90 degree angle, turn arm so forearm points across stomach, then out to the side.

FIGURE 13.2

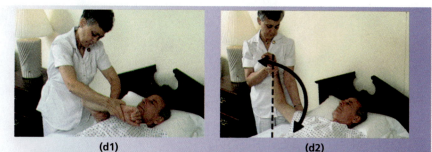

(d1)　　　　　**(d2)**

1 and 2 Shoulder horizontal abduction and adduction. Keeping arm at shoulder level, reach across chest past opposite shoulder, then reach out to the side.

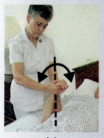

(e)

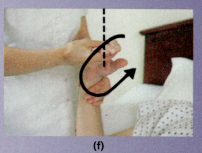

(f)

Elbow flexion and extension. With arm alongside body, bend elbow to touch shoulder, then straighten elbow out again.

Forearm pronation and supination. With arm alongside the body and elbow bent to 90 degrees (a right angle), turn forearm so palm faces first toward head, then toward feet.

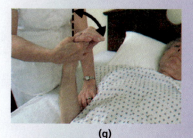

(g)

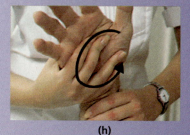

(h)

Wrist flexion and extension. Bend wrist up and down.

Wrist flexion and extension. Bend wrist back and forth and in a circle.

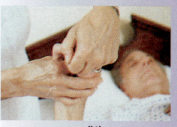

(i1)

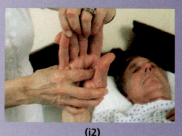

(i2)

1 and 2 Finger flexion and extension. Make a fist, then straighten fingers out together.

FIGURE 13.2　*(Continued)*

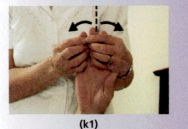

(j1)   **(j2)**

1 and 2 Finger flexion and extension. Touch tip of each finger to its base, then straighten each finger in turn.

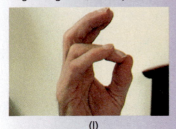

(k1)   **(k2)**

1 and 2 Finger adduction and abduction. With fingers straight, squeeze fingers together, then spread them apart.

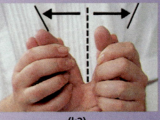

(l)

Finger/thumb opposition. Touch thumb to the tip of each finger to make a circle. Open hand fully between touching each finger.

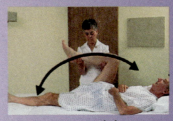

(m)

Hip/knee flexion and extension. Bend knee and bring it up toward chest, keeping foot off bed. Lower leg to bed, straightening knee as it goes down.

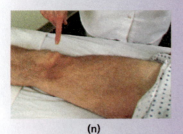

(n)

Quad sets. With leg flat on bed, tighten thigh muscles to straighten the knee, hard, pushing it into the bed. Hold for count of five then relax. Repeat exercise with rolled towel under the knee.

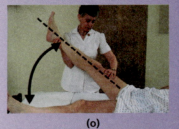

(o)

Straight leg raising. Keeping the knee straight, raise leg up off the bed. Return slowly to the bed, keeping the knee straight.

FIGURE 13.2 *(Continued)*

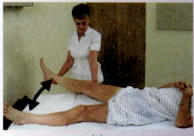

(p)

Hip abduction and adduction. With leg flat on bed and knee pointing to the ceiling, slide leg out to the side. Then slide it back to touch the other leg.

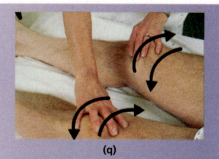

(q)

Hip internal and external rotation. With legs flat on bed and feet apart, turn both legs so knees face outward. Then turn them in so knees face each other.

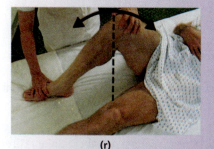

(r)

Hip internal and external rotation (variation). With one knee bent and foot flat on the bed, turn leg so knee moves out to the side, then inward across the other leg. Do each leg separately.

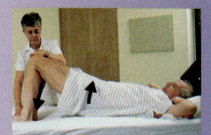

(s)

Bridging. With both knees bent up, feet flat on bed, push on bed with feet to raise hips (as in lifting for a bed pan). Hold for count of five and then relax.

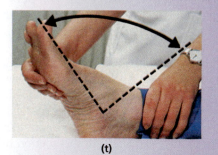

(t)

Ankle dorsiflexion and extension. Bend ankles up, down, and side to side.

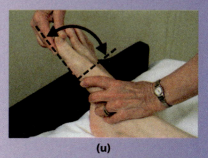

(u)

Toe flexion and extension. Bend and straighten toes.

FIGURE 13.2

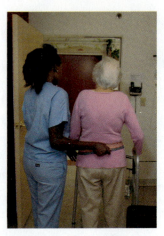

FIGURE 13.3 Using a gait belt protects both you and the patient (Photographer: Patrick J. Watson).

CHOOSING THE CORRECT CHAIR A patient usually spends all or at least part of the day out of his bed. But where does he go when out of bed? Sometimes a patient will sit in a wheelchair, a favorite reclining chair, the sofa, or a kitchen chair. Which is best? Here are several guidelines to follow when choosing a chair:

- The chair should provide good support to the person's back.
- A reclining chair is difficult to get out of, especially when the patient is tired.
- The best type of chair gives the individual the most independence.
- Consider the types of chairs available.
- Use the safest chairs.

A dining room chair or straight-back chair provides a great deal of support. One with arms is best, if it is available (see Figure 13.3). The person should be able to sit with her feet resting on the floor or to place her feet on the floor comfortably without straining. Otherwise, she will not be able to stand safely.

A wheelchair can provide good support while allowing the individual freedom to move around the house. However, a wheelchair is not for everyone. If you think a wheelchair might be useful to your patient, discuss this with the therapist before you suggest it to the patient. If the patient is using a wheelchair, always have the brakes locked when assisting the patient to sit or stand. Never leave a confused patient in a wheelchair with his feet on the foot pedals. The patient may think his feet are on the floor and try to stand up.

TRANSFERRING To transfer a patient means to help him move from one place to another (for example, from his bed to a chair and back again). How well the transfer goes depends on how much confidence your patient has in you. *Know yourself. Know your capabilities. Always stay within your capabilities.* If you feel confident, the person you are caring for will sense this and have confidence in you.

When a person loses the use of a body part, it becomes important to her to control what remains. Use this to your advantage. Observe the patient's abilities and do not help her more than necessary. A gait belt (a strap that buckles around the midsection of the patient) can help you with your patient and give you better control over her center of gravity. Gait belts can be purchased at any pharmacy or medical supply store. The physical therapist will often provide the home health aide with a gait belt to use for safety.

Before a person can move from bed to another place, he must come to a sitting position with legs over the side of the bed (see Procedure 13.2). You can help a person by raising the head of the bed, if possible. This gives him extra assistance. Raise the bed to a high horizontal position so the individual is almost standing when he slides off the bed. Be sure the bed is locked and anchored against a wall so it does not move (see Clinical Alert 13.1).

USING A MECHANICAL LIFT   Some patients are too weak or too heavy to be transferred by another person. Such cases require a mechanical lift. Practice using the model you have available. The manufacturer will often send someone

PROCEDURE 13.2

Helping a Patient to Sit Up

Rationale

Patients who are too weak to adjust their position themselves require assistance. Good body alignment promotes a sense of well-being and prevents fatigue and injury.

1. Wash your hands.
2. Ask any visitor to step out of the room, if appropriate.
3. Tell the patient what you are going to do.
4. Roll the patient on her side, facing you. Bend her knees.
5. Reach one arm over to hold her under the back of her knees.
6. Place your other arm under the neck and shoulder area.
7. Position your feet with a wide base of support and your center of gravity close to the bed.
8. On the count of three, shift your weight to your back leg. While you are doing this, swing the patient's legs over the edge of the bed and pull his shoulders to a sitting position.
9. Remain in front of the patient with both your hands on him for support. Do not leave him until you are sure he is stable.
10. Proceed with the remainder of the transfer. For a patient who requires only a little assistance, the procedure remains the same. Direct the patient through the first nine steps and support him when necessary. Be sure to remain with him in the sitting position until he is stable.

CLINICAL ALERT 13.1

Taking Care of Business

Taking care of business (TCOB) is necessary as you are moving, transferring, and directing patients. Concentrate on what you are doing and be aware of what is going on around you. Dizzy spells, sudden weakness, or loud noises can cause lapses in concentration that in turn can cause a patient to fall or lose his balance. If you are TCOB, you will usually be able to prevent serious injury to the patient and yourself.

to train you in the use of the lift (the contact information is on a sticker attached to the lift). Some lifts differ slightly, but the principles of operation for a mechanical lift using a sling are the same (see Procedure 13.3 and Figure 13.4). If the mechanical lift is a sit-to-stand type of machine, the procedure will be different (contact the manufacturer for details) (see Figure 13.5).

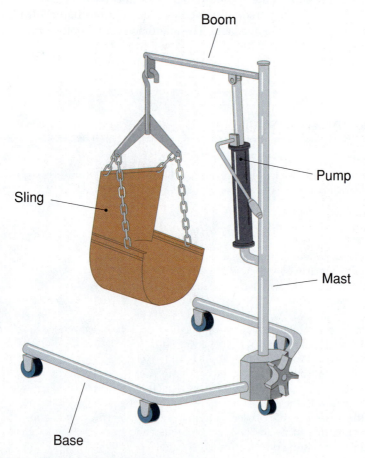

FIGURE 13.4 A mechanical lift using a sling.

PROCEDURE 13.3

Using a Mechanical Lift

Rationale

Some patients may require mechanical assistance to leave bed. Having this assistance available ensures that all patients, regardless of size or condition, can be maintained in good body alignment and moved safely from place to place when needed.

1. Assemble your equipment: mechanical lift, sling.
2. Wash your hands.
3. Tell the patient that you are going to help him out of bed using the portable mechanical patient lift. It is always safer if a second person is available to assist you with the patient.
4. Position the chair next to the bed with the back of the chair in line with the bed's headboard.
5. Cover the chair with a blanket or sheet.
6. Turn the patient from side to side on the bed as you slide the sling under him.
7. Attach the sling to the mechanical lift with the hooks in place through the metal frame facing out.
8. Have the patient fold both arms across his chest, if possible.
9. Using the electric switch, lift the patient from the bed.
10. Guide the patient's legs.
11. Lower the patient into the chair.
12. Remove the hooks from the frame of the portable mechanical lift.
13. Leave the patient safe and comfortable in the chair or wheelchair as appropriate.
14. To return the patient to bed, put the hooks facing out through the metal frame of the sling, which is still under the patient. If the patient is sitting on a specialty cushion to prevent or heal ulcers, the sling will have been removed and need to be slid under the patient for use of the lift again.
15. Raise the patient by using the electrical switch on the mechanical lift. Lift him from the chair into the bed, guiding his legs as you can. If you have a second person to help you, have this person guide the patient's legs.

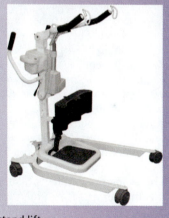

FIGURE 13.5 A sit to stand lift.

16. Lower the patient into the center of the bed.
17. Remove the hooks from the frame.
18. Remove the sling from under the patient by having him turn from side to side on the bed.
19. Put a pillow under the patient's head. Properly position the patient.
20. Remake the top of the bed.
21. Lower the bed to its lowest horizontal position.
22. Wash your hands.

HELPING A PERSON TO STAND AND SIT The procedure for helping an individual stand up can be used with patients who need a great deal of assistance and with those who need little. By using the same sequence of actions each time, you teach the person how to stand up by herself. Help her only when necessary, but remain in good position to guard her as she stands. You may choose to use a gait belt for additional support. Keep your directions short. Memorize the sequence as presented in Procedure 13.4. By memorizing the sequence, you will not need to stop and remember what to say to the patient each time you help them. You should be able to concentrate on how the patient is following your directions, not on trying to remember them yourself (see Procedures 13.5, 13.6, 13.7, and 13.8).

PROCEDURE 13.4

Helping a Patient to Stand

Rationale

Some patients require assistance to stand up and find their balance. Providing this assistance contributes to their independence and sense of well-being. This procedure includes examples of dialogue that normally occurs while assisting a patient from sitting to standing.

1. Instruct the patient sitting on the edge of the bed or in a chair: "Scoot to the front of your chair (or bed). Put your hands on the arms of the chair." As the home health care aide, you should then place your knees between the patient's knees. Your feet should be in a stable position and you should be close to the chair or bed. If the patient has a weak knee, brace it with your knee by putting your knee in front of his knee (see Figure 13.6A).
2. Next, instruct the patient, for example, "Put your right foot flat on the floor slightly back toward the chair (or bed)." *This should be the strongest leg.* You should now bend your knees and lean onto your forward foot to place the same side arm around the patient's waist and place your other hand at the other side of the patient's waist. You have now encircled the patient and are holding him at his center of gravity.
3. The third step involves instructing the patient as follows: "On the count of three, push down with your arms, lean forward, and stand up." The home

(continued)

health aide provides a brace so that the patient remains stable. Remembering to count to three allows you both to know when to start the motion and work as a team. Hold the patient closely. The more assistance needed, the closer you hold the patient. On the count of three, rock your weight to your back foot (see Figure 13.6B).

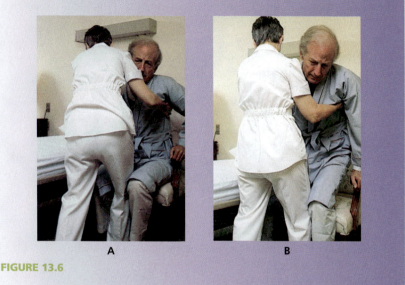

A   B

FIGURE 13.6

Minimal Assistance

As the individual gains strength and confidence, she will require less assistance. You will use the same basic body positioning but will not hold her. You may remain with her for directions and in case you are needed. When minimal assistance is needed, it is best to stand on the weaker side of the patient

PROCEDURE 13.5

Helping a Patient to Sit

Rationale

Some patients require assistance to sit down safely. Providing this assistance contributes to their independence and sense of well-being. Your body mechanics and positioning are the same as in helping the patient to stand. Just reverse the directions.

1. Be sure that the wheels on the bed or chair are locked.
2. Remind the patient to feel the bed or chair with the back of his legs.
3. Direct the patient to reach back for the arms of the chair or the bed.
4. You support and direct the activity as he sits down.

PROCEDURE 13.6

Pivot Transfer from Bed to Chair

Rationale

The pivot transfer provides a safe manner in which to move a patient from one place to another.

1. Prepare the equipment. Place the wheelchair with locked brakes against the bed so the patient can use it for support. Place the chair so that the patient will move toward her stronger side.
2. If you are transferring the patient to a wheelchair, lock the wheels of the chair. If the bed has wheels, lock the wheels of the bed.
3. Wash your hands.
4. Tell the patient what you are going to do.
5. Bring the patient to a sitting position with her legs over the edge of the bed (see Figure 13.7A).
6. Place slippers or shoes on her feet.
7. Explain the procedure to the patient:
   a. She will come to a standing position.
   b. She will then reach for the arm of the chair, pivot, and sit.
   c. You will remain in good support position and guide her.
   d. You will keep your foot near the patient's foot for extra support.
   e. You will use good body mechanics to support her and prevent injury to yourself.
8. When you are sure that the patient understands the procedure, perform the transfer (see Figure 13.7B and C).
9. Secure the patient in the chair. Make her comfortable. Leave her in a safe place.
10. Wash your hands.

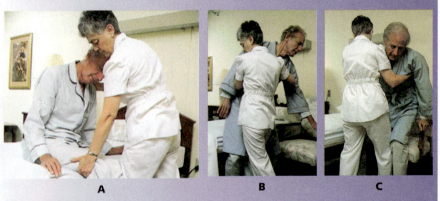

A   B   C

FIGURE 13.7

PROCEDURE 13.7

Transfer from Chair to Bed

Rationale

The pivot transfer provides a safe manner in which to move a patient from one place to another. Your body mechanics and positioning are the same as in helping the patient into the chair. Just reverse the directions.

1. Wash your hands.
2. Prepare the bed.
3. Place the chair at a 45° angle to the bed so the patient moves toward his stronger side.
4. If you are transferring the patient from a wheelchair, lock the wheels of the chair. If the bed has wheels, lock the wheels of the bed.
5. Stand in a good position using a firm base of support and proper body mechanics.
6. Direct the patient to come to a standing position.
7. Direct the patient to reach for the bed and pivot. Help and guide him.
8. Make the patient comfortable.
9. Wash your hands.

and support her with a gait belt. This way, as the patient is changing position, you will be available if she starts to fall or lose balance (see Figure 13.8).

Ambulation Activities

Ambulation refers to the action of walking. If the patient requires a special gait or must learn a new way to walk, the physical therapist will set up a plan for the patient and you to follow. However, the same basic assisting

PROCEDURE 13.8

Going from a Standing Position to a Sitting Position Using Assistive Devices

Rationale

Providing assistance while the patient uses an assistive device is another step toward independence for the patient.

1. Check to see that the chair is secure and safe. Brace it against a wall if possible.
2. The patient then walks to the chair.
3. Direct the patient to turn her back to the chair and feel it with the back of her legs.
4. Direct the patient to let go of the assistive device, reach for the arms of the chair, and slowly lower herself into the chair. (*Note:* The patient may need reassurance.)
5. Guide and support your patient as needed. Remain in front of the patient and in good position to assist her. Always use good body mechanics.

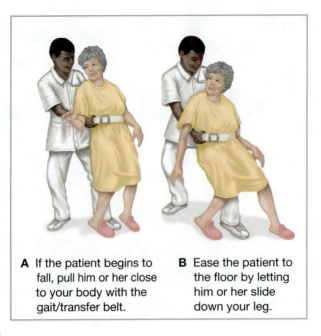

A If the patient begins to fall, pull him or her close to your body with the gait/transfer belt.

B Ease the patient to the floor by letting him or her slide down your leg.

FIGURE 13.8

positions can be used for patients with all types of gaits. Keep the following points in mind:

- Use the proper procedure for the patient to come to a standing position.
- Use a gait belt for extra support.
- Stand on the patient's weaker side and a little behind him.
- One hand should be on the gait belt.

Assistive Walking Devices

Canes, crutches, and walkers help people support themselves while walking. Use of this equipment may be permanent or temporary. An individual may use different pieces of equipment at different times. The decision about which piece of equipment to use will take into consideration the person's needs and abilities. Do not change the equipment or the way in which the person has been instructed to use it. If you have a suggestion or a safety concern, discuss it with the physical therapist (see Guideline 13.2).

Each piece of equipment is prescribed by a physician and fit by a professional nurse or physical therapist to the patient's unique needs. This individualized fit decreases the possibility of accidents. If a piece of equipment is borrowed, check it for fit and make sure that it is safe before it is used.

CANES A patient may use a single-tipped cane, a tripod cane, or a quad-cane (see Figure 13.9). A cane is usually used on the stronger side. That way, the

GUIDELINE 13.2

Using Assistive Walking Devices

- Canes, crutches, and walkers must always have rubber tips on the ends. Tips should not be worn, wet, or torn.
- Screws and bolts should be securely in place. If one is lost, replace it. Do not use the device without the proper screws in place.
- Wooden canes and crutches should be smooth, without cracks.
- Metal canes, crutches, and walkers should have no sharp edges and should be straight.
- To go up stairs, advance the strongest leg to the next step. Bring the cane or crutches and then the weaker leg to the step.
- To go down stairs, advance the cane or crutches to the lower step, followed by the weaker leg and then the stronger one.
- The hand piece of each device should be level with the hip to allow a slight bend at the elbow when the patient is standing.
- All equipment is used after the patient has come to a standing position.
- Do not pull up on a patient's walker or cane when he or she is trying to come to a standing position.

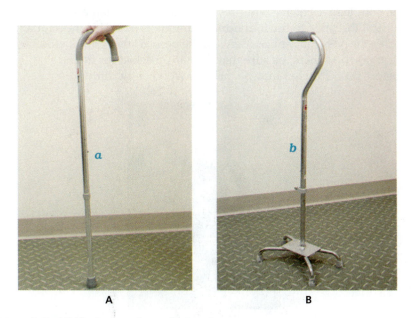

A   B

FIGURE 13.9   (A) Single-tipped cane (B) Quad-cane.

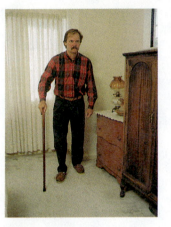 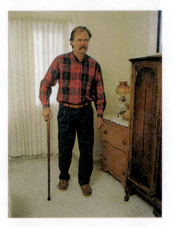

FIGURE 13.10   **FIGURE 13.11**

person's weight is balanced between the cane and the involved side. The base of support will change from that of a normal walking gait. The patient walking with the cane should:

1. place the cane about 12 inches in front on his stronger side (see Figure 13.10)
2. bring the weaker leg forward so that it is even with the cane (see Figure 13.11)
3. bring the stronger leg forward, just ahead of the cane (see Figure 13.12)

CRUTCHES   Crutches assist a person who cannot put complete weight on one or both legs. Crutches are prescribed by a physician and fit by a nurse or physical therapist to the individual's unique needs. This individualized fit decreases the possibility of accidents. If the person has a pair of crutches in the house or borrows them, be sure that they are checked for fit and that they are safe before use. Crutches may be made of wood or aluminum.

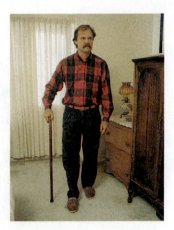

FIGURE 13.12

While using crutches, the patient puts his body weight on his hands and arms, not on the top of the crutch under his arms. Some patients will have to exercise their upper arms before they begin using crutches. The physical therapist, nurse, or physician teaches the patient how to use the crutches and which gait to use. The most common are the swing-to gait or the swing-through gate (see Figure 13.13 and Table 13.1).

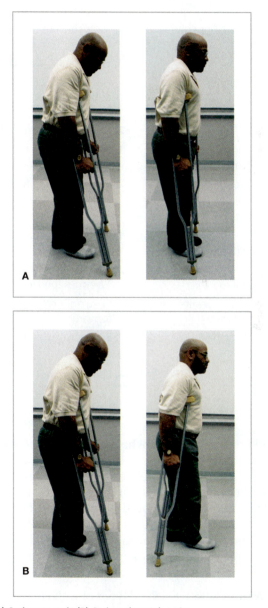

FIGURE 13.13   (A) Swing-to gait (B) Swing-through gait.

TABLE 13.1   Crutch Walking

Gait	Features	Steps
Three-point gait, one non-weight-bearing leg.	One non-weight-bearing leg. Strong upper arms. Client can balance well.	1. Place crutches 8 to 12 inches in front of the body with weaker leg. 2. Bring front leg forward in front of crutches.
Swing-through crutch.	Strong upper arms. Some weight bearing.	1. Place crutches 8 to 12 inches in front of body. 2. Swing body past crutches.
Swing-to crutch.	Strong upper arms. Some weight bearing.	1. Place crutches 8 to 12 inches in front of body while bearing weight on strong leg. 2. Swing body to crutches.
Standard three-point gait.	One non-weight-bearing leg. Strong upper arms. Patient can balance well.	1. Place crutches 8 to 12 inches in front of body with weaker leg. 2. Bring strong leg forward in front of crutches.
Two-point gait.	Weight bearing on both feet. Patient can balance well.	1. Bring right foot and left crutch 8 to 12 inches forward. 2. Bring left foot and right crutch 8 to 12 inches forward.
Four-point gait.	Weight bearing on both feet. Stable gait, slow.	1. Bring right crutch 8 to 12 inches forward. 2. Bring left foot in front of crutch. 3. Bring left crutch in front of left foot. 4. Bring right foot in front of left foot.

WALKER   A walker helps a person who requires support because of greater imbalance or weakness. The walker is safe to push down on only when all four legs are on the ground in a level position. If the walker is being moved, the patient's feet should be stationary. If the walker is stationary, the patient can move his feet. The walker should be picked up and moved, not slid along the ground. It is a good idea to make sure walkways are clear and throw rugs are removed when someone is using a walker. Cluttered walkways and throw rugs can cause difficulty in maneuvering the walker (see Guideline 13.3).

Types of Walkers   There are several types of walkers. The most common is described in the previous section and is used most often when someone needs

GUIDELINE 13.3

Helping with Rehabilitation

- Always apply basic body mechanics.
- Be sure of your patient's abilities before you attempt a procedure. Check each time.
- Use common sense.
- Take care of business (TCOB).
- Know your own abilities. Do not be ashamed to ask for help or additional instruction with a procedure.
- Communicate through words, gestures, and tone of voice.
- Set an example to the patient and his or her family members.
- Use the same procedure each time you assist the patient to set up a routine with which you will both be familiar.
- Apply what you know from one procedure to help you with others.
- Clothing should fit well and not block the patient's view of the floor. Shoes should be flat with nonskid soles.

to push down with her or his weight on the walker to assist in ambulation. Others include the following:

- A walker with skis is designed to allow the patient to push versus lift and set. This walker has skis on the front and wheels on the back. This type of walker is used most often when someone is unable to lift the regular walker to ambulate.
- The rollator walker has wheels in the front and back. It usually comes with a seat basket and brakes. The patient must put on brakes and turn around to sit. This is the most common walker for someone who will use the walker for the rest of his or her life. It requires little effort from the patient and has the added advantages of a sturdy basket to carry items from one place to another. The other advantage is the seat, which is designed for the patient who needs to rest frequently during ambulation (see Figure 13.14).

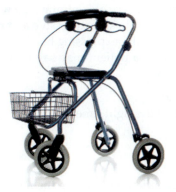

FIGURE 13.14 The rollator walker.

Although walkers can be found in thrift stores or borrowed, it is important to have the walker adjusted to the correct height for the patient's needs. Failure to have the correct adjustment can cause back pain and/or other injuries. The physical therapist will determine which model is the best fit for your patient and can adjust a used walker to accommodate the patient.

SPEECH AND LANGUAGE THERAPY

Speech and language therapy is one of the services provided by the home health team. The speech-language pathologist is the professional who evaluates the need for therapy and who plans the therapy program.

Speech and language therapy is given when the patient has difficulty communicating. It is important to remember that communication involves more than just speaking. Communication also means the ability to understand speech, to read, to write, and to gesture.

A person may need speech and language therapy if she has a disorder that affects the parts of the brain, face, lips, tongue, or throat used to form words. Examples of this kind of disorder are Parkinson's disease, cerebral palsy, and cleft palate. An individual who has had cancer of the tongue or larynx (voice box) may need therapy after the surgeon has removed the cancer.

Aphasia

Injury to the brain may cause a loss of speech or language abilities, called aphasia. Usually, the injury is from a cerebrovascular accident (CVA), often called a stroke. In a cerebrovascular accident, a blood clot, hemorrhage, or vascular spasm in the brain stops oxygen from reaching parts of the brain tissue. When those parts of the brain do not receive oxygen, they stop working. Damage to the brain may also be caused by trauma to the head or by a tumor.

An aphasic person may have difficulty in all areas of communication. It may be hard to speak, understand speech, read, or write. Aphasia may be mild, moderate, or severe. The kind of aphasia is determined by where the brain injury occurs and how much damage is done to the parts of the brain. Aphasia does not mean that the person is unable to make judgments or think. Aphasia only means a person cannot communicate with words.

There are two types of aphasia: expressive and receptive. A person with expressive aphasia has difficulty expressing his thoughts and sometimes communicating in writing. Such a patient may say things involuntarily. He may have difficulty:

- Naming people and things
- Saying yes and no at the right time
- Spelling words
- Counting
- Telling time

Everyone has had the experience of having the name of a person or an object "right on the tip of the tongue." The feeling of knowing what you want to say but not being able to think of the right word is what an expressively aphasic person experiences all day long.

A person with receptive aphasia has trouble receiving, or understanding, what he is hearing, seeing, or touching. For example, he can hear words clearly, but they do not have any meaning for him. It is as if he were listening to a foreign language. He might have the same problem when he looks at words. Some aphasic people even have trouble understanding the use of common objects. They might pick up a comb and not know what to do with it. A person with receptive aphasia may have:

- No interest in watching television or listening to the radio
- No interest in reading the newspaper
- No ability to follow directions
- No ability to answer questions appropriately

The behavior of the aphasic person may seem rude or confusing at times. But think about how *you* might act if you could not say what you wanted to say or if you could not understand what people were saying to you. Always remember that the aphasic person is an intelligent adult. He or she is just as smart as before the brain injury but simply cannot communicate easily. An aphasic person will be most cooperative and least frustrated when you treat her or him as you would any adult.

A patient with aphasia may:

- Tire easily
- Laugh or cry frequently
- Use profanity without meaning to
- Repeat the same word(s) over and over

The speech-language pathologist may teach you the following exercises to practice with the patient. They are often used when the muscles used for speech are weaker. *Never* practice any exercise with a patient that was not taught to him by the speech pathologist.

Exercises

Lips

1. Open mouth as wide as possible, stretch, close tightly and pucker, hold.
2. Pucker lips, hold, move lips to the left, hold, move lips to the right, hold.
3. Reach out with lower lip, hold. Reach out with the upper lip, hold.
4. Smile with lips closed, frown, repeat.
5. Press lips tightly as if you are saying mm.
6. Say ma-me-mi-mo-mu (as clearly and distinctly as you can).

Tongue

1. Put the tongue in the outer left corner of the mouth, move to the right and back. Work for speed and rhythm of movement.

2. Extend the tongue straight forward, then pull back vigorously with the whole tongue.
3. Open mouth wide, lift tongue tip up to the roof of the mouth, down. Do not move your jaw; lift your tongue.
4. Say ta-te-ti-to-tu. Do not move your jaw; lift your tongue.
5. Say da-de-di-do-du. Do not move your jaw; lift your tongue.
6. Say la-le-li-lo-lu. Do not move your jaw; lift your tongue.

Throat

1. Puff up cheeks. Hold air for five seconds—then release air as you blow out.
2. Suck in cheeks—then relax.
3. Puff up cheeks with air—move air from one cheek to the other without letting air escape lips. Alternate from one side to the other.
4. Drink liquids whenever possible through a straw.

YOUR ROLE AS A CAREGIVER

Your role in working with the aphasic patient is important. You will probably spend more time with the patient than any other person on the home health team. You will have a better chance to know the patient and to help him adjust to his new schedule of exercises and activities.

The speech-language pathologist will ask you to do two specific tasks. The first will be to help the patient practice speech or language activities. These activities are always taught first by the speech-language pathologist (speech therapist). Remember that the aphasic person may have various troubles communicating and with different degrees of severity. For this reason, it is always the job of the speech-language pathologist to determine which activities best fit the needs of a particular individual.

If the person has difficulty understanding or using words, you may be taught how to use pictures and printed words to help improve communication. You may be shown how to help your patient practice printing or writing. Sometimes, the patient may have weakened muscles of the face, lips, or tongue. The speech-language pathologist may teach specific exercises to help improve the strength and coordination of those muscles.

The second task will be to observe and report. It is important to observe how the patient makes her needs known and how well she performs the assigned practice tasks. You will want to note in the communication notebook how the patient makes her feelings known to you. Does she point? Shake her head? Use words? You will also want to keep a record of how often the assigned speech or language tasks are performed.

You will be with the patient many more hours during the week than the speech-language pathologist will be. What you report will be useful in planning the therapy program.

Here are some dos and don'ts to keep in mind when you are caring for an aphasic person:.

Do

- Get the attention of the patient before starting to speak.
- Keep instructions and explanations simple. Speak slowly but naturally. Try to limit your conversation to things related to the patient's immediate needs or surroundings.
- Encourage the patient to use common expressions, such as *hello, goodbye,* and *I want.*
- Encourage the patient to be as independent as possible. He is an adult; treat him like one.
- Ask direct questions requiring a simple yes or no answer. For example, ask, "Did you eat lunch?" rather than ""What did you eat for lunch?"
- Give the patient time to reply; allow the patient to show you what he is trying to say.
- Give the patient opportunities to hear speech, such as on the radio and television.
- Meals and dressing times are good opportunities to encourage the patient's attempts to speak. Let him ask for what he needs. He may say the word correctly sometimes and forget it at another time. This is usual for the aphasic person.
- Encourage the patient to use whatever speech ability he has. Counting and singing are good activities. Words such as *up* and *down* or *push* and *pull* can be used during physical therapy exercises.
- Show the patient understanding, but not pity. Help her verbalize her feeling of frustration ("I know it must be difficult for you.").
- By your body language, patience, and attitude of acceptance, create an air of relaxation for the patient. Avoid directions, such as "Relax."
- Sometimes, it will be impossible to understand what the patient is saying. At such times, tactfully try to change the subject or say, "Let's forget it now and come back to it later. The words will probably come when you're not trying so hard."
- You also may encourage the patient to learn the words that go with his personal care. When you are helping the patient bathe, dress, or eat, say the name of each utensil or body part. For example, say, "Fork, you eat with a fork," or "Arm, I'm washing your arm." Your patient may find that he is able to say some of the words with you. If he does, smile and let him know that he has succeeded. If he does not repeat the words, you must not force him. Remember, he wants to talk, and if he could, he would. Talking to him about these activities in the same way each day will help him to relearn what words mean, even if he cannot say them.

Don't

- Don't answer for the patient if she is capable of speaking for herself. Do include the patient in social conversations.

- Don't confuse the patient with too much idle chatter or too many people speaking at once.
- Don't discuss the patient's emotional reactions and problems in his presence.
- Don't interrupt the patient or finish sentences for him. He may require extra time to think of the correct word.
- Don't show your concern about the patient's speech either through words or facial expressions. Do not, under any circumstances, put the patient on display or force her to speak. Remarks such as "Say it for them" can upset and embarrass the patient.
- Don't ridicule or insist that the patient give accurate responses, pronounce correctly, or "talk right." (There is nothing the patient wants more than to do just that.)
- Don't speak to the patient as if she were a child, deaf, or incompetent. She is not deaf (unless a definite hearing loss has been detected). Her problem is generally one of understanding the meaning of your words, as though you were speaking a foreign language. Simplify or rephrase your wording without shouting. Treat her like the adult she is.

If you can show the patient—through your attitude and your work—that you understand his problem and that you want to help him, you will often be rewarded by the gratitude of a more relaxed and comfortable patient. One way to help is to have information readily available on a communication board. A communication board has information important to the patient, such as the day of the week, the name of the caregiver, a picture of his family, names of expected visitors, schedule of care for the day, the weather, and other important information (see Figure 13.15).

HEARING LOSS

You may be caring for an individual with hearing loss. Some are born with hearing loss. Others lose their hearing through exposure to loud noise over a long period of time. Head injuries or ear infections can also cause loss of hearing. Many people lose some ability to hear sounds clearly as they age.

Whatever the cause of the hearing loss, it can be a frustrating problem. The person who is hard of hearing may believe that others are mumbling or speaking unclearly. She may have to work harder to understand what is being said. If it becomes too frustrating to try to follow a conversation, the hard-of-hearing person may begin to avoid social activities. A hearing aid can often be of great help.

Hearing Aid Care

The hearing aid earmold is custom-made to fit the ear. An earmold that does not fit snugly into the ear causes a high-pitched whistling noise when the aid is turned on. The earmold must be kept clean. If earwax or dirt clog the earmold, sound will not pass through. The earmold and aid should be wiped

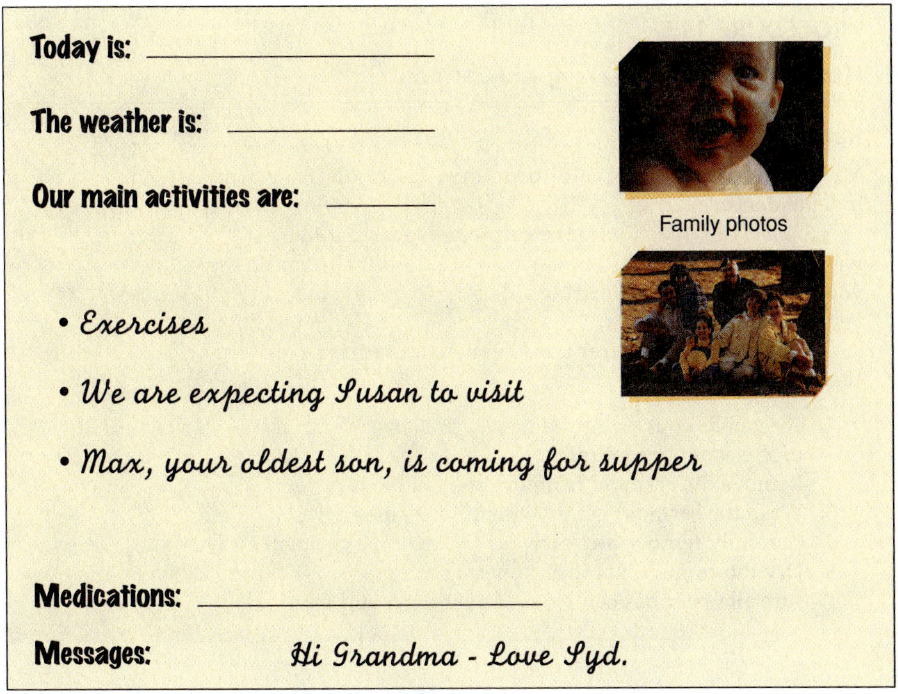

Today is: _____

The weather is: _____

Our main activities are: _____

Family photos

• *Exercises*

• *We are expecting Susan to visit*

• *Max, your oldest son, is coming for supper*

Medications: _____

Messages: *Hi Grandma - Love Syd.*

FIGURE 13.15   Example communication board.

with a dry tissue after each wearing. When not in use, the hearing aid should be kept in a safe place, away from extreme heat or cold (see Procedure 13.9).

BATTERIES MAKE THE HEARING AID WORK   If the hearing aid does not work, the battery may be dead. To insert a new one, match the model number on the battery to the number on the hearing aid case. One battery will last about 125 hours, or ten days. To save battery power, remove the battery from the hearing aid whenever the aid is not being worn. Extra batteries should be stored in a cool, dry place, such as a dresser drawer.

Precautions include the following:

• Keep the hearing aid away from heat sources such as radiators and hair dryers.
• Do not wet the hearing aid.
• Do not drop the hearing aid.
• Do not spray hair spray, perfume, or aftershave lotion on the hearing aid.
• Do not twist the tubing or wires.

If the hearing aid does not work, check to see if:

• the battery is put in correctly and the case is closed tightly.
• the aid is turned on and the volume is loud enough.

PROCEDURE 13.9

How to Clean the Hearing Aid Earmold

Rationale

Maintaining a hearing aid promotes its good function and the patient's independence.

Remember: Wash only the earmold. Never put the body of the hearing aid in water. Never use alcohol or cleaning fluid on the earmold or the aid. Encourage your patient to take the hearing aid off or to protect it during rain and snow to prevent it from getting wet.

Unless manufacturer's instructions are different, follow this procedure to clean the earmold.

1. Assemble your equipment: pan of warm water and mild liquid detergent, pipe cleaner or toothpick.
2. Remove the earmold from the body of the hearing aid.
3. Wash the earmold gently with mild soap and water.
4. Carefully remove any earwax with the pipe cleaner or toothpick.
5. Dry thoroughly. Let it dry overnight, or blow air through the opening to be sure all water has come out of the tubing and earmold.

- there is wax in the earmold (this would need to be cleaned out).
- the tubing or wires are twisted.
- the battery is working.

If all these items have been checked and the hearing aid still does not work, it should go to the hearing aid supplier for repair (the supplier's contact information should be in the hearing aid case).

Guidelines for Talking to a Person with Hearing Impairment

- Get her attention before you start speaking.
- Talk face to face whenever possible. Your patient will understand more of what you say when she can see your face and expression.
- Keep your hands away from your face so they do not block the patient's view of what you are saying.
- Do not chew food when you are speaking; it will make your words unclear.
- Do not exaggerate your words. Speak at a normal rate of speed. You may be asked to speak louder, but do not shout.

OCCUPATIONAL THERAPY

For most of us, the skills and tasks we perform each day do not require conscious effort or awareness of how we do them. We get out of bed, go to the bathroom, bathe, dress, prepare our meals, and feed ourselves. We do not think of the complex movements made by various parts of the body to push; pull; lift; close; zip, hook, and button clothing; or to open or use various objects. Some individuals are unable to perform useful actions with a specific body part, which is called a functional limitation. A person with a functional limitation may have to concentrate to hold and lift a spoon to feed himself. Perhaps his grasp is weak. Perhaps he has lost sensation and cannot feel the spoon in his hand. Anyone who needs help with any or all basic needs such as toileting, bathing, dressing, feeding, grooming, or other day-to-day tasks is a candidate for occupational therapy. This training will help your patient improve her ability to function.

Occupational Therapist (OT) or Registered Occupational Therapist (OTR)

The occupational therapy program focuses on increasing the functional ability of the patient within his familiar environment. The trained person who administers this therapy is a registered occupational therapist (OTR). The individual who is receiving care at home knows what household equipment he has to work with and will learn to adopt new skills in his own home. Being able to learn these skills at home shows the person that he is expected to take an active part in his care. Home is a nonthreatening place for relearning basic skills. An OTR can guide and instruct both the patient and the home health aide in ways to make the transition toward functional independence (see Figure 13.16).

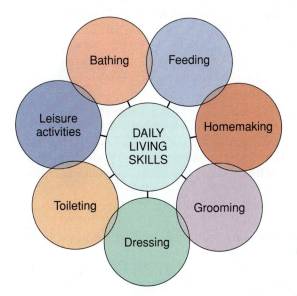

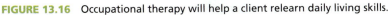

FIGURE 13.16 Occupational therapy will help a client relearn daily living skills.

The OTR works in the following general areas with a homebound patient:

- *Mobilization:* teaching the patient techniques that she can use to change position; to reach, grasp, or turn while sitting; or to maintain balance during an activity.
- *Activities of Daily Living (ADL):* tasks everyone performs each day— toileting, bathing, dressing, feeding, grooming, homemaking, leisure activities.
- *Strength, coordination, and activity tolerance:* the ability to do something without tiring quickly. The individual must learn techniques to conserve his energy, perform the skill task to his own satisfaction, and use his physical resources to the fullest.

YOUR ROLE AS A CAREGIVER

As you begin to assist a person in regaining his or her independence, your role as teacher, helper, and friend becomes important. Remember the following points:

- Your role in each task will be clearly defined by the OTR.
- If you do not understand what the individual you are caring for is supposed to do and what you are supposed to do, ask the OTR to explain more fully. If it is not clear to you, it will not be clear to the patient. It is important for both of you to know what you are expected to do and why you are doing it.
- After each training session with the OTR, you and the patient will have an opportunity to practice what has been demonstrated.
- If the patient finds it difficult and says, "I can't," assist him with part of the routine to help him start. You can say, for example, "You dress your involved arm, and I will help you put on the rest of the shirt."
- If the patient shows signs of pain, tiredness, or discomfort during the activity, stop the routine and report your observations to the OTR or the nurse supervisor.
- Observe which parts of each task the patient can and cannot do. Report your observations to the OTR on her or his next visit.
- Remember, the goal of the patient, OTR, and home health aide is to help the person become functionally independent, in other words, to take care of herself. As she achieves success with each task, your role will change.
- Do not attempt any technique that has not been taught to you and the patient by the OTR.
- Make the environment a safe and helpful one for your patient (see Figure 13.17).
- As the patient begins to regain skills, he may become fearful that he will not be able to manage on his own as well as when you are there to help. Point out positive changes you have observed.

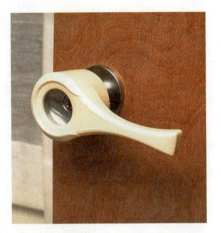

FIGURE 13.17   Extension for door handles.

- Discuss the outside world, the change of seasons, what is happening in the community, the specials at the grocery store, and who won the ballgame. Bring the world into the person's home so the individual can begin to relate to it. Help her to realize that her disability does not have to be her whole world and that it no longer requires her total involvement.
- Observe the patient's daily needs such as his glasses, tissues, a glass of water, the newspaper, and the TV. As early in his rehabilitation as possible, make these items accessible to him. Let him begin to assume responsibility for using them without your help.

Toileting

Taking care of one's own toileting needs is a basic and personal activity. A person who must rely on another person to help with this personal activity often suffers a loss of self-esteem or dignity. A person who assumes responsibility for this part of personal care has taken the first step toward functional independence. Toileting is usually the first skill a patient wishes to learn. Follow the procedure established by the OTR (see Guidelines 13.4, 13.5, and 13.6). Remember, you may assist the patient with toileting, but do not attempt to change the place of toileting until you have been instructed to do so.

Bathing

Bathing stimulates the body. The individual who bathes himself stimulates his involved extremities as he touches and rubs them. He becomes aware that the extremity "is there," even if he cannot really "feel" it. He may become aware that the involved extremity moves when he is using other parts of his body. As he bathes, he moves many parts of his body together. He bends, stretches, reaches, grasps, balances, lifts his arms and legs, turns his head, and shifts his eyes.

GUIDELINE 13.4

Toileting in Bed

- Tell the patient what part of the procedure he will be doing and what you will do.
- Provide a pulling braid (see Figure 13.18). A pulling braid is made from three 4-inch-wide strips of sheeting torn lengthwise and braided together. This braid is tied to the bed frame at one end. The other end is knotted and held by the patient to assist him in sitting or turning in bed.
- Place the bedpan where the patient can reach it. Powder it to prevent the patient's skin from sticking to it.
- Let the patient do as much as he can himself. Assist only if he runs into difficulty.

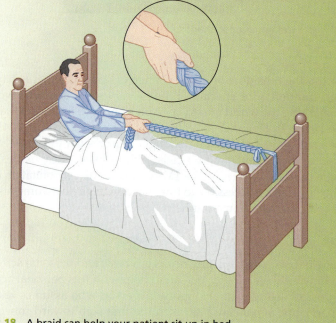

FIGURE 13.18   A braid can help your patient sit up in bed.

It is particularly important that the hemiplegic (a person paralyzed on one side of the body) gives this stimulation to involved extremities. Rubbing the affected body part with the washcloth or towel may arouse sensory nerves lying close to the skin. The brain, receiving these sensations, may send a message down the motor pathways that could trigger an automatic response in the involved arm. When you are bathing the patient, she does not use her own energy output. Her body is not involved with the automatic activity. Therefore, these responses may not be triggered.

GUIDELINE 13.5

Toileting on a Commode

- Before she begins, explain to the patient what she will be doing.
- Be sure the commode is standing securely.
- Place the commode in the position in which the patient was instructed to use it.
- Assist the patient out of bed as you have been instructed.
- Fasten the toilet paper to the commode. Tie the roll with a string or make a holder by stretching out a wire coat hanger and threading the roll onto it and hooking it to the frame. If you use a wire hanger, bend the ends and hook them over the front and back of the commode frame. Tape the ends so they do not scratch the patient (see Figure 13.19).
- Place the roll on the patient's uninvolved side. If she has general weakness, place it on her dominant (most used) side.
- Provide privacy.

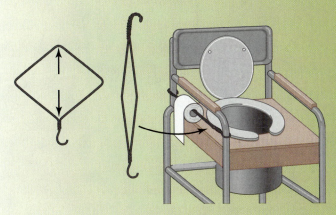

FIGURE 13.19   Use a coat hanger to make the toilet paper easier to access.

The OTR may instruct the patient to bathe in bed or when seated on the commode, on a chair in front of a basin in her room, on a chair at the sink, or on the toilet seat in the bathroom. As the patient regains strength and mobility, the OTR may instruct her in tub bathing or showering using a bench or chair placed in the tub or shower stall. Some states permit the home health aide to supervise and assist patients in showers and tubs; some do not. You will be instructed according to the guidelines in your state (see Guideline 13.7).

Taking a Shower or Bath

By the time the patient can bathe in a tub, he should have mastered skills such as balance, hip flexion, and transfers from sitting to standing with minimal assist-

GUIDELINE 13.6

Toileting in the Bathroom

- Place the commode frame over the toilet as instructed or set the elevated toilet seat in place if the patient uses such a device (see Figure 13.20). If using the commode frame, an 8-by-10-inch sheet of plastic, such as a piece from a garbage or trash bag, can be anchored between the commode seat and frame so it hangs down into the toilet bowl. This will serve as a baffle to prevent urine from splashing out of the toilet bowl. Rinse it off and replace it each time the patient uses the toilet.
- Tell the patient what he will do.
- Allow the patient to do as much as he is safely able to do.
- Assist him with sitting on the toilet as you have been instructed.
- Provide privacy.

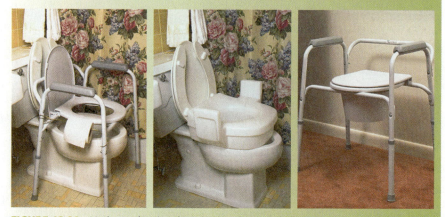

FIGURE 13.20 Various adaptive devices to make toileting easier.

GUIDELINE 13.7

Bathing

- Do not attempt any technique that has not been taught to you and the patient by the OTR. A method that was appropriate for a previous patient may be inappropriate for your present patient.
- Provide a safe environment.
- Assemble everything the patient will need for bathing and dressing. Place all items where she can reach them (see Figure 13.21).
- Thin washcloths and small face towels may be easier for a weak or arthritic patient to handle than thick cloths or large, heavy towels.
- Stabilize the wet soap by placing it on a dampened sponge, face cloth, paper towel, or rubber suction disk where it is less likely to slide.
- The patient should remove her clothing as she was taught by the OTR.

- The hemiplegic patient should wash her involved arm first. She can drape a well-soaped washcloth over the palm of her involved hand, which should be resting palm up on her lap. Then she can lean forward and cradle her uninvolved arm in the hand and slide it back and forth to wash it.
- Remind your patient to rinse off soap and dry each part of her body as she finishes washing it.
- Place nailbrush, bristles up, in the palm of her involved hand resting on her lap, palm up. Your patient can rub her uninvolved fingers across the brush, pushing gently into the palm of the other hand to steady it.
- The patient can also use the nailbrush on the fingers of the involved hand. She may lift the hand into the basin to rinse it, using the other hand for assistance if necessary.
- If the patient is in bed, crank up the bed so that she can see her abdomen and legs. In a regular bed, prop her up with pillows.
- Place the washcloth and towel over the bed rail where the patient can reach them. If she is in a regular bed, use a chair back or the head of the bed.
- Assist the patient with transfers as necessary for safety.
- When the patient is learning to turn on faucets and run water for herself, make sure she turns on the cold first and then the hot. Run cold water through the faucet last so it will be cool if the patient touches it. Certain diseases affect a patient's sense of heat and cold, and she cannot judge temperature. Check the water temperature with your hand before the patient bathes.
- If your patient cannot reach her back, she may use a back brush to extend her reach. If one is not available or your patient cannot use it, you should complete this task.

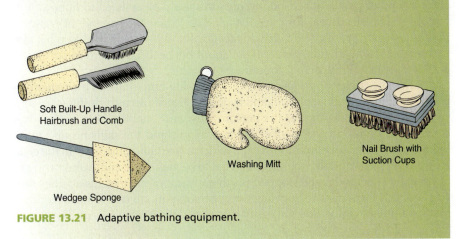

Soft Built-Up Handle
Hairbrush and Comb

Washing Mitt

Nail Brush with
Suction Cups

Wedgee Sponge

FIGURE 13.21 Adaptive bathing equipment.

ance. Your role will be to provide a safe environment and provide assistance as the individual requires it (see Figure 13.22). Remind the patient to transfer to the tub as he has been taught. Be alert for signs of fatigue or weakness.

By the time the patient can shower, he will have mastered most skills necessary for this independent activity. Your role is to continue to remain close to provide assistance as needed. Be alert for signs of sudden weakness.

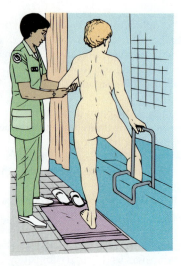

FIGURE 13.22 Assisting a patient into the tub.

Dressing and Grooming

The patient who has been hospitalized or in bed for a long time often starts to feel better about himself when he is dressed in street clothes. Thus, he should be encouraged to get dressed for at least part of every day. Even the wheelchair-bound or partially bed-bound person should be assisted to put on clothing other than sleepwear for part of each day. When the dependent person is up and dressed, it affects not only his feelings of self-esteem, but also his family members' and friends' perceptions about his health. Let him select clothes and do as much of the actual dressing as possible.

Dressing uses many muscle groups. Dressing himself helps the patient improve his coordination, balance, and mobility. Every piece of clothing presents some problem in dressing for the person with functional limitations. However, careful attention to the types of clothing available and the skills needed to put them on may lessen or eliminate many problems (see Guideline 13.8). In the chapter-opening scenario, Mr. Robinson seemed to be gaining strength and caring for himself; however, when he stopped his therapy appointments, his abilities deteriorated. It is important to encourage the person you are caring for to continue therapy until the individual can easily complete daily living skills on his own.

Laundry

It is important for individuals who live alone or are responsible for a family to care for their own basic needs. They should be able to prepare meals, or at least assist in their preparation, and to care for some aspects of housekeeping. Taking care of one's own laundry is a functional activity. Many patients need encouragement to resume this function because they will not do things as neatly and as easily as they once did. Assist the person with handwashing clothes, but let the person do as much as possible. Folding, sorting, and stacking clean clothes can be done slowly and should be adapted to the individual's abilities. Obviously, folding socks and shirts is easier than folding sheets,

GUIDELINE 13.8

Assisting a Patient with Dressing

- Follow the procedure that the OTR has established for your patient.
- Always dress the weak or most involved extremity first.
- Undress the weak or involved extremity last.
- Help the patient select clothing that is roomy and will stretch or give when he puts it on or takes it off. It is easier to put on a garment that opens all the way down the front than one that must be pulled over an involved arm and then pulled over the head.
- Position the patient in front of a mirror. The patient will see with his own eyes that he has missed a button, his collar is turned in, or his pants are pulled to the side.
- Lay out the pieces of clothing where the patient can reach them in the order he will put them on.
- If the OTR has suggested the use of any special tools or adapted equipment for dressing, have them near the patient's clothing (see Figure 13.23). Always use a shoehorn when putting on the patient's shoes. He may use a dressing stick, a buttonhook, or a reacher when he begins to dress himself again.
- Follow the same procedure each time the patient dresses and undresses.

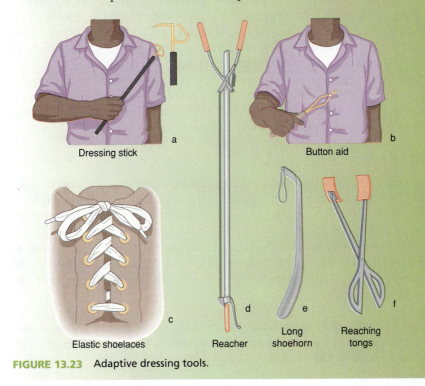

Dressing stick   a

Button aid   b

Elastic shoelaces   c

Reacher   d

Long shoehorn   e

Reaching tongs   f

FIGURE 13.23 Adaptive dressing tools.

CLINICAL ALERT 13.2

Use of Equipment in the Home

Check all equipment, including cleaning equipment, therapeutic aids, and eating implements, for safety before you use it. If you identify an unsafe item and cannot easily fix it, remove it from the patient and alert the therapist and/or family for replacement. Do not use unmarked bottles of anything. If you suspect a bottle does not contain what the label indicates, do not use it.

but stacking sheets is easier than stacking socks. These tasks should be shared as the family members see fit (see Clinical Alert 13.2).

Meal Preparation

If the patient is to take part eventually in meal preparation, assist her in assuming this responsibility slowly. These activities increase her muscular control. Use the devices that the OTR provides. Be sure the individual is instructed by the OTR about the proper use of devices before she uses them. Supervise the patient the first few times she attempts tasks in the kitchen. Praise her and offer support where needed. Point out her successes.

Include the patient in all phases of meal planning and preparation. Use a cutting board with two stainless steel nails projecting from it to hold vegetables, fruits, or meats when paring, scraping, and cutting. Supervise as the patient begins to place the food onto the nails, and help if she has difficulty turning the food or removing it from the spikes.

Use small containers that are easy to handle. Do not fill containers all the way to the top. Use plastic containers instead of glass ones if plastic ones are available. Let the patient assist with the cleanup after the meal—with cleaning off the table, cleaning dishes, and so on (see Figure 13.24).

Feeding

The patient who has difficulty feeding himself, drops utensils, spills food, or chokes and drools when swallowing may feel discouraged. He may refuse to feed himself or to eat as much as he should. He becomes dependent and loses his sense of self-esteem.

Plan mealtimes so that the patient can use his available resources and feed himself successfully. He will eat more and feel better emotionally and physically. He will gain many of the motor skills needed to perform other activities of daily living.

HELPING A PATIENT AT MEALTIME Set up the table or tray so it is convenient and attractive. Give the patient utensils and dishes that she can handle with a minimum of effort. Use cups and glasses light enough for her to lift and silverware she can grasp securely.

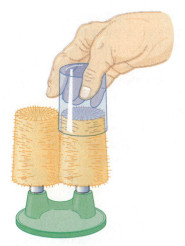

FIGURE 13.24   Adapted dish cleaning tools.

If the individual's dominant side is involved, and she is still trying to eat with that hand, she may lack sensation and the ability to grasp. You can enlarge the fork or spoon handle by wrapping it with paper towels to about an inch in diameter and tape the paper in place. Or slip a foam rubber curler pad over the handle. Either will enlarge the gripping surface so the patient can hold and lift it more easily. The paper towel is temporary and cannot be washed, but the curler can be removed, washed, squeezed dry, and reused on any utensil. Enlarging the handle also makes it easier to use the nondominant hand. If a person has never used her left or right hand to feed herself, she may need the enlarged handle when she first tries.

A rigid plastic cup may be easier and safer for the person to handle than a breakable glass. If the cup has a large hand opening, it will enable the individual to put her fingers or hand around the cup for security (see Figure 13.25).

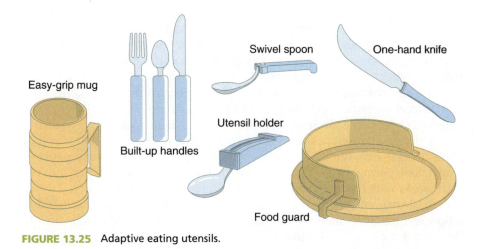

Easy-grip mug

Built-up handles

Swivel spoon

One-hand knife

Utensil holder

Food guard

FIGURE 13.25   Adaptive eating utensils.

A food guard is a plastic ring that slips over the edge of a plate and creates a bumper for the patient to push food against when eating. As food is pushed against an elevated surface, it piles up and spills onto the individual's fork or spoon and enables him to get enough on the utensil to feed himself. Plates, bowls, forks, knives, and spoons with specialty built-up handles make it easier for the patient to grasp and hold onto them while eating.

If a patient's grasp is too weak to hold a fork or spoon without dropping it, a feeding cuff may help. It fits over the person's hand, and the spoon or fork slips into the pocket and allows the individual to lift the utensil without having to grasp it tightly. Cups and glasses with handles open at the bottom can "clip" onto the patient's hand, reducing her need to hold tightly while lifting the cup.

Some patients have visual problems. They may be totally or partially blind. Objects placed to the far right or far left may not be visible to them. These patients may need a reminder to "look to your left (right)" when eating. The OTR may also have you place the plate to the right or left of the person so she can see it more easily.

Other patients may have sensory deficits that affect eating. A patient who lacks sensation and whose facial muscles are weak on one side will have difficulty eating. The individual cannot swallow easily and tends to "pocket" food between his cheeks and teeth on the involved side of the face. Such food buildup can cause gagging and choking. You may have to remind this patient to move his tongue to that side of the mouth to dislodge the food.

Place a shaving mirror in front of your patient and encourage him to glance at it several times during a meal. This technique will enable him to use his eyes to be aware of what occurs when he eats. He may begin to wipe his mouth automatically or to search with his tongue to dislodge stored food or food that remains on his lips.

Leisure Activities

If you can incorporate pleasurable activities into your patient's daily routine, you will contribute to his recovery. Ask the patient and his family what activities were pleasurable before the illness. Although you could try to introduce new activities, it is always better to start with familiar ones. Look for signs that the patient enjoys or at least acknowledges these activities. The patient who used to crochet, knit, or sew may wish to relearn these skills. The OTR will instruct the patient in doing these hobbies again despite the disability and you can reinforce the teaching. Use aids to help patients reach objects safely.

Perhaps a patient has a perceptual deficit and does not see things as they really are. He may not be able to follow the printed lines in a newspaper or read a book because his eyes cannot see the last few words on every line. The OTR works with this patient to help him improve his reading ability.

If pleasurable pastimes are used as therapy tools, you may be asked to follow through with the program. Of course, you will be told exactly how to help in any activity of this kind.

On your own, if you have time to play simple card games with a patient, read aloud to her, or turn on some music for her, it will take her mind off her physical problems and bring her pleasure. Plants and birds—both indoors and outdoors—provide diversion. Pets provide companionship, love, and stimulation to those who enjoy them. Any extra activity that expands the area of interest for a patient is both pleasurable and beneficial. Any activity that stimulates activity and interaction is useful.

Summary

Rehabilitation is vital to recovery of skills or strength lost from illness or an accident. Relearning to complete tasks in a different manner or with different parts of one's body can be the ultimate frustration. To get an idea of what your patient might be experiencing, attempt the same tasks with the same disability; that is, attempt to dress yourself with only one arm, pretending the other is unusable. Your empathy for the patient will guide you in being supportive and encouraging during the recovery process. Remember that sometimes the rehabilitation is to teach a new way of doing a task, and the patient may never recover use of the injured part of his or her body. Exposing the patient to success stories and/or people who have adapted to a disability can also prove helpful.

Chapter 14

Vital Signs

SCENARIO

Mr. Alvarez, a mail carrier, lives with his wife in a house in which they raised their four children. Mr. Alvarez has recently been diagnosed with hypertension and has been given a diet, a series of exercises, and medication. His wife works hard to cook tasty meals that adhere to the diet, but Mr. Alvarez is not fond of them. He does not do his exercises, saying that he walks all day carrying mail and that this exercise enough. He does take the medication but says he feels different when he takes the pills and, because he didn't feel badly before his physical exam, he doesn't understand why he should take them.

VITAL SIGNS

Vital signs are bodily functions that reflect the body's state of health and are easily measurable: body temperature, pulse rate, respiratory rate, and blood pressure. The term is often written as TPR&BP. In some cases, the pulse oxygenation and pain are included in vital signs, which means that you will report the status of the patient's pulse oximeter reading and pain level when you report and record the other vital signs.

When the body is not functioning normally, the measurable rates of vital signs change. Everyone who measures and records a patient's vital signs must be careful and accurate. When you record the reading, write carefully. Be sure your handwriting is clear and easy to read. If you are unsure of your reading, mention this when you report the reading to the nurse or physician.

When to Check Vital Signs

The physician will tell you when and how often to check your patient's vital signs. This decision will be based on the patient's present condition, his past medical history, and his prognosis (probable length of life or illness given the medical condition(s)). Vital signs are not checked in the home as often as they are in the hospital because home care patients are often in a more stable condition.

You should check the vital signs if you observe any change in your patient or after your patient suffers a fall. When you call the health care team to report a change or the fall, they will want you to report the patient's vital signs. This information will assist the appropriate health care team member in making a decision over the telephone. Be sure to record all signs when you take them. If you don't, you might forget.

Adult Normal Vital Signs

- Temperature: 98.6°F or 37°C
- Pulse: 60 to 80 regular beats per minute
- Respiration: 16 to 20 regular breaths per minute
- Blood pressure:
  - Infants: 50/40 to 80/58 mm of mercury
  - Under 18 years old: below 120/80 mm of mercury
  - 18 to 50 years and above: below 140/90 mm of mercury
- Pain: none

These rates are given to you as a guide. A person can have a reading that varies from these figures and be healthy. But if you took thousands and thousands of TPR&BPs, you would have these rates as average readings. On an individual basis, it is more helpful to compare several of your patient's readings than to compare hers with the average rates.

Reporting Vital Signs

When you are assigned to take a patient's vital signs, the physician will tell you when you should call her or him with the readings. In the home, you may often take vital signs without reporting them each time. It is most important, however, for you to know when to report your findings. Ask for guidance. If you are in doubt, report. It is far better to report an unnecessary reading than not to report one that is necessary.

Communicating with the Patient About Vital Signs

There was a time when hospitals and doctors did not share information with patients, but this is no longer the case. Especially in a person's home, you will be expected to share the vital sign readings with your patient. Please communicate promptly. If you do not, the patient may think you are hiding something from him. Remember, it is his body you are caring for and he has the right to know how it is working. If a patient does not wish to know his vital signs, do not force the information on him.

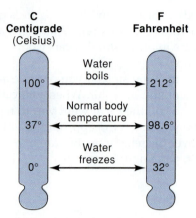
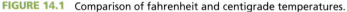

FIGURE 14.1 Comparison of fahrenheit and centigrade temperatures.

BODY TEMPERATURE

Body temperature is a measurement of the amount of heat in the body. The balance between heat produced and heat lost is the body temperature. The normal adult body temperature is 98.6°F or 37°C. There is a normal range in which a person's body temperature may vary and still be considered normal (see Figures 14.1 and 14.2).

Body Temperature Range

- Oral: 97.6 to 99°F (36.4 to 37.2°C)
- Rectal: 98.6 to 100°F (37.0 to 37.8°C)
- Axillary: 96.6 to 98°C (35.9 to 36.7°C)

For recording the patient's temperature, three symbols are used:

1. °: degree or degrees
2. F: Fahrenheit
3. C: Centigrade or Celsius

Record the patient's temperatures according to the method used by the physician. Fahrenheit temperature can be written in two ways:

98.6°F or 98°F

If you are using a centigrade (Celsius) thermometer, the temperature would be written as follows:

37.3°C or 37°C

Write an *R* with the temperature reading if a rectal temperature was taken. Write an *A* beside the temperature reading if an axillary (under the armpit) temperature was taken.

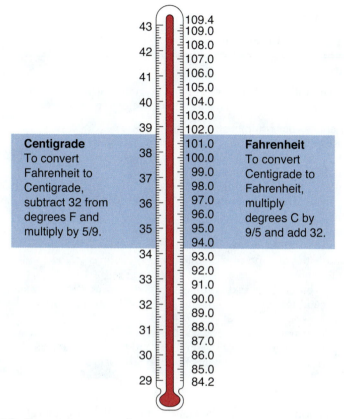

Centigrade
To convert
Fahrenheit to
Centigrade,
subtract 32 from
degrees F and
multiply by 5/9.

Fahrenheit
To convert
Centigrade to
Fahrenheit,
multiply
degrees C by
9/5 and add 32.

FIGURE 14.2 Temperature conversions.

The body temperature is measured with an instrument called a thermometer. A thermometer is a delicate, hollow, glass tube with a liquid sealed inside that is sensitive to temperature. The liquid expands when the temperature rises and contracts when the temperature goes down. Even if the temperature rises only slightly, the liquid will expand and travel up the tube, indicating the change. The outside of the glass thermometer is marked with lines, or calibrations, and numbers. These markings make it possible to measure exactly the change in the liquid.

Types of Thermometers

There are several different types of thermometers:

- Glass
- Battery-operated, electronic, digital readout
- Chemically treated paper

Each kind of battery-operated and chemical thermometer is slightly different. Read the instructions carefully before using any thermometer.

PROCEDURE 14.1

Shaking a Glass Thermometer

Rationale

The material inside the thermometer must be in the correct place for the temperature reading to be accurate and for the thermometer to be ready for the next use.

1. Assemble your equipment: glass thermometer.
2. Wash your hands.
3. Before using the thermometer, check to make sure that it is not cracked and that the bulb is not chipped.
4. Hold the thermometer firmly between your fingers and your thumb at the stem end farthest from the bulb. The bulb is the end inserted into the patient's body.
5. Stand clear of any hard surfaces such as counters and tables to avoid striking and breaking the thermometer while you shake it. For practice, you might stand with your arm over a pillow or mattress in case you accidentally drop the thermometer.
6. When you are sure that you have a good hold on the thermometer, shake your hand loosely from the wrist. Do it as if you were shaking water from your fingers.
7. Snap your wrist again and again. This will shake the liquid down to the lowest possible point—below the numbers and lines (calibrations).
8. Always shake a thermometer before and after using it.

This section is related to the standard glass thermometer: the most dangerous type of thermometer found in the home. Glass thermometers come in three types (see Procedures 14.1, 14.2, 14.3 and 14.4):

1. *Oral:* An oral thermometer is used to measure the patient's temperature by mouth and is also used in measuring the axillary temperature. The bulb is long and thin so that it contacts as much of the mouth lining as possible (see Procedure 14.5).

PROCEDURE 14.2

Reading a Fahrenheit Thermometer

Rationale

Reading a thermometer correctly is an important part of patient care.

1. Assemble your equipment: Fahrenheit thermometer, probe cover (if appropriate), gloves.
2. Using your thumb and first two fingers, hold the thermometer at the stem.
3. Hold the thermometer at eye level. Turn the thermometer back and forth between your fingers until you can see the column of liquid clearly.

4. Notice the scale or calibrations. Each long line stands for one degree.
5. Four short lines are marked between each of the long lines. Each short line stands for two-tenths (0.2) of a degree.
6. Between the long lines that represent 98° and 99°, look for a longer line with an arrow directly beneath it. This special line points out normal body temperature.
7. Look at the end of the liquid. Notice the line or number where the liquid ends. If it is one of the short lines, notice the previous longer line toward the silver tip that goes into the patient's mouth. The temperature reading is the degree marked by that long line plus two-, four-, six-, or eight-tenths of a degree. If the liquid ends on the fourth short line after the line marked 97, the temperature is 97.8°F. If the liquid ends between two lines, use the line closer to the silver tip (see Figure 14.3).
8. Write down the patient's temperature right away, using the figure you read on the thermometer. Some people write 97.8°F. Others write 97.8F. Be consistent with the method you use. Always indicate if the reading is oral, rectal, or axillary.

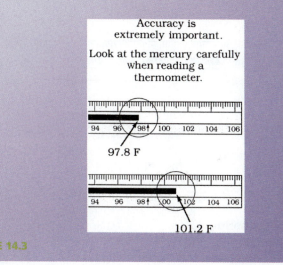

Accuracy is extremely important.

Look at the mercury carefully when reading a thermometer.

97.8 F

101.2 F

FIGURE 14.3

PROCEDURE 14.3

Reading a Centigrade (Celsius) Thermometer

Rationale

Reading a thermometer correctly is an important part of patient care.

1. Assemble your equipment: Celsius thermometer, probe cover (if appropriate), gloves.
2. Using your thumb and first two fingers, hold the thermometer at the stem.
3. Hold it at eye level. Turn the thermometer back and forth between your fingers until you can see the column of liquid clearly.

(continues)

4. Notice the scale or calibration. Each long line shows one degree.
5. Nine short lines are marked between each number. These short lines are one-, two-, three-, four-, five-, six-, seven-, eight-, and nine-tenths of a degree. If the liquid ends after the line marked 36 and on the third short line, the temperature reading is 36.3°C. If the liquid ends after the long line marked 37 and on the eighth short line, the temperature reading is 37.8°C. If the liquid ends after the line marked 37 and on the fifth short line, the temperature reading is 37.5°C (see Figure 14.4).
6. Write down the patient's temperature right away. Some people write 37°C. Others write 37.5C. Be consistent with the method you use. Always indicate if the reading is oral, rectal, or axillary.

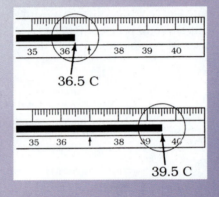

FIGURE 14.4

PROCEDURE 14.4

Cleaning a Glass Thermometer

Rationale

Proper cleaning of a thermometer is an important part of infection control in the home.

1. Assemble your equipment: glass thermometer, tissue and/or cotton balls, soap, disposable gloves, cool running water.
2. Wash your hands and put on gloves. Wipe the thermometer off from the stem to the bulb. Throw away the tissue.
3. Soap a tissue.
4. Holding the thermometer, rotate the soapy tissue around the thermometer from the stem to the bulb.
5. Holding the thermometer under cool running water, repeat the process.
6. Discard the tissue.
7. Dry the thermometer with a dry tissue. Discard the tissue.
8. Put the thermometer into a case, bulb first.
9. Dispose of gloves and wash your hands.

PROCEDURE 14.5

Measuring an Oral Temperature

Rationale

Taking a patient's temperature correctly is an important part of patient care.

1. Assemble your equipment: clean oral thermometer, tissue or paper towel, gloves, paper and pen, a watch with a second hand.
2. Wash your hands.
3. Tell the patient that you are going to take her temperature orally.
4. Ask the patient if she has recently had hot or cold liquids or if she has smoked. If the answer is yes, wait ten minutes before taking her temperature.
5. The patient should be in bed or sitting in a chair. Do not take a temperature while the patient is walking.
6. Take the thermometer out of the container and inspect it for cracks or chips. Do not use it if you see any.
7. Shake the liquid in the thermometer down until it is below the calibrations.
8. Run the thermometer under cool water to make the thermometer more pleasant in the patient's mouth.
9. Ask the patient to lift her tongue. Place the bulb end of the thermometer under her tongue. Ask her to keep her lips gently closed around the thermometer without biting it. (If the patient cannot close her mouth, take the temperature by another method, such as rectal or axillary) (see Figure 14.5).

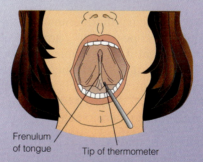

Frenulum of tongue   Tip of thermometer

FIGURE 14.5

10. Leave the thermometer in place for eight minutes. The latest research shows that oral temperature is more accurate when the thermometer remains in the mouth for eight minutes. If you are using a digital thermometer, however, just wait until the machine beeps, which tells you it is finished.
11. Stay with your patient if you think that she cannot keep her mouth closed. (Wear gloves.)
12. Wash your hands and put on gloves. Take the thermometer out of the patient's mouth. Hold the stem end and wipe the thermometer with a tissue from the stem toward the bulb.
13. Read the thermometer.
14. Record the temperature and your observations concerning the patient during this procedure.

(continues)

15. Shake down the liquid in the thermometer.
16. Clean the thermometer.
17. Make the patient comfortable.
18. Remove gloves and wash your hands.

2. *Security:* A security thermometer has a strong construction. It is used for taking an infant's rectal temperature. If a glass thermometer is used at a physician's office, the security or stubby type with a red knob at the stem is for rectal temperatures and the one with a green knob at the stem is for oral temperatures.

Mercury

Mercury, the silver metal that, until recently, has been used in thermometers and blood pressure cuffs, is now known to be a poison when it is inhaled, ingested, or comes in contact with skin. If it remains in the thermometer or blood pressure cuff, it poses no danger, but if either instrument breaks, the incident and the area must be treated as a hazardous waste spill.

You are strongly advised not to use a thermometer that contains mercury. If you should find one in a home, suggest to the patient and her or his family that they obtain a nonmercury thermometer. .

- Do not discard a mercury thermometer in the trash. Ask your health care team about the proper way to discard it. One suggestion is to wrap it in paper towels, seal it in a double bagged plastic bag, and call the local health department or department of public works for assistance with disposal. Departments of public works often schedule hazardous waste collection days for different type of household hazardous waste, including the mercury in thermometers.

If a mercury thermometer should break in the house, open the windows immediately to decrease the amount of vapor that is inhaled. Do not touch the mercury! Do not use a vacuum cleaner to clean the spill. Sweep it onto cardboard, put the mercury, the glass, and the cardboard into a double bagged plastic bag and call the local health department or department of public works for assistance with disposal (see Guideline 14.1 and Clinical Alert 14.1).

Using a Plastic Sheath over a Thermometer

A plastic thermometer cover, or sheath, may be used to protect the thermometer from the patient's secretions and to aid in thermometer cleanup and reading. Use of a sheath on a glass thermometer does not mean that you do not have to wash the thermometer after each use; it only makes the washing easier. Be sure to read the directions for each type of sheath because they can differ (see Procedures 14.6 and 14.7).

GUIDELINE 14.1

Safety Considerations While Using Thermometers

- Do not expect a patient to talk with a thermometer in his mouth.
- Glass thermometers break and shatter easily. Handle them with care. Be especially careful to avoid breaking a thermometer while it is in a patient's mouth or rectum.
- Keep each thermometer in a case. Do not leave any thermometers loose in a pocket, drawer, or dresser.
- Never clean a glass thermometer with hot water. The liquid will expand so much that the thermometer will explode.
- If the patient thinks that he may be about to sneeze, he should remove the thermometer.

CLINICAL ALERT 14.1

Wash all glass thermometers with warm soapy water before use. If you think a thermometer was used to take a rectal temperature, do not use it for an oral temperature, no matter how you wash it. Digital thermometers must also be cleaned after each use and after they have stayed in a drawer for several days (unless they will be used with a probe cover).

PROCEDURE 14.6

Using a Thermometer Sheath

Rationale

Using protective equipment correctly is an important part of infection control in the home.

1. Assemble your equipment: glass thermometer, thermometer sheath, trash bag, tissues, disposable gloves.
2. Wash your hands.
3. Shake down the thermometer.
4. Hold the sheath so that you can insert the thermometer into the plastic between the paper covering and the plastic (see Figure 14.6).
5. Withdraw the thermometer, now covered with the clear plastic sheath. Be sure the sheath covers the entire thermometer and does not hang off the end (see Figure 14.7).
6. Take the patient's temperature using the standard procedure.
7. Put on gloves. Remove the thermometer from the patient.
   a. Method A: Remove the sheath with a tissue and discard it in the trash.
   b. Method B: Insert the sheath back into the package outer sleeve. Remove the thermometer, leaving the contaminated sheath in the sleeve. Discard it in the trash (see Figure 14.8).

(continues)

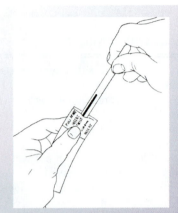

FIGURE 14.6

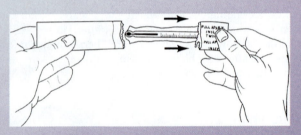

FIGURE 14.7

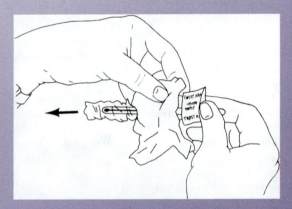

FIGURE 14.8

8. Read the thermometer and record the temperature.
9. Wash and store the thermometer according to the standard procedure.
10. Remove gloves and wash your hands.

PROCEDURE 14.7

Measuring an Axillary Temperature

Rationale

Taking a patient's temperature correctly is an important part of patient care.

1. Assemble your equipment: oral thermometer, tissue or paper towel, paper and pen, a watch with a second hand.
2. Wash your hands.
3. Ask visitors to leave the room, if appropriate.
4. Tell the patient that you are going to take her temperature by placing a thermometer under her arm.
5. Remove the thermometer from its case and shake down the liquid so that it is below the calibrations.
6. Inspect the thermometer for cracks or chips. Do not use it if you see any.
7. Remove the patient's arm from the sleeve of her clothing. If the axillary region is moist with perspiration, pat it dry with a towel.
8. Place the bulb of the oral thermometer in the center of the armpit in an upright position (see Figure 14.9).

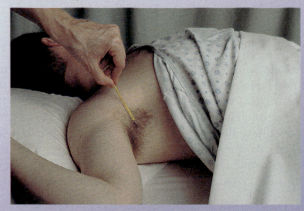

FIGURE 14.9   Photographer: Patrick Watson.

9. Put the patient's arm across her chest or abdomen.
10. If the patient is unconscious or too weak to help, you will have to hold the arm in place.
11. Leave the thermometer in place 10 minutes. Stay with the patient.
12. Remove the thermometer. Wipe it off with a tissue from the stem to the bulb.
13. Read the thermometer.
14. Record the temperature and your observations concerning the patient during this procedure. (Note that this is an axillary temperature by placing an A next to the reading.)
15. Shake the liquid down until it is below the calibrations.
16. Clean the thermometer.
17. Replace the thermometer in its case.
18. Make the patient comfortable.
19. Wash your hands.

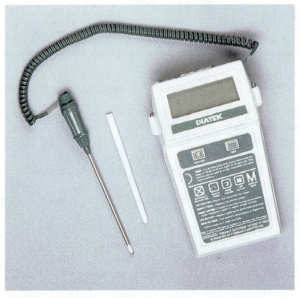

FIGURE 14.10 An electronic thermometer and probe cover.

Digital or Electronic Thermometers

Digital thermometers come in several types. It is important that you receive instructions on how to use the model that you have. These models are designed to be used in or on a specific part of the body and may not be used in any other place on the body (see Figure 14.10). Others may be used interchangeably as oral, rectal, or auxiliary thermometers, depending on the probe attached (see Procedure 14.8). Some thermometers are made specifically for use in the ear. These aural or tympanic thermometers measure temperature from the blood vessels on the tympanic membrane of the ear (see Procedure 14.9).

- All thermometers have on/off buttons that activate/deactivate the battery. Be sure the battery is good and the thermometer is working before you use it.
- All digital thermometers have number readouts. That is, they give you the exact temperature they are measuring. You do not have to read calibrations.
- All thermometers have probes. Electronic thermometers have red probes for rectal use and blue probes for oral use. A cover is used over every probe and is changed after each use.
- Be sure you know how the thermometer signals that it has measured the patient's temperature. Usually, the whole process takes about ten to fifteen seconds.
- Observe the same safety precautions with a digital thermometer as you would with a glass one.
- If the battery is not working, check the instructions for the type of battery needed and follow the instructions for changing it.
- You may or may not wear gloves for taking a patient's temperature.

PROCEDURE 14.8

Measuring an Oral Temperature Using an Electronic or Digital Thermometer

Rationale

Using a thermometer correctly helps produce an accurate measure of a patient's temperature.

1. Assemble your equipment: electronic thermometer, correct sheath, trash bag.
2. Wash your hands.
3. Tell the patient you are going to take his temperature orally.
4. Insert the electronic probe firmly into the probe cover.
5. Ask the patient to wet his lips and lift his tongue.
6. Place the probe under the patient's tongue on one side of his mouth. Ask him to close his lips. You may have to hold the probe.
7. Leave the probe in place until the thermometer signals it is finished.
8. Gently remove the probe and read the temperature on the digital display.
9. Discard the probe cover without touching it.
10. Return the probe to its holder.
11. Return the unit to its holder or charging station.
12. Wash your hands.

PROCEDURE 14.9

Measuring a Temperature Using an Aural/Tympanic Thermometer

Rationale

Using a thermometer correctly helps produce an accurate measure of a patient's temperature.

1. Assemble your equipment: aural/tympanic thermometer, probe cover or sheath, trash can (see Figure 14.11).
2. Wash your hands.
3. Tell the patient that you are going to take his temperature using his ear and that it will not hurt.
4. Insert the cone-shaped probe into the probe cover.
5. Position the patient's head so that it is directly in front of you.
6. For children under the age of three, gently pull the ear straight back (see Figure 14.12). For people three and older, gently pull the outer ear up and back to open the ear canal (see Figure 14.13).
7. Gently insert the probe into the ear canal. You may have to use a gently rocking motion to help the probe slip into the canal and seal the ear canal.
8. Hold the thermometer in place until it signals it is finished.
9. Gently remove the probe and read the digital display.
10. Eject the probe into the trash.
11. Position the patient in a safe, comfortable position.
12. Return the thermometer to its holder or charging station.
13. Wash your hands.

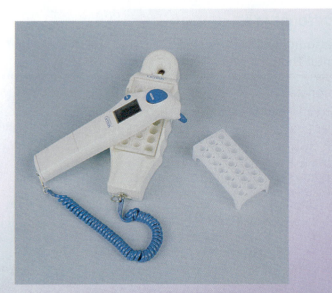

FIGURE 14.11 An infrared (tympanic) thermometer used to measure the tympanic membrane temperature.

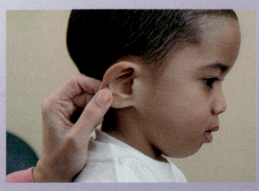

FIGURE 14.12 Pull the pinna back and down for a child under age 3.

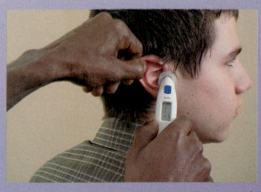

FIGURE 14.13 For someone over the age of three pull the top of the ear up and back.

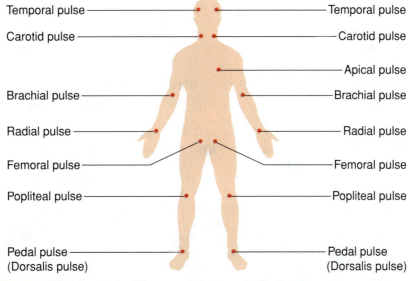

Temporal pulse —————————————————— Temporal pulse

Carotid pulse ——————————————————— Carotid pulse

————————————— Apical pulse

Brachial pulse ——————————— Brachial pulse

Radial pulse ——————————— Radial pulse

Femoral pulse ————————— Femoral pulse

Popliteal pulse ————————— Popliteal pulse

Pedal pulse ———————— Pedal pulse
(Dorsalis pulse) (Dorsalis pulse)

FIGURE 14.14 Pulses can be felt at many places on the body.

TAKING A PULSE

Each time the heart beats, it pumps blood into the arteries, which causes the arteries to expand. Between heartbeats, the arteries contract and return to their normal size. The heart pumps the blood in a steady rhythm. The rhythmic expansion and contraction of the arteries, which can be measured to show how fast the heart is beating, is called the pulse. Measuring the pulse is one method of observing how the circulatory system is functioning.

The pulse measures how fast the heart is beating. At certain places on the body, the pulse can easily be felt under your fingers (see Figure 14.14). One of the easiest places to feel the pulse is at the wrist. This is called a radial pulse because you are feeling the radial artery (see Procedure 14.10). When taking the pulse, you must be able to report accurately the following pieces of information:

- *Rate:* number of pulse beats per minute
- *Rhythm:* regularity of the pulse beats, that is, whether the length of time between the beats is steady and regular
- *Force:* strength of the beat (weak or bounding)

You use a stethoscope to listen to the apical pulse. The apical pulse is the pulse measured at the apex of the heart. The stethoscope is an instrument that makes it possible to listen to various sounds in a patient's body. The stethoscope is a tube with one end that picks up sound when it is placed against a part of the

PROCEDURE 14.10

Measuring the Radial Pulse

Rationale

Measuring a patient's pulse correctly is an important part of care.

1. Assemble your equipment: watch with a second hand, paper and pen.
2. Wash your hands.
3. Tell the patient that you are going to take her pulse.
4. If the patient is standing, ask her to sit down, or have her lying in a comfortable position in bed for five minutes before you measure the pulse.
5. The patient's hand and arm should be well supported and resting comfortably.
6. Find the pulse by placing the tips of your middle three fingers on the palm side of the patient's wrist, in line with her thumb directly next to the bone. Press lightly until you feel the beat. If you press too hard, you may stop the flow of blood and then you will not feel a pulse. (Never use your thumb. Your thumb has its own pulse, and you would count it instead of the patient's.) When you have found the pulse, notice the rhythm. Note if the beat is steady or irregular. Notice the force of the beat (see Figure 14.15).

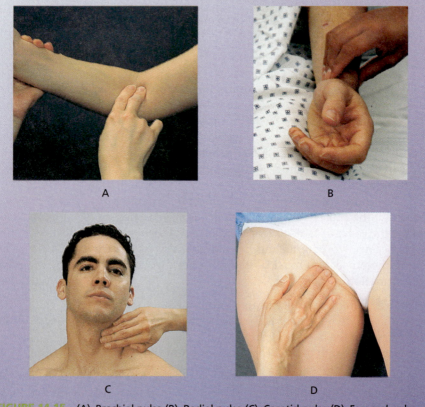

A   B

C   D

FIGURE 14.15   (A) Brachial pulse (B) Radial pulse (C) Carotid pulse (D) Femoral pulse.

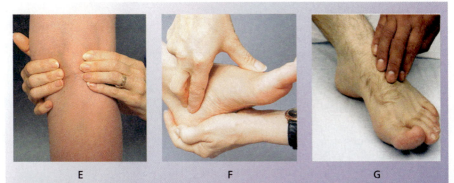

E   F   G

FIGURE 14.15 (*CONTINUED*) (E) Popliteal pulse (F) Posterior tibial pulse (G) Dorsalis pedis pulse.

7. Look at the position of the second hand on your watch. Start counting the pulse beats (what you feel) until the second hand comes back to the same number on the clock.
   a. Method A: Count the pulse beats for one full minute and report the full-minute count. This is always done if the patient has an irregular beat.
   b. Method B: Count for thirty seconds, until the second hand is opposite its position when you started. Then multiply the number of beats by two. This answer is the number you record. For example, if the count for thirty seconds is thirty-five, the count for sixty seconds (one minute) is seventy beats.
8. Record the pulse rate, rhythm, and force immediately.
9. Make the patient comfortable.
10. Wash your hands.

body. This end is either bell-shaped (and called a bell) or it is round and flat (and is called a diaphragm) (see Figure 14.16).

The apical-radial deficit is the difference between the pulse count at the apex of the heart and the pulse count at the radial artery. Noting this difference is one way to see if the circulatory system is working properly (see Procedures 14.11 and 14.12).

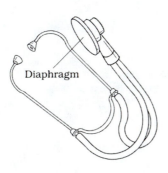
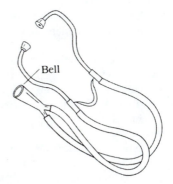

Diaphragm

Bell

FIGURE 14.16 The stethoscope.

PROCEDURE 14.11

Measuring the Apical Pulse

Rationale

Measuring a patient's pulse correctly is an important part of care.

1. Assemble your equipment: stethoscope, antiseptic swabs, watch with a second hand, paper and pen.
2. Wash your hands.
3. Ask visitors to leave the room, if appropriate.
4. Explain to the patient that you are going to take his apical pulse.
5. Clean the earpieces of the stethoscope with antiseptic solution. Put the earpieces facing forward in your ears.
6. Uncover the left side of the patient's chest. Avoid overexposing the patient.
7. Locate the apex of the patient's heart by placing the bell or diaphragm of the stethoscope under the patient's left breast. Be sure this is the place you hear the heart beating the loudest.
8. Count the heart sounds for a full minute.
9. Write the full-minute count. Also record the rhythm and the quality of the sounds and your observations concerning the patient during this procedure.
10. Cover the patient and make him comfortable.
11. Clean the earpieces of the stethoscope. Return the equipment to its proper place.
12. Wash your hands.

PROCEDURE 14.12

Measuring the Apical-Radial Deficit

Rationale

Measuring a patient's pulse correctly is an important part of care.

1. Assemble your equipment: stethoscope, antiseptic swabs, watch with a second hand, paper and pen.
2. Wash your hands.
3. Ask visitors to leave the room, if appropriate.
4. Explain to the patient that you are going to take her pulse both apically and radially.
5. There are two methods of taking the apical pulse deficit:
   a. Method A: Two people do this procedure together at the same time. One counts the radial pulse and the other counts the apical pulse for one full minute. The difference between the two pulses is known as the apical-radial deficit.
   b. Method B: The caregiver first takes the apical pulse, then takes the radial pulse. The difference between the two pulses is known as the apical-radial deficit. Because the readings are not taken at the same time, method B is not considered as accurate as method A.

6. Count the apical pulse and the radial pulse for a full minute, and record both figures.
7. Record the figure for the pulse deficit and your observations concerning the patient during this procedure.
8. Make the patient comfortable.
9. Clean the equipment and return it to its proper place.
10. Wash your hands.

MEASURING RESPIRATIONS

The human body must have a steady supply of air. When you breathe in, air is drawn into the lungs. The waste products from this process are removed from the body as you exhale. Respiration is the process of inhaling and exhaling. One respiration includes breathing in once and breathing out once. When a person breathes in, her chest expands. When she breathes out, her chest contracts.

When you count respirations, watch a person's chest rise and fall as she breathes. Or feel her chest rise and fall with your hand. Either way, you should count respirations without the patient knowing it. If she thinks her breathing is being counted, she will not breathe naturally. What you want to count is her natural breathing. Besides counting respirations, you will be noticing whether the patient seems to breathe easily or seems to be working hard to breathe. When a person is working hard to breathe, it is called labored respiration. You must also notice whether her breathing is noisy (see Procedure 14.13).

Normally, adults breathe sixteen to twenty times a minute. Children breathe more rapidly. The elderly breathe more slowly. Exercise, digestion, emotional stress, disease conditions, some drugs, stimulants, heat, and cold can all affect the number of times a person breathes per minute.

Abnormal Respiration

While you are counting the patient's respirations, it is important to observe and make note of anything about his breathing that appears to be abnormal. Different types of abnormal respiration that you should be familiar with include the following:

- *Stertorous respiration:* The patient makes abnormal noises such as snoring sounds when he breathes.
- *Abdominal respiration:* The patient mostly uses his abdominal muscles to breathe.
- *Shallow respiration:* The patient breathes using only the upper part of the lungs.
- *Irregular respiration:* The depth of breathing changes and the chest rise and fall rate is not steady.

PROCEDURE 14.13

Measuring Respirations

Rationale

Measuring a patient's respirations correctly is an important part of a patient's care.

1. Assemble your equipment: watch with a second hand, paper and pen
2. Wash your hands.
3. Ask visitors to leave the room, if appropriate.
4. Hold the patient's wrist just as if you were taking his pulse. This way he will not know you are watching his breathing. Count the patient's respirations, without his knowing it, immediately after counting his pulse rate.
5. If the patient is a child who has been crying or is restless, wait until he is quiet before counting respirations. If a child is asleep, count his respirations before he wakes up. Always count a child's pulse and respirations before you measure his temperature. Most children become upset when you measure their temperatures.
6. One rise and one fall of the patient's chest count as one respiration.
7. If you cannot see clearly the chest rise and fall, fold the patient's arms across his chest. Then you can feel his breathing as you hold his wrist.
8. Check the position of the second hand on the watch. Count one when you see the patient's chest rising as he breathes in. The next time his chest rises, count two. Keep doing this for a full minute. Report the number of respirations you count.
9. You may be permitted to count for thirty seconds. Count the respirations for thirty seconds and then multiply the number you counted by two. For example, if you count eight respirations in thirty seconds (one half-minute), your number for a full minute is sixteen.
10. If the patient's breathing rhythm is irregular, always count for a full minute. Observe the depth of the breathing while counting the respirations.
11. Immediately write down the number you counted.
12. Note whether the respirations were noisy or labored and your observations concerning the patient during this procedure.
13. Make the patient comfortable.
14. Wash your hands.

- *Cheyne-Stokes respiration:* At first, the breathing is slow and shallow; then the respiration becomes faster and deeper until it reaches a kind of peak; then the respiration slows down and becomes shallow again. The breathing may then stop completely for 10 seconds and then begin the pattern again. This type of respiration may be caused by certain cerebral (brain), cardiac (heart), or pulmonary (chest) diseases or conditions. It frequently occurs before death.

MEASURING BLOOD PRESSURE

Blood pressure is the force of the blood pushing against the walls of the blood vessels. When you take a patient's blood pressure, you are measuring the force of the blood flowing through the arteries. There is always a certain amount of pressure in the arteries because the heart, by pumping, is constantly forcing blood to circulate. The amount of pressure in the arteries depends on two factors: the rate of heartbeat, and how easily the blood flows through the blood vessels.

The heart contracts as it pumps the blood into the arteries. When the heart is contracting, the pressure is highest. This pressure is called the systolic pressure. As the heart relaxes between each contraction, the pressure decreases. When the heart is most relaxed, the pressure is lowest. This pressure is called the diastolic pressure. When you take a patient's blood pressure, you are measuring these two pressures (see Procedure 14.14).

PROCEDURE 14.14

Measuring Blood Pressure

Rationale

Measuring a patient's blood pressure correctly is an important part of patient care.

1. Assemble your equipment: sphygmomanometer (blood pressure cuff), stethoscope, antiseptic pad to clean the earpieces of the stethoscope, paper and pen.
2. Wash your hands.
3. Tell the patient that you are going to take her blood pressure.
4. Wipe the earpieces of the stethoscope with the antiseptic pad.
5. Have the patient resting quietly. She should be either lying down or sitting in a chair.
6. If you are using the mercury apparatus, the measuring scale should be level with your eyes.
7. The patient's arm should be bare up to the shoulder or the patient's sleeve should be well above the elbow.
8. The patient's arm from the elbow down should be resting fully extended on the bed, the arm of the chair, or your hip, well supported, with the palm upward.
9. Unroll the cuff and loosen the valve on the bulb. Then squeeze the compression bag to deflate it completely.
10. Wrap the cuff snugly and smoothly around the patient's arm above the elbow. Do not wrap it so tightly that the patient is uncomfortable from the pressure.
11. Leave the area clear where you will place the bell or diaphragm of the stethoscope.
12. Be sure the manometer is in position so you can read the numbers easily.
13. With your fingertips, find the patient's brachial pulse at the inner side of the arm above the elbow. Hold the bell or diaphragm there and inflate the cuff until the pulse disappears. Note the reading on the indicator. Quickly deflate the cuff. This is the approximation of the patient's systolic reading and is called the palpated systolic pressure.

Source: This procedure is based on the article "Hypertension—What Can Go Wrong When You Measure Blood Pressure," *American Journal of Nursing* 8, no. 5 (1980): 942–945.

(continues)

14. Put the earpieces of the stethoscope into your ears and place the bell or diaphragm of the stethoscope on the brachial pulse. Hold it snugly but not too tightly. Do not let the stethoscope touch the blood pressure cuff.
15. Tighten the thumbscrew of the valve to close it. Turn it clockwise. Be careful not to turn it too tightly. If you do, you will have trouble opening it.
16. Hold the stethoscope in place. Inflate the cuff until the dial points to 30 mm above the palpated systolic pressure.
17. Open the valve counterclockwise, which allows the air to escape. Let it out slowly until the sound of the pulse comes back. A few seconds must go by without sounds. If you do hear pulse sounds immediately, you must stop the procedure. Then completely deflate the cuff. Wait a few seconds. Then inflate the cuff to a much higher calibration above 200. Again, loosen the thumbscrew to let the air out. Listen for a repeated pulse sound. At the same time, watch the indicator.
18. Note the calibration that the pointer passes as you hear the first sound. This point indicates the systolic pressure (or the top number).
19. Continue releasing the air from the cuff. When the sounds change to a softer and faster thud or the sounds disappear, note the calibration. This is the diastolic pressure (or bottom number).
20. Deflate the cuff completely. Remove it from the patient's arm.
21. Record your reading on the patient's chart.
22. After using the blood pressure cuff, roll it up over the manometer and replace it in the case.
23. Wipe the earpieces of the stethoscope again with an antiseptic swab. Put the stethoscope back in its proper place.
24. Wash your hands.
25. Record the blood pressure and your observations concerning the patient during this procedure.

When a person's blood pressure is higher than the normal range for his or her age and condition, it is referred to as high blood pressure, or hypertension (see Tables 14.1 and 14.2). When a patient's blood pressure is lower than the normal range for his or her age and condition, it is referred to as low blood pressure, or hypotension. One reading of high blood pressure does not mean that a person has hypertension. This diagnosis can be made

TABLE 14.1 Blood Pressure Guidelines

New Classification (2003)		Previous Classification
140/90 or above	Hypertension	High blood pressure >140/90
120/80 to 139/89	Prehypertension	Borderline 130–139/85–89
119/79	Normal	Normal 129/84 or below
		Optimal 120/80 or below

Source: From *Pearson's Comprehensive Medical Assisting, Administrative and Clinical Competencies,* Second Edition, by Beaman Fleming-McPhillips, Routh, Gohsman, and Reagan, p. 715, Table 35-11.

TABLE 14.2 Average Normal Blood Pressure Readings

Patient's Age	Average Normal Blood Pressure Reading
Newborn	75/55
6–9 years of age	90/55
10–15 years of age	100/65
16 years to adulthood	118/76
Adult	120/80

Source: From *Pearson's Comprehensive Medical Assisting, Administrative and Clinical Competencies*, Second Edition, by Beaman, Fleming-McPhillips, Routh, Gohsman, and Reagan, p. 716, Table 35-12.

only by a physician after a complete medical evaluation. Variations in blood pressure occur for many reasons; for example, when someone is angry, excited, or anxious, her or his blood pressure may be higher than normal. In addition, some medications and chemicals, such as caffeine or nicotine, can raise blood pressure.

Instruments for Measuring Blood Pressure

The easiest way to measure someone's blood pressure is by using the automatic machines that can be found at the local drugstore. Each machine is different; some strap around the wrist; others wrap around the arm like a traditional blood pressure cuff. Follow the instructions on the enclosed pamphlet that comes with the machine. In these cases, a monitor gives you a digital reading of the person's blood pressure.

In addition to the store-bought machines, a patient's blood pressure can be taken using an instrument called a sphygmomanometer. Sphygmomanometer is a combination of three Greek words:

1. *Sphygmo,* meaning "pulse"
2. *Mano,* meaning "pressure"
3. *Meter,* meaning "measure"

This instrument is usually called simply the blood pressure cuff. The four main parts of this instrument are the manometer, valve, cuff, and bulb (see Figure 14.17).

Two kinds of instruments are used for taking blood pressure. One is the mercury type. The other is called the aneroid (dial) type. Both kinds have an inflatable, cloth-covered rubber bag or cuff. The cuff is wrapped around the patient's arm. Both kinds also have a rubber bulb for pumping air into the cuff. The procedure for measuring blood pressure is the same, except for reading the measurement. When you use the mercury type, watch the level of a column of mercury or liquid on a measuring scale. When you use the dial or aneroid type, watch a pointer on a dial.

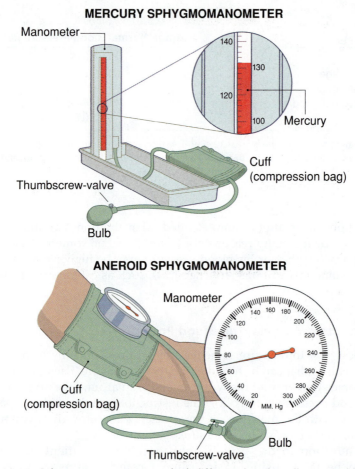

FIGURE 14.17 Sphygmomanometers may look different, but they all measure blood pressure accurately.

When you take a patient's blood pressure, you do two tasks at the same time. Listen to the brachial pulse as it sounds in the brachial artery in the patient's arm. Also watch an indicator (either a column of mercury or a dial) in order to take a reading.

Use a stethoscope to listen to the brachial pulse. It is important to note the first tapping sound you hear and the last sound you hear. Sometimes, you will hear a tapping sound, then silence, then a tapping sound again. The true reading is the first sound you hear. Often, the first sound is missed through improper technique, and only the second sound is heard and recorded. By carefully following the procedure in this book, you will not miss the first sound and will record an accurate and truthful blood pressure.

If you should hear the tapping noise all the way to the "O" on your indicator, try to listen for a change in the sound and record the patient's blood pressure reading as follows:

142/72/0

142   systolic reading; first tapping sound heard

72   diastolic reading; change in sound

0   last sound heard

PULSE OXYGENATION

The measurement of pulse oxygenation is referred to as the pulse ox or PO_2 and is recorded as a percentage (i.e., PO_2 90 percent). The pulse ox is measured by a clamp-type device that is clamped on or secured on one of the fingers. The device indirectly measures the oxygen saturation in the blood. An average pulse ox is above 93 percent. Many factors, such as stress, exercise, anesthesia, infection, or disease, can cause a drop in one's pulse ox. Oxygen is normally used until a person can keep her or his pulse ox reading above 90 percent on room air. When you take a pulse ox reading, include whether the person was on oxygen or not, and if so, how many liters. For example, PO_2 92 percent RA means the pulse oximeter read 92 percent and the person was on room air (meaning no oxygen). If the person was on two liters of oxygen, the pulse ox would be recorded as PO_2 92 percent 2L. Because there are no other vital signs given in percentages, the PO_2 is often left off the recording (i.e., 92 percent 2L).

PAIN

Pain Management

Every person has the right to be free of pain. Thus, we as health professionals have the responsibility to identify, record, and report the presence of pain and take steps to manage the pain. Everyone experiences pain daily and responds differently to it. Response to pain is an intricate and personal experience. It is the result of personal experiences, health status, and cultural norms. Other influencing factors could be age, family dynamics, and time of day.

Do not compare one person with another. Some people accept pain as normal, some think it is a punishment, and some think it indicates they are getting better. Be objective and nonjudgmental when the patient discusses her personal experience.

At times patients in pain are unable to participate in rehabilitation, interact with others, or maintain a feeling of control or well-being.

Acute and Chronic Pain

Acute pain is usually short in duration. It has a beginning and an end. An example is pain after an operation. The pain starts after the surgery and eventually goes away.

Chronic pain is always present. The condition that causes this pain is also usually chronic. An example would be arthritis pain. This pain can be relieved and may even disappear for a time, but it will return. For more information on pain management, see the Resource Page at the end of this book.

Medication

Each health professional and each patient has a different point of view about pain medication. It is important for you to know your point of view of pain and pain medication. Be nonjudgmental when your patient and the patient's family members discuss the situation in the house. If you are not comfortable with the plan, discuss this with the appropriate members of the health care team. Keep the following points in mind:

- Be consistent. Follow the plan. Do not change the plan without discussing it with the physician.
- Plan your care around administration of medication so that the individual you are caring for will be most comfortable. Discuss this with the patient; together you will determine the best schedule for care and medication.
- Observe your patient's reaction to the medication. If the reaction is not what is expected, report it to the physician immediately!
- If the patient is taking more of the medication than was ordered, report this to the physician immediately!

Family Dynamics

The way in which people within a family interact affects their tolerance of and reaction to pain. Some families shun people in pain, some families cater to people in pain, some people see acceptance of pain as "manly," and some people see acceptance of pain as part of life and do nothing about it. It is important to try to understand how family members treat a person in pain. This helps in determining the best plan of care for the patient in his or her family unit.

Measuring Pain

The reporting of pain is strongly subjective. Each person has her or his own definition of what is mild pain, bearable pain, and horrible pain. A scale used within the health care industry to quantify pain goes from 1 to 10, with 10 being the worst pain imaginable (see Figure 14.18). When someone cannot read or is unable to comprehend a 1-to-10 pain scale, you can assess pain with pictures of faces depicting pain levels instead of numbers. Figure 14.xx is a face scale developed by Baker-Wong and is used in most medical facilities as an alternative to asking the patient to rate his or her pain on a 1-to-10 scale. When asking the patient if he is in pain, ask him to rate the pain on this scale. Then report that number. Be sure to record the time of day, the number, and when the last pain medication was given. It may also be important to record

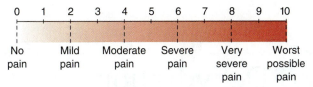

FIGURE 14.18   Numerical pain scale.

what the patient was doing. Having this record will let you compare one day with the next and help point out any noticeable changes.

It is also important to note other changes in the patient that indicate the status of his pain:

Breathing pattern	Facial expression, jaw position
Skin: dry, clammy, or sweaty	Tone of voice
Body position and movement	

For more information on pain medications, see Chapter 3.

Summary

The support and reinforcement you give the patient are your most important activities. Your careful observation and reporting of changes in the patient's vital signs or pain help the plan of care remain current. Encourage the patient to tell you when she experiences changes in her breathing or temperature, or when she senses an increase in heart rate. Also, encourage her to discuss her reaction to pain. Encourage her to continue to try medications prescribed by the physician for pain and other methods, such as relaxation, to relieve the pain. Continually observe the patient and the environment to be sure it is safe. Some patients try alternative methods for pain control. They buy machines, eat unusual foods, or practice rituals. Discuss these alternative methods with the physician to determine if they are safe and if there is any contraindication with the medications prescribed.

Chapter 15

Preventing Fluid Overload and Dehydration

SCENARIO

Mrs. Oates, an elderly widow, lives with her older sister, Ms. Davis, in the family home on a large piece of land. Living in this rural area has been a family tradition, and both Mrs. Oates and her sister will not discuss leaving the house or hiring help to maintain it. Several nieces and nephews live in the city about 50 miles away and visit infrequently. Mrs. Oates is receiving chemotherapy for cancer and seems to be tolerating it well. She is grateful to the Red Cross person who drives her to the city every week for the treatment. Ms. Davis, although she is older, appears able to cook the meals and do the laundry. A local church member does the shopping weekly and brings it to the sisters. The sisters enjoy listening to the radio; watching television; and talking to their dog, Lucky.

FLUID BALANCE

Water is essential to human life. Next to oxygen, water is the most important nutrient the body requires. A person can lose half his body protein and almost half his weight and still live, but losing only one-fifth of his body fluid will result in death.

Through eating and drinking, the average healthy adult will take in about 3½ quarts of fluid every 24 hours. This is called fluid intake. The average adult eliminates about 3½ quarts of fluid every 24 hours, which is called fluid output. The human body has several ways of keeping the amount of fluid it eliminates balanced with the amount of fluid it takes in. This balance is what allows the body to continue to function in a healthy state. When this balance is disturbed, the body is said to be in a state of fluid imbalance (see Figure 15.1). In some medical conditions, fluid may be held by the body tissues, which causes swelling and is called **edema**. In other medical conditions,

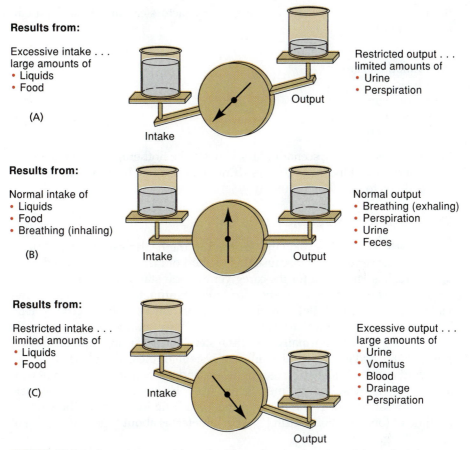

Results from:

Excessive intake . . .
large amounts of
• Liquids
• Food

(A)

Intake

Output

Restricted output . . .
limited amounts of
• Urine
• Perspiration

Results from:

Normal intake of
• Liquids
• Food
• Breathing (inhaling)

(B)

Intake

Output

Normal output
• Breathing (exhaling)
• Perspiration
• Urine
• Feces

Results from:

Restricted intake . . .
limited amounts of
• Liquids
• Food

(C)

Intake

Output

Excessive output . . .
large amounts of
• Urine
• Vomitus
• Blood
• Drainage
• Perspiration

FIGURE 15.1   (A) Intake exceeds output; (B) Intake equals output; (C) Intake is less than output.

much fluid can be lost, which is called dehydration. Fluids can be discharged from the body through the:

- kidneys in the form of urine
- skin in the form of perspiration
- lungs during breathing
- intestinal tract

When to Keep Records of Fluid Balance

When a person is healthy, the fluid balancing system works by itself; however, when a person is ill or disabled, this system often does not function to its maximum. When a change in a patient's condition occurs, fluid imbalance may be the first sign that something is wrong. Thus, keeping accurate records of an individual's intake and output provides data about how the person's fluid balancing system is functioning. Many factors can affect the fluid balance system:

- Medication
- Emotional stress
- Exercise
- Nourishment
- Weather
- General health

In the chapter-opening scenario, Mrs. Oates's chemotherapy likely makes her vomit and/or feel like not eating or drinking, yet it will be important that she drinks fluids to avoid dehydration.

The Metric System of Measurement

MEASURING FLUID Many quantities used in the health care field are measured in cubic centimeters. Because this method of measurement is used more and more, it is important for the caregiver to understand what it means.

The term *cc* is an abbreviation for "cubic centimeter" and *ml* is an abbreviation for "milliliter." Both are units of measurement in the metric system. The metric system of measurement is used in many countries of the world. In the United States, we normally use one system for measuring liquids (ounces, pints, quarts, and gallons) and a different system for measuring length (inches, feet, yards, and miles). Scientists, engineers, and many health care professionals use the metric system for measuring liquid, length, and weight. The basic unit of measurement is the meter, which is a little longer than the yard. A centimeter (one one-hundredth [$^1/_{100}$] of a meter) is about four-tenths ($^4/_{10}$) of an inch long.

A cubic centimeter can be thought of as a square block, with each edge of the block one centimeter long. If we filled this block with water, we would have a cubic centimeter (1 cc) of water. Note: Using the notation *cc* or *ml* is the same, and people often use *ml* versus *cc* because it is so easy to mistake the written *cc* for zeros. The list in Figure 15.2 includes liquid amounts with which you are probably familiar. It also gives the same approximate amounts in cubic centimeters.

RECORDING INTAKE AND OUTPUT

The amounts of intake and output (I&O) can be written on a log called an intake and output sheet. The form can be provided by the physician or medical clinic, or you can make your own. Figure 15.3 shows an example sheet that you can make to record I&O. The intake and output sheet is divided into two parts, intake on the left and output on the right. After measuring intake and output, record the amount in the proper column. You also indicate the time and what was drunk or expelled. The amounts in each column are totaled every twenty-four hours.

U.S. CUSTOMARY LIQUID MEASURE WITH EQUIVALENT METRIC MEASUREMENTS

cc	=	cubic centimeter
ml	=	milliliter
oz	=	ounce
1 cc	=	1 ml
1/4 teaspoon	=	1 cc
1 teaspoon	=	4 cc
30 cc	=	1 oz
60 cc	=	2 oz
90 cc	=	3 oz
120 cc	=	4 oz
150 cc	=	5 oz
180 cc	=	6 oz
210 cc	=	7 oz
240 cc	=	8 oz
270 cc	=	9 oz
300 cc	=	10 oz
500 cc	=	1 pint
1,000 cc	=	1 quart
4,000 cc	=	1 gallon
pt	=	pint
qt	=	quart
gal	=	gallon

FIGURE 15.2 Liquid measurement conversions.

Client name _____ Date _____

INTAKE			OUTPUT		
Time		Amt.	Time		Amt.
Total			Total		

FIGURE 15.3 Example intake and output sheet.

Starting an Intake and Output Record

A twenty-four-hour intake record is started with the first fluids the person drinks in the morning. The first urinary output of the morning, however, is considered part of the previous day's I&O because the fluid that formed the urine was consumed within the previous twenty-four hours. Therefore, the first urine recorded on the output sheet will actually come from the second urination of the day.

Responsibility for Keeping an I&O Record

The responsibility for keeping an accurate I&O record is a shared one. A family member must be taught to keep the record when you are not in the home. It is most important that all people who write on the sheet use the same procedure; otherwise, the total will not be accurate. If you are asked to keep additional information, such as the amount of solid food the patient eats, the physician or nurse will show you how to record this information. You will need to teach the patient's family members how to keep a simple I&O record, answer any questions they may have, and reinforce the teaching as needed.

FLUID INTAKE

Although solid foods also contain liquid, most fluids in the body are taken in when a person drinks liquids. A patient's intake includes all liquids.

Measuring with a Container

A container or measuring cup is used to measure intake and output. It is marked or calibrated with a row of short lines and numbers. These markings show the amount of liquid in both cubic centimeters and ounces. You can use a regular measuring cup. Another calibrated container may be a baby bottle. Be sure that you use one container to measure intake and a different one for output (see Procedure 15.1).

PROCEDURE 15.1

Measuring the Capacity of Serving Containers

Rationale

Knowing the capacity of serving containers aids accurate planning for patient intake.

1. Assemble your equipment: complete set of dishes, bowls, cups, and glasses used by the patient; measuring cup; water; pen and paper.
2. Fill the first container with water.
3. Pour this water into the measuring cup.
4. Look at the level of the water and determine the amount in cubic centimeters (cc).
5. Write this information on the paper. For example, a carton of milk equals 240 cc.
6. Repeat these steps for each dish, glass, bowl, or cup used by the patient.

Now you have measurements for the various items used by the patient on a daily basis.

To record accurately the exact amounts of fluids taken in by the patient, you will have to measure the amount of liquid contained in each serving container, bowl, glass, and cup the patient uses. It is helpful to make a list of how much each one contains. Then you can refer to it rather than measuring the liquid each time you fill the container.

Measuring Fluid Intake

Tell the patient that his intake is being measured. Encourage him to help you as much as he can by asking him to keep track of how much liquid he drinks. Record the fluid intake as soon as the individual has consumed the fluids. Do not wait or you will likely forget. Think about fluid intake every time you remove a tray, glass, or cup.

When measuring fluid intake, you will have to note the difference between the amount the person drinks and the amount he leaves in the serving container. It is a good idea to list the intake and output in the same unit of measurement. If you keep the output in cc, record the intake in cc, too. If you keep the output in ounces, record the intake in ounces.

FLUID OUTPUT

Measuring Fluid Output

Fluid output is the total of liquids that come out of the body. Most fluid is discharged from the body as urine. Other terms for this bodily function are *void* or *pass water*. Output also includes emesis (vomitus), drainage from a wound, loss of blood, and excessive perspiration. Every time your patient uses the urinal, emesis basin, or bedpan, the urine and other fluids must be measured (see Procedure 15.2).

PROCEDURE 15.2

Determining the Amount of Fluid Consumed

Rationale

Measuring and recording intake correctly assists in determining the patient's ability to process fluid.

1. Assemble your equipment: measuring cup, pen and paper, and leftover liquids in serving containers.
2. Pour the leftover liquid into the measuring cup.
3. Look at the level and determine the amount in cc.
4. From your list, determine the amount in the full serving container.
5. Subtract the leftover amount from the full container amount. This figure is the amount the patient actually drank.
6. Immediately report this amount on the intake side of the intake and output sheet.

You should tell the patient that her output is being measured and ask her to cooperate. All patients who are measuring their output must urinate in a bedpan, urinal, or container. Ask the individual not to place toilet paper in this container. Provide a plastic bag for this purpose. Then dispose of the tissue in the toilet. If at all possible, ask your patient not to move her bowels while urinating.

Documenting Fluid Output

It is important to notice all qualities about the urine when you measure it. Changes in the urine are also important and should be reported immediately. Some medications can change the color of urine. Some foods can change the odor of urine. Discuss this with the physician so you know what to expect and what is usual for your patient with regard to:

- the color of urine
- the odor of urine
- urine with particles or urine that is clear
- urinary increase or decrease in amount

Fluid Output from an In-Dwelling Catheter

Sometimes, a patient has a catheter (tube) inserted into his urinary bladder by the physician or nurse. This catheter drains all of the patient's urine into a plastic urine container, which hangs below the level of the urinary bladder (see Figures 15.4 and 15.5). *Remember, you learned in Chapter 11 that*

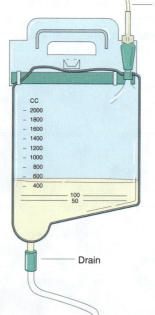

Tubing from the client

- Check tubing for obstructions.
- Be sure client is not lying on tubing.
- If amount of urine remains the same or increases rapidly, report to nurse.

CC
— 2000
— 1800
— 1600
— 1400
— 1200
— 1000
— 800
— 600
— 400
100
50

Drain

FIGURE 15.4   A plastic urine collection container should be hung on the bed frame below the level of the bladder.

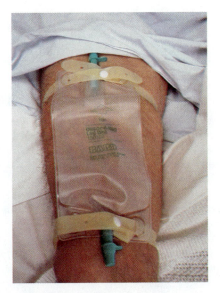

FIGURE 15.5 Leg drainage bag for ambulatory patients.

the patient should not be lying on the catheter tubing because it could cause skin sores. To measure the urine, the caregiver empties the plastic urine container into a hard plastic container, measures the urine for amount, and records the amount. This procedure is always done whenever the container is full and always before the time the caregiver leaves the home. Measurement is always taken once the urine has been transferred to the hard plastic container because this provides the more accurate measurement (see Procedure 15.3).

FLUID OUTPUT FROM THE INCONTINENT PATIENT   If the patient is incontinent (he or she cannot control bowels and/or urine), you should record each time the bed is wet on the output side of the I&O sheet. Even though the urine cannot be measured, it will be obvious that the patient's kidneys are functioning.

Measuring Fluids Other Than Urine

Vomitus and diarrhea are also measured according to the procedure for measuring urinary output. Be sure to indicate on the I&O sheet what fluid you are recording.

If a patient bleeds a great deal, has wound discharge, or perspires heavily, indicate these details on the I&O sheet. Include the following in your recording:

- What was wet
- How wet (damp, dripping, etc.)
- Size of the wet area
- Time it occurred

PROCEDURE 15.3

Measuring Urinary Output

Rationale

Measuring urinary output is one way to assist in assessing the body's ability to maintain fluid balance.

1. Assemble your equipment: bedpan and cover or urinal or container for urine, disposable gloves, measuring container, paper and pencil.
2. Wash your hands and put on gloves.
3. Pour the urine from the bedpan or urinal into the measuring container.
4. Place the container on a flat surface for accuracy in measurement.
5. At eye level, carefully look at the container to see the number reached by the level of urine. Remember it.
6. Rinse and return the measuring container to its proper place (pour the urine and the rinse water into the toilet).
7. Rinse and return the urinal or bedpan to its proper place (pour the rinse water into the toilet).
8. Remove gloves and dispose of them. Wash your hands.
9. Record the amount of urine in cc and the character of the urine on the output side of the I&O sheet.

BALANCING FLUID INTAKE

Patients who need fluids added to their normal intake are told to increase their fluid intake. As the caregiver, you will be responsible for encouraging your patient to take in extra fluids. Fluids should never be forced or restricted without the patient's consent. Be sure you know how much fluid the patient is to have within a twenty-four-hour period. You can encourage the patient to drink the adequate amount of fluids in any of the following ways:

- Show enthusiasm and be cheerful.
- Provide different kinds of liquids that the individual prefers, as permitted.
- Offer liquids without being asked.
- Offer hot and cold drinks.
- Offer liquids in divided amounts; for example, 800 cc every 8 hours means the person ought to drink 100 cc an hour.

On the intake side of the I&O, record the amount taken in by the patient in cc. Report to the physician if the patient is consistently unable to drink the amount required.

In some cases, it is healthier for patients to restrict their fluid intake. This includes patients with congestive heart failure, hyperparathyroidism, edema, and kidney disease. At times patients will feel more comfortable if they consume less fluid. Some mental illnesses have an accompanying uncontrollable thirst as part of the disorder. Often physicians will suggest fluids are limited to a certain amount. Follow orders and measure accurately. Your calm and reassuring attitude can make a big difference in how the patient feels and reacts to decreasing fluid intake. Keep the following points in mind:

- Know the reason for decreasing fluid intake so you can explain the risks of fluid overload.
- Record the amount of intake on the intake side of the I&O sheet.
- More frequent oral hygiene is a helpful addition to stimulate the mouth.
- Assist the patient with budgeting her fluid intake throughout the day so she doesn't feel deprived.
- Discuss with the physician the patient's reaction to this restriction.
- If the restriction is severe, the patient may be permitted to suck on ice chips or candy. Check with the physician before you start this type of alternative.

STRAINING URINE

You may be asked to strain urine after you have measured it or you may be instructed not to measure but just strain it (usually if the physician is concerned about kidney stones). In either case, you will collect the urine in the same manner as if you were to measure it. Be sure the patient knows she is to save all her urine and has a container available. The toilet tissue should not be dropped into the container with the urine but rather disposed of in a plastic bag (see Procedures 15.4 and 15.5).

PROCEDURE 15.4

Emptying a Urinary Collection Bag from an In-Dwelling Catheter

Rationale
Periodically emptying a collection bag is an important step in determining the patency of the catheter and in preventing infection.

1. Assemble your equipment: measuring container, paper towels, paper and pencil.
2. Wash your hands.
3. Protect the floor with paper towels.
4. Open the drain at the bottom of the plastic urine container and let the urine run into the measuring cup. Then close the drain. Be sure the urine does not touch the floor. Be sure the tubing from the catheter bag does not touch the floor.
5. Place the measuring container on a flat surface for accuracy in measurement.
6. At eye level, carefully look at the container to see the level of urine. Remember it.
7. Rinse the measuring container and put it in its proper place (put the urine and rinse water into the toilet).
8. Wash your hands.
9. Record the time, amount in cc, and anything unusual concerning the urine on the output side of the I&O sheet.

PROCEDURE 15.5

Straining Urine

Rationale

Collecting the sediment in urine is important for noting calculi (kidney stones).

1. Assemble your equipment: disposable paper strainers or gauze that fits into the container, specimen container with label, urine specimen, disposable gloves.
2. Wash your hands.
3. Put on gloves.
4. Pour the urine through the strainer into a calibrated container.
5. Put the strainer with any particles into the specimen container. Do not remove any particles.
6. Record the amount of urine measured, if appropriate. Record the date and time of the collection.
7. Discard the urine.
8. Clean the containers.
9. Put the specimen in the appropriate place until it can be sent or taken to the laboratory.
10. Remove gloves and wash hands.

Summary

Recording fluid intake and output is not always necessary, but you will be required to record such information when the data can help indicate if the body is functioning properly. For some conditions, the physician will want fluid intake and output recorded regularly. If this is the case, use the system discussed in this chapter to document your findings. Because fluid is such a dynamic part of bodily functions, it is important to report any significant changes you notice.

Chapter 16

Specimen Collection

SCENARIO

Mr. Hogan lives with his wife and son, Ronald, in a large house. Ronald suffered a diving accident when he was fifteen and has been mentally disabled since then. Although he can care for himself when reminded, he cannot live independently. The Hogans have a housekeeper who has been with them for many years. She does the cooking and the cleaning. Now that Mr. Hogan is becoming more forgetful, the housekeeper and Mrs. Hogan share the work and the care of Mr. Hogan and Ronald.

SPECIMEN COLLECTION

As one of its natural functions, the human body regularly rids itself of various waste materials. Most of the wastes are discharged in the form of urine and feces. The body also discharges waste in sputum, which is coughed up from the lungs.

Bodily wastes can be tested in the laboratory to detect changes in the bodily function. The doctor uses this information to decide on an appropriate treatment for the patient. Specimens are samples of bodily products that are collected and sent to the laboratory for examination.

When you are collecting a specimen, you must be accurate in following the procedure and labeling of the specimen. You have to collect the specimen at exactly the right time. The name of the patient, her address, the date, and the time of specimen collection should be printed on the label in clear letters. This label must be attached securely to the specimen container. All laboratories throw away unlabeled specimens. If this happens, another one will have to be collected, resulting in extra time and cost for the patient.

Many times specimens must be stored in the home for a short period until they are taken to the laboratory. It is your responsibility to be sure of the correct storage procedure for a specimen.

Urine specimens must be free of fecal matter. They must also be free of menstrual blood. If the person you are caring for is menstruating, a vaginal tampon must be in place while the urine specimen is collected. Before you suggest this, however, discuss it with the physician.

Obtaining a Specimen

Tell your patient that a urine specimen will be needed next time he uses the bathroom. Some individuals are embarrassed by the procedures involved in obtaining certain types of specimens. The person you are caring for will be calm and cooperative if you show understanding and assist him when necessary. If the individual understands the procedure and is physically able, he should be able to obtain the specimen himself with some direction.

Human waste material has many names. Street language uses one set of terms. Many cultures use other sets of terms. Many people do not know the correct English words for human waste material. It is usually a good idea to try to use the words that the patient and his family use (this is especially true for children). If these words are offensive to you, tell your patient what words you will be using to describe the waste materials.

Importance of Accuracy

When obtaining a specimen it is important to follow all the "rights":

- *The right specimen:* as ordered by the doctor.
- *The right time:* when the specimen should be collected.
- *The right amount:* the amount needed for the laboratory to test.
- *The right container:* the correct cup for each specimen.
- *The right label:* filled out properly and neatly.
- *The right method:* procedure by which you collect the specimen.
- *The right asepsis:* washing your hands before and after collecting the specimen and using disposable gloves.
- *The right attitude:* how you approach and speak to the patient.

Infection Control in Collecting a Specimen

Asepsis means "free of disease-causing organisms." When collecting specimens, it is important to use good medical aseptic techniques to prevent contamination. Wash your hands carefully before and after collecting each specimen. Handwashing before you collect the specimen prevents contamination of the specimen by anything that may be on your hands. Handwashing after you perform this procedure prevents bacteria from the specimen from remaining on your hands.

URINE SPECIMEN COLLECTION

Routine

Routine collection is a single sample of urine taken from the patient as she urinates, also known as voiding. No special precautions are taken. At times, you will be told to take a specimen of the first urine of the day, but if you are not given time instructions, this specimen may be taken when it is convenient. Be sure that the patient's perineal area or penis is clean before obtaining the specimen (see Procedure 16.1).

A Patient with a Foley Catheter

A urine specimen from a patient with a Foley catheter in place takes time to collect. A Foley is a flexible plastic tube (a catheter) that is inserted into the bladder to provide continuous urinary drainage. Be sure the patient has had fluid to drink before you attempt the collection. Tell the patient what you will be doing because he will be unable to see the procedure or take an active part in it. It is imperative that the specimen be labeled properly. Include the fact that the specimen was obtained from a catheter (see Procedure 16.2).

Midstream Clean-Catch Urine Collection

A special method is used to collect a patient's urine when the specimen must be totally free from contamination. This special type of specimen is called a midstream clean-catch urine specimen. *Clean-catch* refers to the fact that the urine is not contaminated by anything outside the patient's body. The procedure requires careful washing of the genital area. Midstream means catching the urine specimen between the time the patient begins to void and the time he stops.

All the equipment and supplies necessary for this specimen are usually found in a special kit that the laboratory sends to the patient. If you are unable to obtain such a kit, sterilize a jar to use for catching the urine. Wash the genital area with a nonirritating, sterile cleansing solution and sterile gauze. Be sure all soap is off the area before collecting the specimen (see Procedure 16.3).

Twenty-Four Hour Collection of Urine

A twenty-four-hour urine specimen is a collection of all urine voided by a patient over a twenty-four-hour period. All urine is collected for twenty-four

PROCEDURE 16.1

Collecting a Routine Urine Specimen

Rationale

A properly collected specimen allows a laboratory to evaluate the chemical structure of the urine and evaluate for possible further testing.

1. Assemble your equipment: bedpan or urinal, disposable gloves, measuring container for measuring output, urine specimen container and lid, paper or plastic bag for toilet tissue, label, wet washcloth, towel.
2. Prepare the label. Write clearly the patient's name and address, the date, and the time. Also write what type of specimen is being collected, for example, *routine urine*.
3. Wash your hands and put on gloves.
4. Ask visitors to leave the room, if appropriate.
5. Tell the patient a urine specimen is needed. Explain the procedure to him. If he can collect the specimen himself, he should do so.
6. If the patient is able, he can urinate directly into the container. If he is not, ask him to urinate into the bedpan or urinal. Remind the patient to put toilet tissue into a paper bag or a plastic bag, not the bedpan. You can discard the tissue in the toilet and the bag in the trash, or place the bag with the tissue in the trash. Remove gloves and wash your hands.
7. If the patient requires assistance with washing his hands, offer the patient a washcloth and towel to wash his hands each time he voids. Otherwise, remind the patient that he should always wash his hands after urinating.
8. Make the patient comfortable.
9. Put on gloves and take the bedpan or urinal into the bathroom.
10. If the patient is on intake and output (I&O) logging, pour the urine into a clean measuring container and note the urine amount on the I&O sheet.
11. Pour the urine into the specimen container. Fill it three-quarters full or to the indicated line on the specimen cup.
12. Put the lid on the container. Wipe off the outside of the container. Secure the label to the container.
13. Pour the urine remaining in the bedpan, urinal, or measuring container into the toilet.
14. Clean the equipment (i.e., bedpan, urinal, or measuring container) by washing with soap and water, rinsing, and air drying. Then return these items to their proper place.
15. Remove gloves and wash your hands.
16. Store the specimen, as directed by the physician or lab, in the correct place until it is taken to the laboratory.

hours, usually from 7 A.M. on the first day to 7 A.M. the following day (see Figure 16.4).

When you obtain a twenty-four-hour urine specimen, you must ask the patient to void and discard his voided urine at 7 A.M. because this urine has been in the bladder an unknown length of time. The test should begin with

PROCEDURE 16.2

Obtaining a Urine Specimen from a Patient with a Foley Catheter

Rationale

A properly obtained urine sample allows a laboratory to evaluate the chemical structure of the urine and evaluate for possible further testing.

1. Assemble your equipment: specimen container and lid, measuring container, label, disposable gloves, padding to protect the bed, protective cap for drainage tubing or sterile gauze pads.
2. Prepare the label. Write clearly the patient's name and address, the date, and the time. Write the type of specimen and how it was obtained.
3. Wash your hands.
4. Explain the procedure to the patient.
5. Put on gloves.
6. Clamp an in-dwelling urinary catheter below the port by folding the plastic tubing in half and applying a metal or plastic clamp.
7. Wait no more than fifteen minutes for a small amount of urine to collect in the tubing above the port.
8. Insert a sterile syringe gently into the port (after swabbing with alcohol). Take care not to poke the needle through the tubing (see Figure 16.1).

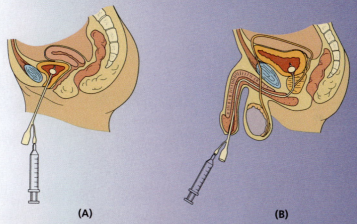

(A)   (B)

FIGURE 16.1   (A) Female foley catheter urine collection (B) Male foley catheter urine collection.

9. Withdraw approximately 10 cc of urine.
10. Insert the urine into a sterile specimen cup. Take care not to touch the rim or inside cover of the cap to prevent contamination of the specimen.
11. Unclamp the tubing and straighten it out. Be sure that the urine is now freely flowing.
12. Apply the correct lab label to the specimen cup and bag, according to policy.
13. Report the results of the procedure to the appropriate health care team member.
14. Remove gloves and wash your hands.
15. Store the specimen in the correct place, as directed by the physician or lab, until it is taken to the laboratory.

PROCEDURE 16.3

Collecting a Midstream Clean-Catch Urine Specimen

Rationale

A properly collected sample allows a laboratory to evaluate urine free from bacteria.

1. Assemble your equipment: clean-catch kit or sterilized jar, sterile cleansing solution, sterile gauze, disposable gloves, bedpan or urinal (if the patient is unable to go to the bathroom), wet washcloth, towel, waste bag.
2. Prepare the label by writing clearly the patient's name and address, the date, and the time. Write the type of specimen and how it was obtained.
3. Wash your hands.
4. Ask visitors to leave the room, if appropriate. You may want to explain this procedure to a family member.
5. Tell the patient you need a midstream clean-catch urine specimen.
6. Explain the procedure. If the patient is able, she may collect the specimen herself.
7. If the patient is not able to collect the specimen, assist her with the procedure.
8. Open the disposable kit.
9. Put on the gloves. Remove the towelettes and the urine specimen container. Do not put your hand inside the container or lid.
10. For female patients:
    a. Separate the folds of the labia and wipe with one towelette from the front to the back along one labia. Throw away the towelette. The labia must be separated during cleansing and collection of the specimen.
    b. Wipe the opposite labia with the second towelette. Throw it away.
    c. Wipe down the middle using the third towelette. Throw it away (see Figure 16.2).
11. For male patients:
    a. If the male is not circumcised, pull the foreskin of the penis back before cleansing the penis. Hold it back during urination.
    b. Use a circular motion to clean the head of the penis. Use all three towelettes. Discard each one after use (see Figure 16.3).

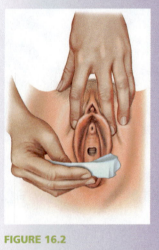

FIGURE 16.2

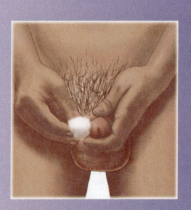

FIGURE 16.3

12. Ask the patient to start urinating into the bedpan or the toilet. Then ask him to stop. Place the sterile urine container under the stream of urine and ask the patient to start urinating again. Fill the container one-half to three-quarters full. The remaining urine may be discarded.

13. If the patient is on intake and output (I&O) logging, all the urine must first be voided into a sterile measuring container and measured, then put into the sterile specimen container provided. Be sure to note on the I&O sheet the amount of urine sent as a specimen.

14. Cover the urine container with the proper lid. Be sure not to touch the inside of the lid or the container. Wipe off the outside of the container.

15. Take off your gloves.

16. Wash your hands.

17. Make the patient comfortable. Offer the patient a wet washcloth and towel to wash her hands.

18. Clean the equipment and replace it.

19. Wash your hands.

20. If the patient requires assistance with washing her hands, offer the patient a washcloth and towel to wash her hands each time she voids. Otherwise, remind the patient that she should always wash her hands after urinating.

21. Store the specimen in the correct place, as indicated by the physician or lab, until it is taken to the laboratory.

the bladder empty. For the next twenty-four hours, save all the urine voided by the patient. On the following day at 7 A.M., ask the patient to void and add this specimen to the previous collection. This way, the doctor can be sure that all of the urine for the test came into the urinary bladder during the twenty-four hours of the test period (see Procedure 16.4).

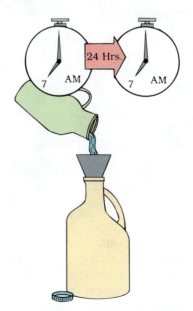

FIGURE 16.4 Write down the 24 hours in which you are collecting the urine.

PROCEDURE 16.4

Collecting a Twenty-Four-Hour Urine Specimen

Rationale

A properly collected sample allows a laboratory to evaluate the chemical structure of the urine and evaluate for possible further testing.

1. Assemble your equipment: large container (usually a one-gallon bottle that the laboratory often supplies), bedpan or urinal, disposable gloves, funnel (if the neck of the bottle is small), measuring container for measuring output if the patient is on I&O, label for the container, wet washcloth, towel.
2. Fill out the label. Clearly write the patient's name and address, the date, and the time the collection started.
3. Wash your hands and put on gloves.
4. Ask visitors to leave the room, if appropriate.
5. Tell the patient that a twenty-four-hour specimen is needed. Explain the procedure to him and his family. Discuss the placement and care of the gallon container of urine.
6. You may be instructed to refrigerate the urine. If so, one way is to keep it in a bucket of ice. This ice must be changed as it melts. It may, of course, be kept in the refrigerator if that is acceptable to the patient and his family.
7. During the collection of the specimen, ask the patient to use the bedpan or urinal each time he voids. Remind him not to throw toilet tissue into the bedpan or urinal and to try to urinate without moving his bowels at the same time. Provide a waste bag for the toilet tissue. When the procedure is completed, discard the tissue promptly in the toilet or trash.
8. If you are logging the patient's output of urine, measure all urine each time and write it on the I&O sheet. If the patient collects the urine himself, have him give you the sample so you can measure it prior to putting it in the larger container of collected urine.
9. When the collection starts, have the patient urinate. *Throw away this first urine* to be sure that the bladder is completely empty as the collection starts. If this urine is discarded at 7 A.M., the collection will continue until 7 A.M. the following morning.
10. For the next twenty-four hours, all of the patient's urine should be saved. At the end of the collection, the time the collection stopped should be written on the label. Store the bottle in the proper place until it is sent to the laboratory.
11. If the patient requires assistance with washing his hands, offer the patient a washcloth and towel to wash his hands each time he voids. Otherwise, remind the patient he should always wash his hands after urinating.
12. Be sure to clean all equipment *after each urination* by washing with soap and water, rinsing thoroughly, and letting it air dry.

The patient and his family must understand the importance of collecting *all* urine voided within the twenty-four-hour period. If one urination is accidentally discarded, the test is not accurate and must be repeated.

It is your responsibility to be sure of the correct placement of the twenty-four-hour urine collection bottle. Some specimens must be kept on ice and others are not. If you are not sure how to store the urine for the twenty-four-hour urine catch, be sure to ask the lab.

Collecting Urine from an Infant

It is often difficult to collect urine from an infant because he cannot cooperate and void when asked. Therefore, it is important to gather the specimen correctly the first time. This is accomplished by cleaning the genital area, securing the urine collection container to the infant, and putting the diaper on the infant and over the container. The procedure may appear uncomfortable to the child, but it does not hurt him. Reassure the child's parent or guardian that you are not hurting the child and that the information the doctor will have after the laboratory examination of the urine will help in the child's care. Be kind, efficient, and thoughtful of both child and parents (see Procedure 16.5).

PROCEDURE 16.5

Collecting a Urine Specimen from a Child Who Is Not Toilet-Trained

---

Rationale

A properly collected sample allows a laboratory to evaluate the chemical structure of the urine and evaluate for possible further testing.

1. Assemble your equipment: urine specimen bottle or container, plastic disposable infant urine collector, gloves.
2. Prepare a label. Write the patient's name and address, the date, and the type of specimen. Fill in the time when the actual specimen is obtained.
3. Wash your hands.
4. Ask visitors to leave, except the parent or guardian of the infant.
5. Explain to the child and her parent that you want to collect a urine specimen. A toddler who is not yet toilet-trained often can understand language and is more likely to cooperate if she knows what is expected of her. Use language the child understands and is familiar with.
6. Put on gloves and take off the child's diaper.
7. Clean the genital area. Be sure it is dry or the collector bag will not stick (see Figure 16.5).
8. Remove the outside piece that surrounds the opening of the plastic urine collector. Be sure the skin is not folded under the sticky part as you apply it. Place the opening of the bag around the male penis or the female meatus. Do not cover the rectum. The specimen is useless if it is contaminated with fecal matter.
9. Put the child's diaper on as usual.
10. Check every half-hour to see if the child has voided. You cannot feel the diaper. You must look inside the diaper.
11. When the child has voided, remove the urine collector gently. Do not spill the urine. Pour the urine into a specimen container.

(continued)

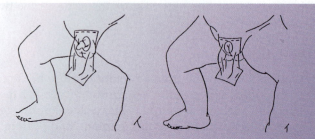

FIGURE 16.5

12. Wash off any excess sticky material on the genitalia. Make the baby comfortable.
13. Remove gloves and wash your hands.
14. Store the specimen in the correct place until it is taken to the laboratory.

COLLECTING A STOOL SPECIMEN

"The solid waste from a person's body has many names: *stools, feces, fecal matter, excreta, excrement, B.M.,* and *bowel movement.* They all mean the same thing. The doctor sometimes requires a sample of the patient's feces to assist him or her in diagnosing the patient's illness or in monitoring the patient's progress. A feces sample is called a stool specimen. Certain tests must be performed only on a warm stool. You will be told whether the specimen is to be warm or cold (see Procedure 16.6).

PROCEDURE 16.6

Collecting a Stool Specimen

Rationale
Determine if blood, parasites, or foreign bodies are present in the stool.

1. Assemble your equipment: bedpan, stool container, disposable gloves, label, wooden tongue depressor, washcloth, towel.
2. Fill in the label with the patient's name and address, the date, and the type of specimen. Fill in the time when the actual specimen is obtained.
3. Wash your hands and put on gloves.
4. Ask visitors to leave the room, if appropriate.
5. Tell the patient that a stool specimen is needed. Explain that he is to call you whenever he can move his bowels. If this doesn't occur during your time at the home, then see if you can teach the collection procedure to a family member. You should do so to prevent delay in obtaining the specimen.
6. Have the patient move his bowels in the bedpan. If the patient is unable to use the bedpan, place several layers of toilet tissue in the bottom of the toilet and have the patient move his bowels on the paper. This way, you will be able to obtain a specimen easily.

7. Ask the patient not to urinate into the bedpan and not to put toilet tissue into the bedpan. Provide him with a plastic bag to dispose of the tissue temporarily. Then discard the tissue in the toilet or the entire bag and tissue into the trash.
8. After the patient has had a bowel movement, take the bedpan into the bathroom.
9. Remove gloves and wash your hands.
10. If the patient requires assistance to wash his hands, offer the patient a wash-cloth and towel to wash his hands each time he voids. Otherwise, remind the patient he should always wash his hands after defecating.
11. Make the patient comfortable.
12. Put on gloves. Using the wooden tongue depressor, take 1 to 2 tablespoons of stool from the bedpan and place it into the stool specimen container.
13. Cover the container. Do not touch the inside of the container or the top of it.
14. Wrap the depressor in a piece of toilet tissue and discard it into a plastic or paper bag.
15. Empty the remaining feces into the toilet.
16. Clean the bedpan and return it to its proper place.
17. Remove gloves and wash your hands.
18. Store the specimen in the correct place, as indicated by the physician or lab, until it is taken to the laboratory.

COLLECTING A SPUTUM SPECIMEN

Sputum is a substance collected from a patient's lungs. It contains saliva, mu-cous, and sometimes blood or pus. It is usually clear in color but can be gray, yellow, green, or red. The best time to collect a sputum specimen is in the morning, right after the patient awakens (see Procedure 16.7).

PROCEDURE 16.7

Collecting a Sputum Specimen

Rationale

A properly collected sample allows a laboratory to determine the presence of dis-ease-causing bacteria or blood.

1. Assemble your equipment: sputum container with lid, tissues, disposable gloves (see Figure 16.6).
2. Label the container with the patient's name and address, the date, and the type of specimen. Fill in the time when the actual specimen is obtained.
3. Wash your hands and put on gloves.
4. Ask visitors to leave the room, if appropriate.
5. Tell the patient a sputum specimen is needed.
6. If the patient has eaten recently, have her rinse out her mouth. If she wants oral hygiene at this time, help her as necessary.
7. Give her the sputum container. Ask her to take three consecutive deep breaths. On the third breath, ask her to exhale deeply and cough. She should be able to bring up sputum from within the lungs. Explain to her that saliva is not adequate for this test.

(continued)

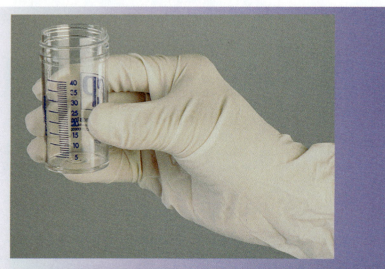

FIGURE 16.6 Sputum container.

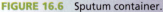

8. Have the patient spit the sputum directly into the specimen container.
9. Cover the container immediately. Be careful not to touch the inside of either the container or the cover.
10. Offer the patient oral hygiene.
11. Make the patient comfortable.
12. Remove gloves and wash your hands.
13. If the patient requires assistance to wash her hands, offer the patient a wash-cloth and towel to wash her hands each time she collects sputum. Otherwise, remind the patient she should always wash her hands after collecting sputum.
14. Store the specimen in the correct place, as indicated by the physician or lab, until it is taken to the laboratory.

Summary

Specimen collection is not the easiest part of being a caregiver; however, it is necessary for monitoring or diagnosing certain conditions. Be sure to ask questions of the physician to get all the details for collecting the specimen (i.e., amount needed, storage until delivered, container to be used, time to be collected, etc.). Most of all, reassure the person during the collection process. Such reassurance is especially important in situations similar to the chapter-opening scenario, when a patient may be mentally impaired.

Chapter 17

Special Procedures

SCENARIO

Mrs. Collins, a retired nurse, lives in a boarding house. She shares a small kitchen with her neighbor. The refrigerator is small, and periodically food goes missing. The bathroom is shared by three people. Mrs. Collins does not leave her room unless she goes to the doctor or the corner store where she buys her groceries. She spends her days in her chair looking out of the window and watching television. Her family does not live nearby, and she has no friends who visit. Mrs. Collins has some savings, but she is frugal because she does not know how long her money will last. Her two big expenses are her medication and her food. She has recently accepted oxygen, but you are not sure how much she uses it.

ASSISTING WITH MEDICATION

Medication is prescribed by a physician; dispensed by a pharmacist; and administered, or given without patient assistance, by a nurse. All these professionals are licensed by the state to perform their duties. These duties are specific. Failure to stay within the state guidelines can result in a legal action ending in a fine, revocation of a license to practice the profession, and possibly jail time. In addition, these people are paid for their services. As a caregiver, you are not licensed to administer medication. You are expected, however, to assist your patients as they take their own medication. When you *administer* to patients, you take all responsibility that goes along with giving medication. When you *assist* patients, they share the responsibility.

Prescription drugs are prescribed by a physician and cannot be obtained without a prescription. Over-the-counter drugs can be purchased without a prescription. As a caregiver, you will not administer either type of drug but you will assist the patient with those drugs that have been prescribed by the physician.

YOUR ROLE AS A CAREGIVER

As a caregiver, you will probably spend more time with the patient than any other member of the health care team. During this time, you will often be assigned to assist the patient with medication (see Procedure 17.1). To assist the patient with medication correctly, you will have to have certain information. Without this information, an accident could happen. Accidents involving medication are serious because they can cause the patient pain, delay recovery, and sometimes even cause death.

The physician and/or the pharmacist will provide all information about the patient's medication(s). Then a medication plan is formed for the patient and reviewed with the caregiver and the patient. If available, a home health nurse can assist in educating the patient and his or her family members about medication. As the caregiver, you must be sure to have all the information needed to perform your duties to the best of your ability.

To perform the duties associated with medication, it is important for you to know the five rights of medication, as outlined in Figure 17.1. You

---

PROCEDURE 17.1

Assisting a Patient with Medication

Rationale

Correct assistance with medication is an important part of patient care.

1. Assemble your equipment: medication, spoon, water or juice, dressings if medication is applied to the skin, tissues or cotton balls.
2. Wash your hands.
3. Ask visitors to leave the room, if appropriate.
4. Remind the patient it is time for her medication.
5. Check the five rights of medication.
6. Place the medication within reach of the patient. Loosen the tops of bottles or tubes.
7. Assist the patient as necessary:
   a. *Oral medication:* Hold patient's hand if necessary and assist her with any liquid.
   b. *Ointments:* Assist the patient as needed with medication and dressing.
   c. *Eye drops:* Guide her hand and wipe excess liquid or ointment from under the eye: from the nose to the outer corner of the eye.
8. Make the patient comfortable.
9. Put the medication in its proper place. Dispose of the used equipment.
10. Wash your hands.

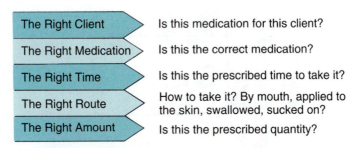

The Right Client	Is this medication for this client?
The Right Medication	Is this the correct medication?
The Right Time	Is this the prescribed time to take it?
The Right Route	How to take it? By mouth, applied to the skin, swallowed, sucked on?
The Right Amount	Is this the prescribed quantity?

FIGURE 17.1 The Five Rights of Medication must be observed every time a client takes medication.

should also know the side effects of your patient's medication, how to store the medication, and how it reacts with food. If you observe any side effects after your patient has taken the medication, report them immediately to the physician. Some of the most common side effects are identified in Figure 17.2. However, any change in behavior associated with the taking of medication should be noted.

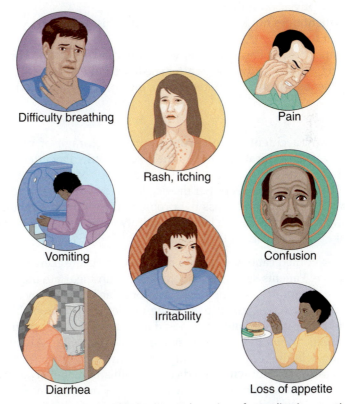

Difficulty breathing

Rash, itching

Pain

Vomiting

Irritability

Confusion

Diarrhea

Loss of appetite

FIGURE 17.2 Changes in usual behavior can be a sign of a medication reaction. Report these immediately to the physician.

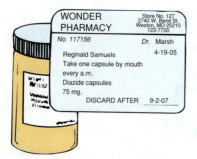

FIGURE 17.3 The label on the medication bottle must be checked every time the client takes the medication.

As you spend time in your patient's house, you will observe many details and events. Here are a few of the observations you should report to the physician immediately:

- Your patient is not taking the medication exactly as it has been prescribed (see Figure 17.3).
- Your patient is taking medication (prescription or over the counter) of which the physician is unaware.
- Your patient does not know why he is taking his drugs, and you cannot explain it to him.
- Your patient experiences nausea, vomiting, diarrhea, itching, difficulty breathing, a rash, or hives soon after she takes her medication.
- Your patient's orientation, concentration, memory, and/or mood changes.

Medication Storage

Each year, many accidents result from improper storage of medication. Medications have an expiration date on the box or bottle. Pay attention to all expiration dates and discard medications that are expired. Tour the patient's house and observe how she keeps her medication. If it is poorly stored, correct this situation. If you cannot discuss the problem directly with the individual you are caring for, discuss it with her or his family members or physician and together make a plan to correct the situation.

- Patients save medications, but some medications change chemical makeup as they age. Patients save medication so they can medicate themselves if they have symptoms—yet the same symptoms can be caused by a different physical problem. The practice of saving medication is extremely dangerous. Old medication should be disposed of with the patient's permission.
- Many medications have similar names and look alike. Always store medications in the container in which they came.
- Do not assist a patient with a medication from an unlabeled container.
- Do not change the place your patient stores his medication without his permission. People do not always read labels but take medications from the places they expect to find them.

- Keep medication out of reach of children and confused, forgetful patients. Refer to Chapter 4 for suggestions about safe medication storage in this situation.
- Keep medication away from extreme heat, extreme cold, or bright light.

It is important to dispose of medication in a safe manner that does not promote environmental pollution, such as flushing it down the toilet or leaving the medication for other people or animals to access. For the best disposal method, contact your local health department or local department of public works.

ASSISTING A PATIENT WITH OXYGEN THERAPY

Oxygen is considered a medication. The same rules and responsibilities that apply to you when you assist an individual with medication apply when assisting a patient with oxygen. Oxygen is prescribed by a physician. It is delivered to the home by a special company.

The three main kinds of oxygen storage are:

- *Portable oxygen tank:* This small tank is intended to be used for short time spans, usually outside the house. It is filled from a larger tank inside the house.
- *Stationary cylinder tank:* Several different types of cylinders are all designed to remain stationary and deliver oxygen over several days. The tubing connected from the cylinder to the patient can be adjusted in length to increase patient mobility.
- *Oxygen concentrator:* This device removes oxygen from the air and delivers it, through tubing, to the patient. The tubing length can be adjusted.

The company delivering the oxygen is responsible for refilling the tank, servicing the equipment, and teaching the patient and his family members how to use the equipment. The company should provide a telephone number to call in case of an emergency. This contact information is normally located on the tank, too. Although the oxygen may be dispensed in several ways, all oxygen is dispensed from a tank to the patient through a plastic tube connected to a nasal cannula or face mask. Oxygen is extremely drying, so a container filled with water or medication usually is attached to the tank. The oxygen passes through the water and takes on moisture before it is delivered to the patient.

The following are important parts of oxygen delivery systems:

Nasal cannulas: Nasal cannulas, or tubes, are used to give oxygen to a patient. The cannulas are inserted into the person's nostrils. The plastic cannula is a half-circle length of tubing with two openings in the center. It fits about one-half inch into the individual's nostrils. Nasal cannulas are held in place by plastic tubing around the person's head or under the chin and are connected to the source of oxygen by a length of plastic tubing.

Face mask: A face mask is a piece of plastic shaped like a cup that covers the individual's nose and mouth and has holes in it. A tube connects the mask to the oxygen tank or concentrator, and a piece of elastic material holds the mask securely to the person's face. This mask is used when the patient requires more oxygen than can be given by cannula. The mask must be removed for the individual to eat. A person can say a few words with the mask in place but usually removes it to speak.

Humidification container: A humidification container is attached to the oxygen tank or concentrator that adds moisture to the oxygen flowing to the patient. This process helps avoid the drying of the patient's nostrils.

Regulator: The regulator shows the amount of oxygen being distributed to the individual.

Meter: A meter that shows the percentage of oxygen left in the tank is often present.

Safety Measures

Because oxygen is extremely flammable, follow these safety measures:

- Put up "No Smoking" signs in the rooms where the patient uses the oxygen. *Enforce this rule without exception!*
- Report to the physician if the patient uses the oxygen other than as prescribed.
- Use cotton bedclothes to decrease static electricity.
- Do not use electric shavers or hair dryers while oxygen is running. Keep electric plugs to these devices out of wall outlets while oxygen is running. If an electric plug is pulled from an outlet while oxygen is running, a spark could cause an explosion. Use a three-pronged plug, if possible.
- Do not use flammable products (i.e., aerosol sprays, paint thinner, and cleaning fluids) while the patient is using oxygen.
- Do not use oxygen near candles, fireplaces, barbeques, space heaters, or other open flames in the room (if it is used outside, keep oxygen twenty feet from the source of a flame, like that in a barbeque).
- Avoid combing a person's hair while she or he is receiving oxygen. A spark of electricity from the individual's hair could set off an explosion.
- Ask for careful instructions about which valve turns the oxygen on and off.
- Do not change the setting on any oxygen equipment. The setting has been chosen by the physician. Too much or too little oxygen can cause the patient to change his breathing pattern, his heart rate, and his speech pattern. Call the physician immediately if you notice any of these signs. *Do not change the oxygen setting unless instructed to do so.*
- Keep a fire extinguisher in the home near the oxygen tank. Make sure the fire department knows there is an oxygen tank in the home. Stickers can be obtained from the oxygen company to post on the door to the home.
- Keep oxygen tanks upright. Lying a tank down or knocking one over can be dangerous.

Indications that the patient is receiving too much oxygen are as follows:

- Sleepiness or difficulty waking up
- Headache
- Difficulty speaking
- Slow, shallow breathing

Indications that the patient is receiving too little oxygen are as follows:

- Tiredness
- Blue fingernails and/or lips
- Anxiety, restlessness
- Irritability
- Unusual confusion

NONSTERILE DRESSING CHANGES

At times your patient may have wounds or areas on the body that must be covered by a bandage or dressing. Dressings that do not require sterile techniques or application of medication to the wound will often be accomplished by you. These dressings are called nonsterile. When applying a dressing, it is important to keep the following in mind:

- Protect the wound.
- Protect the surrounding tissue.

The type of dressing used will address these issues. Sometimes a dressing will use tape to secure it, sometimes additional bandage material will be wrapped around the area, and sometimes an occlusive dressing will be used.

When changing a dressing, always note the color, odor, amount, and consistency of the drainage (discharge) on the old dressing. Also note how big the wound is and the condition of the skin surrounding the wound. Note any change in the wound since you last saw it. If the nurse is scheduled to visit, be sure and save the old dressing for her to see. Each dressing is somewhat different, but Procedure 17.2 contains general rules for changing all nonsterile dressings.

CATHETER CARE

In-Dwelling Catheter

The in-dwelling urinary catheter is the most common kind of catheter used for taking fluids out of the body. This catheter is made of plastic or rubber and is inserted by a nurse or physician through the patient's urethra into his bladder. A catheter may be used when an individual is unable to urinate naturally, or it may be used to measure the amount of urine left in the bladder after a person has urinated naturally. It may also be used to help keep an incontinent

PROCEDURE 17.2

Changing a Nonsterile Dressing

Rationale

Dressing a wound correctly prevents infection and contributes to the patient's comfort.

1. Assemble your equipment: clean dressing, tape, cleansing solution, disposable gloves, paper bag or plastic bag for old dressings, medication that the patient will apply.
2. Wash your hands and put on gloves.
3. Ask visitors to leave the room, if appropriate.
4. Tell the patient you will change his dressing.
5. Open the paper bag.
6. Open the clean dressings without touching the center of them. Prepare the tape in a convenient place.
7. Position the patient so that you have clear access to the wound and the old dressing.
8. Remove the old dressing. Note the drainage for amount, color, odor, and consistency. Note the size of the wound and the condition of the surrounding skin. Place the soiled dressing in the paper or plastic bag.
9. Cleanse the wound and the skin as you have been instructed. Use circular motions and clean from the clean areas to the dirty. The wound is considered clean and the skin dirty. Discard cleaning materials in the paper or plastic bag.
10. Allow the patient to assist you as much as possible.
11. If a medication is to be applied to the wound, assist the patient with the application, as needed.
12. Apply clean dressings. Hold all dressings by the corners as you apply them. Do not contaminate the center of the bandages. Tape the dressing in place, leaving the edges free. Do not put tape completely around the edges of the bandage (see Figure 17.4).

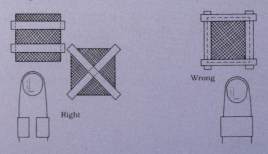

FIGURE 17.4

13. Make the patient comfortable.
14. Close the bag and discard it in a covered container, preferably outside. If possible, put the paper or plastic bag into another plastic bag to prevent leakage and contamination of the large trash can.
15. Remove gloves and wash your hands.
16. Make a notation in the patient's communication notebook that you changed the patient's dressing. Also note your observations of the patient during this procedure.

GUIDELINE 17.1

In-Dwelling Urinary Catheter

It is normal for urine to change from light yellow to dark yellow, depending on the concentration and the amount of fluid the patient has consumed.

- Check from time to time to make sure that the level of urine has increased. If the level stays the same, call the physician.
- If the patient says that he feels that his bladder is full or that he needs to urinate, call the physician.
- If the patient is allowed to get out of bed for short periods, the bag goes with him. It must always be held lower than the patient's urinary bladder to prevent the urine in the tubing and bag from draining back into the urinary bladder.
- Check to make sure the catheter and tubing flow freely and without obstruction.
- Be sure the patient is not lying on the catheter or the tubing. This position would stop the flow of urine.
- Be sure the tubing from the bed to the bag is always straight.
- The catheter should be secured at all times to the patient's inner thigh or, in the case of male patients, the abdomen (if a supra pubic catheter is used). This position keeps the catheter from being pulled on or being pulled out of the bladder. Either tape or special straps made for this purpose can be used.
- Most patients with urinary drainage through a catheter are on intake and output measurement.
- If urine leaks around a catheter, report this to the health care team.
- A male patient may have an erection while the catheter is in place, which is a natural occurrence. Assure him there is nothing the matter with him, and maintain a concerned attitude. Encourage the patient to talk to his physician if he has questions.
- Empty the collection bag frequently and from the correct port. Protect the floor from spillage. Collection bags come in many types. If you find one that is new to you, ask the health care team for assistance.
- Clean the collection tubing and the bag as instructed by the physician. Some medical providers suggest discarding collection equipment after a specified amount of time. Some will give you a cleansing procedure.
- Keep the patient's urinary opening clean. Even though he is not urinating, mucous and perspiration collect in the area.
- Be sure the tubing is free of fecal matter and mucous.
- Cover the exposed ends of tubing only with sterile covers.
- Notify the physician if you see sediment or blood in the tubing or collection bag.

patient dry. An incontinent patient is one who cannot control her urine or feces (see Guideline 17.1).

Sometimes a urinary catheter is used for only one withdrawal of urine. Sometimes it is kept in place in the bladder for days or even weeks. This type of catheter is called an in-dwelling catheter or Foley catheter. This catheter is specially made so that it will stay in the bladder. It has two tubes, one inside the other. The inside tube is connected at one end to a balloon. After

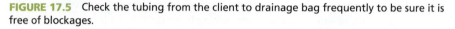

Plastic Urine Container
Hung on Bedframe

Tubing from client.
Check tubing for blockages.
Be sure client is not lying on tubing.

Check level in container for
increase in level. If level remains
the same or increases rapidly,
report to your supervisor.

Drain for Emptying the Container

FIGURE 17.5 Check the tubing from the client to drainage bag frequently to be sure it is free of blockages.

the catheter has been inserted, the balloon is filled with water or air so the catheter will stay in place. Urine drains out of the bladder through the outer tube and collects into a container. The container is attached to a point lower than the person's urinary bladder. An in-dwelling catheter is always a closed system, which means it is never opened except when the urine collecting bag is emptied.

In males, the catheter is sometimes surgically placed directly into the bladder, this type of catheter is referred to as supra pubic. The tubing is secured to the abdomen to reduce the pressure on the catheter and provide the straightest route for the urine to drain.

Urinary in-dwelling catheters drain by straight drainage from the patient into a bag (see Figure 17.5). This type of drainage gets its name from the fact that the tubing from the bed to the bag must be kept straight and all other tubing must be kept above the tubing from the bed to the bag. When the tubing is in its proper position, the urine drains freely into the bag. If the tubing is not in the proper position, the urine could back up into the bladder or the kidneys (see Procedure 17.3).

Leg Drainage Bag

A leg bag is a small plastic collection bag worn on the individual's leg. This apparatus allows the patient to be more active than when using the traditional straight drainage technique. It cannot be used when the person is lying down because the urine cannot drain properly in that position.

Use the same techniques to prevent infection when changing a straight drainage bag as you use for putting on a leg bag (see Procedure 17.4). Be sure to double-check that the bag is aligned correctly, with the top facing upward so the urine drains properly. Empty the bag immediately after it is removed or when it is full. If the patient is on intake and output (I&O), record the amount of urine collected.

PROCEDURE 17.3

Catheter Care

Rationale

Correct catheter care decreases the risk of infection and contributes to the patient's overall comfort.

Note: This procedure may be incorporated into the morning bath routine. Be sure you use clean water for this procedure.

1. Assemble your equipment: basin of water and mild soap or cleaning solution, washcloth or gauze pads, paper or plastic bag for waste, disposable gloves.
2. Wash your hands.
3. Ask visitors to leave the room, if appropriate.
4. Tell the patient you are going to give him catheter care.
5. Position the patient on his back so the catheter and urinary meatus are exposed. Put on your gloves.
6. Wash the area gently. Do not pull on the catheter, but hold it with one hand while wiping it with the other (see Figure 17.6).

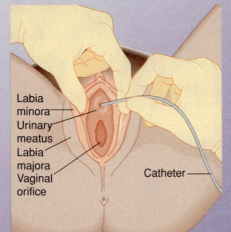

Labia
minora
Urinary
meatus
Labia
majora
Vaginal
orifice

Catheter

FIGURE 17.6 Be sure to keep the entire perineum clean in female clients to prevent irritation and infection.

7. Observe the meatus for redness, swelling, or discharge.
8. Wipe away from the meatus. Wipe from the meatus to the anus.
9. Wipe one way and not back and forth.
10. Remove your gloves.
11. Dry the area.
12. Apply lotion or powder in small quantities to the thighs. Ask the physician if this area should be kept dry or moist.
13. Make the patient comfortable.
14. Dispose of the dirty water in the toilet. Clean your equipment and put it in its proper place.
15. Wash your hands.

PROCEDURE 17.4

Changing a Catheter from a Straight Drainage Bag to a Leg Bag

Rationale

Changing correctly to and from a leg bag increases the patient's comfort and mobility and decreases the risk of infection.

1. Assemble your equipment: leg bag with straps, disposable gloves, alcohol wipes or antiseptic solution, sterile cover for straight drainage tubing, and sterile 4 × 4 bed protector.
2. Wash your hands and put on gloves.
3. Ask visitors to leave the room, if appropriate.
4. Tell the patient you are going to put on his leg bag.
5. Expose the end of the catheter and the drainage tubing. Put the bed protector under this area.
6. Disconnect the drainage tubing from the catheter and allow it to drain. Put a sterile cover on the end of the tubing, and place it out of the way but not on the floor. Do not put the catheter on the bed.
7. Wipe the attachment tube of the leg bag with an alcohol swab and insert the tube into the catheter.
8. Secure the leg bag to the patient's thigh.
9. Make the patient comfortable.
10. Empty the drainage bag. If the patient is on intake and output (I&O), measure the urine and note it on the log.
11. Remove gloves and wash your hands.

Uses of External Urinary Drainage Systems

When a male is incontinent, the nurse may suggest the use of a temporary drainage system that collects the urine and keeps the patient dry. One end of the catheter is kept in place at the end of the penis and one end is connected to a tube that hangs straight down into a collection container (see Procedure 17.5).

This straight drainage system should not be left on for more than twenty-four hours at a time. It must be removed at least that often so that the penis may be washed and inspected). If there is any change in the skin and the individual complains of pain or discomfort or the catheter does not drain, remove the catheter and drainage container, discard it, and call the physician. Observe the patient shortly after the catheter has been applied and then frequently when you are with him.

INTRAVENOUS THERAPY

Intravenous therapy (IV) is prescribed by a physician and administered by a registered nurse. During this procedure, the nurse inserts a needle into one of the patient's veins to provide a way to give fluids or medication. The medication or fluids are given by single injection and continuous drip slowly from a bag

PROCEDURE 17.5

External Urinary Drainage

Rationale

Correct application of external drainage decreases the risk of infection and skin breakdown, and increases the patient's general well-being and dignity.

1. Assemble your equipment: external urinary system (consisting of a condom, a catheter, and a straight drainage system), material to secure condom to penis (tape, strap, or adhesive foam), soap, water, towel, disposable gloves.
2. Wash your hands.
3. Ask visitors to leave the room, if appropriate.
4. Tell the patient you are going to put on an external urinary collection device. Put on gloves.
5. Position the patient on his back so that the penis is exposed. Cover the patient so he is not exposed.
6. Wash the entire penis and dry thoroughly. Observe the penis for any discharge or redness.
7. Roll the condom onto the entire length of the penis.
8. Secure the condom. Be sure the strap is tight enough to hold the condom in place but not so tight as to hurt the patient.
9. Attach the catheter to the condom and to the straight drainage. Secure the collection bag on a bed or chair.
10. Make the patient comfortable.
11. Dispose of the dirty water in the toilet. Clean your equipment and put it in its proper place.
12. Remove gloves and wash your hands.

or pump that regulates the flow of medication or nourishment through a tube secured to the needle. The following are types of IV infusion:

- *Continuous infusion:* Fluid and/or medication is always running. This type of therapy is most often prescribed for an individual who has a family member or friend who can assume responsibility for the insertion site and care of the IV bags.
- *Intermittent infusion:* Small amounts of fluid or medication are given for short times. Each time a dose is needed, the IV must be started again.

There are three types of intravenous therapy:

- *Peripheral line:* Veins, usually of the upper extremities, are used.
- *Central venous line:* A catheter is surgically implanted into one of the large veins. This type of catheter is used when the medication is irritating to the blood vessels or must be given frequently, or when large amounts of medication must be given. The end of the catheter used for medication administration is visible on the chest area. Family members and the caregiver should be taught by the physician or nurse prior to

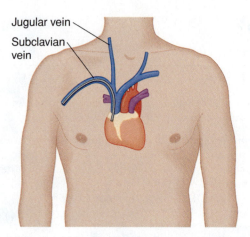

FIGURE 17.7   Central lines should be cared for as prescribed by the physician. Be sure to immediately report to your supervisor any discomfort the patient describes.

performing catheter care. Do not touch the catheter until you have received instruction in how to use it (see Figure 17.7).

- *Peripherally inserted central venous catheter (PICC):* This catheter is inserted at the bedside by a specially trained nurse or physician. The tube is inserted directly from the arm vein to the heart. The PICC line is used for long-term use of antibiotics. The care of this catheter and the dressing can be taught to the caregiver and family members by the physician or nurse. Do not remove the dressing unless you have been instructed to do so and how to do so.

YOUR ROLE AS A CAREGIVER

Be observant and supportive. Support the patient and her or his family members as they learn to care for the equipment. A patient who has a continuous infusion may walk around as long as the IV bag of fluid is above the insertion site and does not pull on the tubing. Remind the patient not to sit or lean on the tubing.

Central venous lines are covered by a dressing when not in use. A peripheral line sometimes has a cap on it when it is not in use. This cap is usually covered by a dressing. The caregiver is responsible for making sure that the dressing stays dry and clean. The dressing should be checked at least every eight hours to be sure it is secure. You should also be alert to changes in the site and report them immediately. Report to the physician if:

- the patient complains of pain in the area
- the area is red, hot, and/or swollen
- you can see blood or any drainage from the area
- the patient removes the needle or tubing, or if the needle or tubing falls out
- the tubing contains blood

- the level of fluid in the bag does not decrease
- the bag breaks

Be sure to document when you check the dressing. Write down that you checked the area and the condition of the dressing and the skin.

CAST CARE

A patient who has broken a bone or sprained or strained a muscle may have a cast or splint placed on the body part to immobilize it. The procedure provides support to the injured part and prevents deformity by keeping it in the correct body alignment. Splints and casts are temporary. Permanent support to the bones in the form of pins, plates, and replacement of joints may also be necessary.

Plaster casts are, in reality, a form of bandage. They are used as a support to hold injured bones in alignment while they are healing. Casts are wet when applied, then allowed to dry. Once they are hardened, the casts should be kept dry. Plastic or fiberglass casts perform the same task but are lighter, cleaner, and easier to use and remove.

While a plaster cast is drying, the patient's position must be maintained and the cast left uncovered. It is normal for the cast to feel hot to the touch as it is drying. Pillows can be placed to support the cast so it will not move while it is still soft.

Keep the following points in mind when caring for a patient who is wearing a cast:

- A cast should not restrict circulation to the part of the body in the cast.
- A cast should not cause pain. The pain should be only from the healing bone or muscle.
- The skin under a cast frequently itches. Do not put anything into the cast because you might cause a scratch that can lead to a skin infection.
- If the body part that is casted swells, the cast can become too tight and create pressure areas. If this occurs, contact the physician immediately.

YOUR ROLE AS A CAREGIVER

Keep the cast clean and dry. It should be protected while a patient is using the bedpan or toilet and when bathing. Do not wash a plaster cast because it will crumble. A plastic grocery bag can be tied around the cast to protect it from becoming wet.

Some casts can be wet and allowed to air dry. Check with the patient and the physician about the care for each cast. Just because casts look alike does not mean that they are cared for in the same way.

Encourage your patient to take an active part in his cast care. Some people feel restricted in a cast and do not use the part of the body in a cast as much as they are able. This unnecessary restriction of activity leads to a feeling of uselessness and loss of muscle tone.

Frequent and careful checking of the cast and the injured body part helps prevent complications. Call your supervisor if you notice any of the following:

- Patient complaints of numbness or tingling in toes or fingers
- Discoloration of the toes or fingers
- Swelling of the limb at the edge of the cast
- Unusual odors coming from the cast
- Rough or cracked edges on the cast
- A loosely fitting cast
- Discolorations on the cast

A patient may ask you how much movement she will have when the cast is removed. Tell her that you will learn the answer for her. Then call the physician and discuss what to tell the patient. Do not promise the patient that she will be fine unless that is what the physician has told her. Beware of telling her that everyone who has a broken arm is eventually back to normal because everyone heals differently.

OSTOMY CARE

The creation of an ostomy is a surgical procedure. An ostomy is a new opening in the abdomen for the release of wastes from the body. The opening is called a stoma. This operation is necessary when the colon or urinary system is diseased or injured. Ostomies are created for many reasons, not only because a patient has cancer. Sometimes, the surgery is done to allow the colon to heal following an injury. Some ostomies are temporary and others are permanent. The word *ostomy* means "opening into." A colostomy is an opening into the colon. An ileostomy is an opening into the ileum. An ureterostomy is an opening into the ureter. The opening is from the abdominal wall to the affected organ. The visible part is the stoma, which looks like a pink rosebud (see Figure 17.8).

There are several types of colostomies. The specific name of a colostomy comes from the placement of the stoma. It can be in the ascending, descending, or transverse colon. It can have one opening (single barrel) or two openings side by side (double barrel). The surgeon decides which type of colostomy is made.

A person with an ostomy must wear an appliance to collect the matter released through the stoma. This collection bag is held over the stoma by special paste, adhesive, and/or a belt (see Figure 17.9). Some ostomy appliances are permanent, which means that they are reused after they are cleaned and dried. Some bags are disposable and used only once (see Figure 17.10).

Undergoing an ostomy is a life-alerting experience and is usually a traumatic occurrence. It requires a big change in the way the person excretes either urine or fecal matter. It requires changes in the daily routine of the individual and often of family members. An ostomy changes the person's body image.

Every patient and his or her family members react differently to this experience. Some people learn the new routines and return to their previous

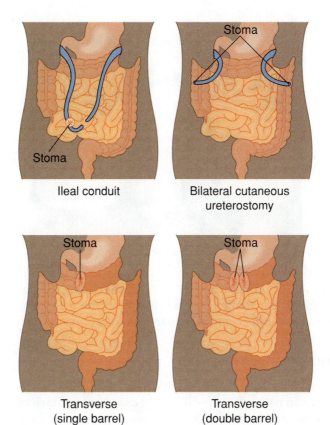

Ileal conduit

Bilateral cutaneous ureterostomy

Transverse (single barrel)

Transverse (double barrel)

FIGURE 17.8   The physician determines the placement and type of ostomy before surgery.

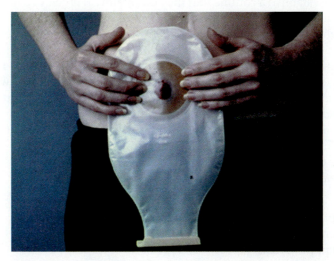

FIGURE 17.9   The choice of collection device is a personal one.

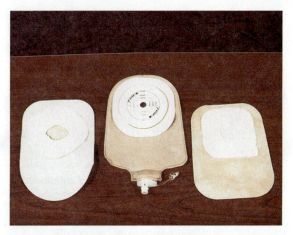

FIGURE 17.10 There are various types of ostomy appliances.

lifestyles. Some individuals do not. Be alert to the coping mechanisms of your patient and his or her family members. Support them as they learn how to care for the ostomy and become familiar with the appliances.

YOUR ROLE AS A CAREGIVER

When you receive your assignment, the patient's physician will explain why the patient has an ostomy. You will be told exactly how much of the patient's care you will be responsible for. You will also be told what the patient knows about her operation.

Your patient's goal is to be as self-sufficient as possible. If the patient cannot assume her total care, you will assist the patient and her family members as they establish a routine that they can maintain when you are no longer in the home.

If, while you are caring for a patient, that patient must have an operation for an ostomy, the patient and his family members may want to discuss this operation with you. They will ask you questions. Do not lie to them. If they ask you questions that you cannot answer, assure them you will get the answers from the physician. If the patient asks you questions about death, recovery, and the future and you are uncomfortable discussing this information with the patient, discuss these topics with the health care team social worker or nurse. Frequently, a patient or family member will ask you the same question many times, which is a way of confirming that the first answer you gave was the real one.

All ostomy care is based on several considerations:

- Aseptic technique (rules of cleanliness)
- Patient's and family members' reactions to the procedure
- Patient prognosis
- Frequent changing of the collection bag

A collection bag must be changed when it is full or when the adhering seal is broken. Some patients will be well enough to sit in the bathroom on the toilet to do this procedure. Also, many patients will be learning to do this procedure independently, in which case you will assist them less and less.

Some patients irrigate their colostomy as part of their routine. Irrigating a colostomy is like giving an enema into the ostomy. After you have received the appropriate instruction, you may assist the patient as he carries out this procedure.

As a caregiver, you will be assisting patients and their family members in many phases of ostomy care. Patients are often afraid of or disgusted by this procedure. Be patient and understanding. Let the person and the family members express their feelings. Listen. Although most ostomy patients are encouraged to assume their own care, they do so at different paces. Respect the individual's feelings and wishes. Discuss with the health care team your patient's reactions and your own feelings about the tasks you are performing. In this way, you will gain a better understanding of your patient and yourself (see Procedure 17.6).

PROCEDURE 17.6

Assisting with an Ostomy

Rationale

Assisting with ostomy care contributes to the patient's independence and overall well-being, and decreases the risk of skin irritation.

Note: Each patient has his own routine for caring for his ostomy. Procedure 17.6 is a general guide.

1. Assemble your equipment: bedpan, disposable bed protector, bath blanket, clean ostomy belt (adjustable ostomy appliance), toilet tissue, basin of water, soap or cleanser, washcloth, disposable gloves, towels, lubricant or skin cream (as ordered), plastic waste bag.
2. Wash your hands.
3. Ask any visitors to leave the room, if appropriate.
4. Tell the patient that you are going to assist him with changing his ostomy appliance.
5. Cover the patient with the bath blanket. Ask the patient to hold the top edge of the blanket. Without exposing the patient, fan-fold the top sheet and bedspread to the foot of the bed under the blanket.
6. Place the disposable bed protector under the patient's hips to keep the bed from becoming wet or dirty.
7. Place the bedpan within easy reach.
8. Put the washbasin, soap, washcloth, and bath towels near the bed. Put on gloves.
9. Open the belt. Protect it if it is clean and can be used again. If the belt is dirty, remove it. It must be replaced with a clean one.
10. Remove the soiled plastic stoma bag from the belt carefully.

(continued)

11. Put the soiled plastic bag into the bedpan. Wipe the area around the ostomy with toilet tissue to remove any loose feces. Place the dirty tissue in the plastic bag. Flush the tissues down the toilet later.
12. Wet and soap the washcloth. Wash the entire ostomy area with a gentle circular motion.
13. Dry the area gently with a bath towel.
14. Apply a small amount of lubricant or protective cream (if ordered) around the area of the ostomy. The lubricant is to prevent irritation to the skin around the ostomy. Wipe off all excess lubricant so that the ostomy device will adhere to the skin.
15. If using a wafer, secure it around the stoma. Be sure the wafer is the correct size (see Figure 17.11).

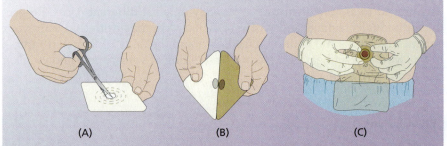

(A)	(B)	(C)
Cut the hole in the center of the wafer 1/8-inch larger than the stoma.	Peel the backing from the wafer.	Place the wafer around the stoma and attach a clean bag.

FIGURE 17.11

16. Put a clean adjustable belt, if the patient wears one, on the patient. Place a clean stoma bag through the loop.
17. Remove the disposable bed protector. Change any damp linen.
18. Replace the top sheet and bedspread, and remove the bath blanket.
19. Make the patient comfortable.
20. Remove all used equipment. Dispose of waste material into the toilet. Do not throw the plastic collection bag down the toilet; place it into the plastic liner in the wastebasket.
21. Clean the bedpan and put it in its proper place.
22. Empty the washbasin in the toilet. Wash it thoroughly with soap and water. Rinse and dry it and return it to its proper place.
23. Remove gloves and wash your hands.

Other Ostomies

Other types of ostomies involve surgical openings directly into various parts of the upper gastrointestinal tract. Which organ is opened depends on the disease or injured part of the gastrointestinal tract of the patient. Here are some examples:

- Gastrostomy is an opening to the stomach through which nutrients in liquid form are provided to the person. A bolus feeding is one in which the liquid is injected through the tube once or at intervals throughout

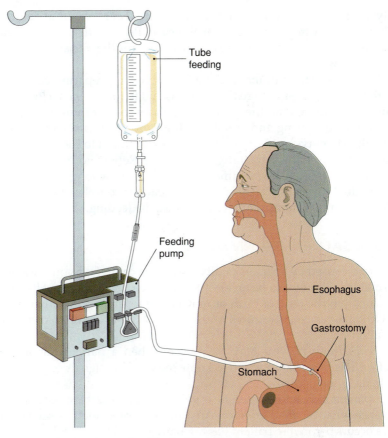

Tube feeding

Feeding pump

Esophagus

Gastrostomy

Stomach

FIGURE 17.12   A pump keeps the tube feeding drain at a predetermined rate.

the day, or it is continuous, which means that a feeding pump (similar to an intravenous [IV] pump) is connected all or most of the day and provides a continuous flow of nutrients to the patient.

- Duodenostomy is an opening to the abdomen directly at the duodenum (the beginning of the small intestine). This ostomy is also used for giving the patient nutrients via a tube. These feedings have to be continuous or the feeding might back up into the lungs.
- Jejunostomy is another ostomy surgically inserted into the small intestine and used for continuous tube feeding.

These incisions are kept open by the presence of a tube or a screw cap. The patient will receive part or all of his nourishment through this opening. He may also take his medication through this opening (see Figure 17.12).

YOUR ROLE AS A CAREGIVER

Your role in working with a patient who has one of these openings is to assist him in feedings and in the care of the area. You will not be given complete responsibility for the procedure because it is important that a family member be able to assist the individual when you are not there. Cleanliness is an important part of the care. Be sure that the patient's or family member's hands are clean before caring for the site and before starting the feeding.

Assist the patient in making the feeding or in preparing commercially prepared feeding. Be sure to read directions and to follow them closely. When mixing the solution, date the container with important information such as date and time of mixing and initial use. It is wise to discard any feeding that is more than twenty-four hours old. Warm the solution to room temperature. Observe how the patient tolerates the feeding. Report your observations to the health care team. Note the time of the feeding, how long it lasts, and how the individual tolerates it. Also note if the patient complains of any nausea, vomiting, diarrhea, cramps, or sweating after the feeding.

SEIZURE-SAFE ENVIRONMENT

A seizure is caused by an abnormality within the central nervous system. This abnormality is thought to be an electrical problem in the nerve cells. Seizures can occur from the time of birth or may be the result of a head injury or disease. Often, the cause of seizures is unknown. Seizures are often controlled by medication.

As a caregiver, you may be present when a patient has a seizure. Therefore, it is important for you to know the warning signals of a seizure and what to do if one occurs.

A patient may know when he is going to have a seizure because he may experience what is called an aura. An aura may be a smell or sensation that always occurs before the patient has a seizure.

There are two types of seizures: grand mal and petit mal. The latter is a partial-body seizure.

The grand mal seizure may include stiffness of the total body, followed by a jerking action of the muscles. Usually, the patient becomes unconscious. The patient may bite her tongue or become incontinent. These seizures can last for several minutes.

In the petit mal seizure, the patient may appear to be daydreaming. Her eyes may roll back and there may be some quivering of the body muscles. The petit mal seizure usually lasts less than thirty seconds. The patient usually has no memory of the seizure. A patient who has been diagnosed as having epilepsy or who has seizures due to other diseases often leads a normal, productive life. Other people's ignorance about seizures is the patient's biggest enemy.

YOUR ROLE AS A CAREGIVER

Your role as a caregiver in caring for a patient having a seizure is to prevent the patient from injuring himself. If you are present at the beginning of a seizure, you may turn the patient's head to the side. If the patient's jaw is already tight or his teeth are clenched, *do not try to pry his teeth apart.* Help the patient lie down on the floor. Loosen his clothing and move any furniture that he might hit as he moves. Place a pillow or something soft under his head. *Turn his head to the side to promote drainage of saliva or vomitus. Never try to move or restrain the patient.* Protect the patient from people who may stare at him. Protect him from embarrassment.

Comfort the patient after the seizure. Clean him of any saliva, urine, or fecal matter. Assist him with mouth care and care of his body after the seizure. After the patient is comfortable and safe, contact the physician.

BLOOD SUGAR TESTING

Testing urine provides an accurate and easy method of checking how much acetone may be present. These procedures are usually conducted for diabetic patients (see Chapter 18) and may be done with patients who have other disorders. The Acetest or Ketostix reagent strip determines the amount of acetone or ketones in the urine. The physician will prescribe when the test should be done and what equipment to use.

For each test, use either a reagent strip or a reagent tablet. A reagent is a substance used in a chemical reaction to determine the presence of another substance. The names of these tablets or strips vary greatly according to geographical area and the pharmaceutical company that makes them. Instructions for these tests are on the package of reagent strips or reagent tablets. Be sure to follow the instructions exactly. All tablets and strips used for these tests are poisonous. Always put equipment in a safe place where children or confused adults cannot reach them. Be sure to wash and dry all equipment between tests and keep bottles tightly closed. Some readings are recorded as percentages and some as "plus" (+, ++, +++, etc.). Be sure you ask how the patient reports her readings.

For testing the urine, a small amount of fresh specimen is needed. The word *fresh* is used to refer to urine that has accumulated recently in the patient's urinary bladder. The word *fractional* is used to refer to a small portion of the urine voided. To obtain fresh urine, it is necessary to discard the first urine voided because this urine has remained in the bladder for an unknown length of time. One-half hour after discarding the urine, collect a fresh urine specimen (the urine that has recently accumulated in the urinary bladder) for the test.

The amount of glucose in the blood indicates the amount of medication and food the diabetic person must have. Diabetic patients are taught how to monitor their blood glucose by using one of several testing devices (see Procedure 17.7). They are also instructed how to record their findings and how to adjust their medication. The device and the timing of the tests are prescribed by the physician and may be different for each patient.

DEEP BREATHING

Shallow breathing takes place in the upper lobes of the lungs, which are surrounded by bony areas on all sides. The lungs cannot expand much in the bony enclosure, so they cannot take in much oxygen or exhale much carbon

PROCEDURE 17.7

Testing Blood for Glucose

Rationale

Testing blood correctly contributes to the patient's general well-being and assists with ongoing monitoring of her medication, diet, and exercise regime.

1. Assemble your equipment: One-Touch profile meter, test strips, penlet and lancet, disposable pipette, disposable gloves, band-aid.
2. Wash your hands.
3. Explain to the patient that you are going to test her blood sugar.
4. Make the patient comfortable and wash her hands with soap and water.
5. Put on disposable gloves.
6. Match the code on the test strips to the number on the meter. Check the expiration date on the test strips. Discard them if they have expired. The code number may have to be reset. Follow the manufacturer's instructions.
7. Remove test strip from container. Close the container. Do not touch the white area of the strip.
8. Press the power button and insert the strip into the meter (see Figure 17.13).

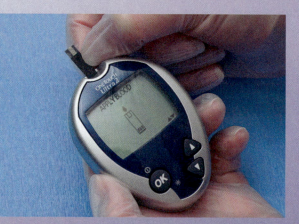

FIGURE 17.13 Make sure the monitor is turned on and insert the test strip into the glucometer in the designated slot.

9. Insert the lancet into the penlet (if applicable) according to the manufacturer's directions.
10. Place the end of the lancet firmly against the side of a fingertip of the patient.
11. Press the button on top of the penlet.
12. Squeeze the finger gently to obtain a large drop of blood, which is discarded.
13. Obtain a second drop of blood and apply it to the testing strip.
14. Wait a short time for the results to appear on the blood glucose meter.
15. Apply a band-aid to the patient's finger.
16. Remove disposable gloves and wash your hands.

PROCEDURE 17.8

Helping a Patient with Deep-Breathing Exercises

Rationale

Teaching the patient deep-breathing exercises helps reduce anxiety and promotes overall mental wellness.

1. Assemble your equipment: equipment for mouth care following this procedure, tissues, basin or specimen container, plastic bag for waste.
2. Wash your hands.
3. Ask visitors to leave the room, if appropriate.
4. Tell the patient you are going to help him with deep-breathing exercises.
5. Direct the patient to breathe in deeply through his nose.
6. Direct the patient to blow out through his mouth with his lips pursed, as though he were blowing out a match.
7. Repeat steps 1 to 6 ten times.
8. Offer the patient mouth care.
9. Dispose of the tissues into a plastic bag.
10. Make the patient comfortable.

dioxide. People who have had lung disease for a long time have barrel chests. The chest cavity has taken on this shape in an attempt to make the lungs inhale more oxygen.

Deep breathing helps people inhale more air with less effort than their usual type of breathing. When people breathe deeply, the lower lobes of the lungs push the soft tissue of the abdomen out of the way and expand to take in more air. People who have lung disease continue to breathe with shallow breaths because of fear and misinformation about how their bodies work. You can help your patient trust deep breathing by explaining how the lungs work (see Procedure 17.8).

YOUR ROLE AS A CAREGIVER

A patient who is learning to breathe deeply is often frightened. Be patient and gentle. Praise the person and point out small successes. Continue to reinforce the reasons why deep breathing is important.

When the patient takes a deep breath, his shoulders and chest should *not* move. His abdomen should expand. When he exhales his abdomen should become *flat*. If the individual is confused about how to do breathe deeply, tell him to cough. The squeezing of the abdominal area will make him aware of where the muscular activity should take place. Coughing is forced expiration. Deep breathing sometimes produces a coughing response, especially if the lungs are congested. Keep a basin, tissue, or specimen container (if ordered) near the patient. Collect any mucous he may bring up. Encourage him to spit it out. Note the color, amount, and odor.

Protect the patient from visitors and friends when he is coughing. Deep breathing is frequently unpleasant, although it is important. Because it can also make people cough and bring up mucous, plan this exercise between mealtimes so you will not cause vomiting or loss of appetite.

The physical or respiratory therapist will instruct you about how often to do this exercise. She may also give you special instructions for your patient. Remember, all patients are different. Although the exercise may look the same for two people, it may be done for different reasons. The physical therapist will also tell you of any special observations you are to make while you help the patient.

Even though you are trained to do these exercises, do not start them until the therapist says that the patient is ready to progress to such exercises. The aim of teaching patients deep breathing, also called abdominal breathing, is to change their breathing habits permanently.

MAKING NORMAL SALINE

Normal saline is a solution of salt and water that has many uses. Its chemical makeup is close to that of the fluids in the body. It is usually used to wash open areas or to clean sore bony prominences or bedsores. It may also be used by a nurse to irrigate a Foley catheter. Procedure 17.9 gives the recipe and instructions on creating normal saline at home.

SITZ BATH

The term *sitz bath* means "seat bath" or a "bath taken while seated." The area bathed is the perineal area. Such a procedure may be ordered to promote healing of the area, to decrease pain following surgery or a procedure, and to increase relaxation of the muscles in the perineal area. The patient can take a sitz

PROCEDURE 17.9

Making Normal Saline

Rationale

Making normal saline decreases the need for the patient to purchase saline and contributes to infection control in the home.

1. Assemble your equipment: large pot, sterilized one-quart jar and lid, two teaspoons of salt, one quart of water, source of heat (stove, sterno, fire).
2. Wash your hands.
3. Measure one quart of water into the pot. Add two teaspoons of salt. Boil, covered, for ten minutes.
4. Pour the sterile saline into the sterilized jar, and replace cover. Allow the solution to cool.
5. The solution may be used up to forty-eight hours after preparation.

bath either in a specially designed bath that fits into the toilet or commode or in a bathtub that has had a covered rubber ring placed in it so that the perineal area is suspended off the tub floor.

Safety Considerations

Be sure the water is the correct temperature. It should be comfortable to the touch and measure between 95° and 110°F or between 35° and 43°C. Water that is too hot will burn the patient, and water that is too cold will cause the muscles to tighten up rather than relax.

Help the patient start and finish the procedure. Safely getting on and off the commode or in and out of the tub should be done slowly and at the patient's speed. Protect the patient from slipping and falling on towels, clothes, or dressings.

Maintain the water temperature by adding warm water when necessary.

Help the patient keep track of the time. The usual length of time for a sitz bath is between ten and fifteen minutes. You will be told how long and how often your patient should have a sitz bath by the physician. Check on your patient frequently and tell her how long she has yet to go. Ask your patient how she feels and also observe her.

YOUR ROLE AS A CAREGIVER

Your role as a caregiver is to help the patient take his sitz bath as it has been ordered. If you find the patient deviates from the order, report those changes to the physician.

You will also be responsible for cleaning the sitz bath or the bathtub following the procedure. Be sure that the bath area is clean and dry and ready for the next time the patient must bathe. Assist the patient with dressings that he may have to apply and dispose of soiled dressings in plastic bags in the outside trash.

Following the procedure, and after the patient is comfortable and the area is clean, you can note any of the following elements, as necessary:

- The patient's reaction to the bath
- A description of any drainage from the wounds
- How the patient finished the procedure—new dressing, returned to bed, and so on

TOTAL PARENTERAL NUTRITION

Patients who are severely malnourished and who are unable to eat may receive their nutritional requirements by means of total parenteral nutrition (TPN). For long-term administration, a catheter is surgically placed in a large vein and the nutrition is administered directly into the bloodstream. A physician orders the exact dose of the supplement, which must be mixed by a pharmacy. A pharmacy or company specializing in this service has the responsibility for delivering the correct feeding to the patient every twenty-four hours. The catheter used for the feeding is used for no other purpose. Some bottles or bags must be kept refrigerated. Some must be at room temperature. If the delivery does not arrive on time or you notice that the feedings are stored improperly, call the physician. Do not discard any unused feedings. Return them to the pharmacy.

Patients may receive this treatment for a short amount of time or for several years. Some patients receive their feedings in the evening, thus making it possible for the person to go to work during the day. Others receive feedings over a twenty-four-hour period. Patients who receive this treatment must be able to assume responsibility for feedings or have responsible family members who can perform this task. This teaching usually takes place in the hospital and is reinforced in the home by the company that brings the feedings. Be sure you and the patient have the emergency telephone numbers to call with questions. The professionals from the supply company are responsible for checking the pump and the catheter insertion site. If family members have any questions between visits, they should be encouraged to contact the suppliers via the emergency telephone numbers. You will not be asked to administer the feedings or change the dressings on the catheter, but you will be responsible for assisting with preparation and/or patient self-administration of the feedings.

YOUR ROLE AS A CAREGIVER

You will care for the patient's personal needs during administration of the TPN and help the family members incorporate this task into their regular routine. Look for any changes in the patient. Report these changes immediately to the physician. If you are to keep a record of intake and output, vital signs, and weights, do so accurately. Keep the following points in mind:

- Report any shortness of breath, tingling in the patient's arms or feet, weakness, or temperature change.
- Report any irritation or drainage near the catheter site.
- Report any change(s) in the patient.
- Help the patient maintain a comfortable position during the feeding. The tubes should be straight and not under the patient's body. Help the patient identify the place in the house where he or she prefers the feeding to be administered.

HOT AND COLD COMPRESSES

Compresses are used to decrease swelling, increase circulation, and manage pain. Procedure 17.10 indicates how to apply a hot compress. It is important to note that a container specially designed for hot fluid or chemicals that create heat should be used for this procedure. For cold compresses, ice is often used and should be in a leak-proof container that is flexible to lay on the designated area of the body. Procedure 17.11 reviews how to apply a cold compress.

PROCEDURE 17.10

Applying a Hot Compress

Rationale

Use of a hot compress can decrease swelling, promote healing, and manage pain.

1. Assemble your equipment: hot pack, thermometer, water, heating pad or physician-recommended chemical pack or solution.
2. Wash your hands.
3. Make sure the patient is in a comfortable position.
4. Expose the area where the hot compress will be used.
5. Prepare the compress by heating per instructions on the pack or by heating water to a temperature between 105°F and 110°F. Dry off the water pack. If using a chemical pack, make sure there are no holes in the package to avoid chemical leakage. Follow the instructions on the pack to activate it.
6. Test the compress on your skin to ensure it will not burn the patient.
7. Slowly place the compress directly to the skin of the desired area. Check the temperature of the water; when the water cools, replace with warm water. Do not leave a hot compress for more than fifteen to thirty minutes total or as otherwise directed by the physician.
8. Observe the area for any redness, swelling, or pain. Stop the procedure if any discomfort occurs.
9. Empty the water (if used) and dry the container (if reusable). If using a chemical pack, discard it in the trash after use. If using a heating pad, make sure it is unplugged and put it away after the treatment.

PROCEDURE 17.11

Applying a Cold Compress

Rationale

Cold compresses are used to prevent or decrease swelling, manage pain, and decrease body temperature.

1. Assemble equipment: ice pack, chemical cold pack, towel.
2. Wash your hands.
3. If you are using an ice pack, fill the ice pack only to the point where it is still flexible enough to fit on the area where it will be applied. Dry off the pack.
4. If you are using a cold chemical pack, ensure that there are not holes in the package to prevent the chemical from leaking. Follow the instruction on the pack to activate it.
5. Apply to the affected area. Cold can be applied directly to the skin; however, a towel is often used between the cold pack and the skin at first to allow the skin to adjust to the cooling temperature.

(continued)

6. Frequently ask the patient if the temperature is adequate or too cold for comfort. If the pack becomes warm before the treatment is done, empty the water and refill with ice.
7. If any redness, irritation to the skin, swelling, or pain occurs, remove the cold compress.
8. Do not use a cold compress longer than fifteen to thirty minutes at a time.
9. Empty the melted ice and dry the container if it is reusable. If using a chemical pack, discard it in the trash.

Summary

The procedures discussed in this chapter are the most commonly performed at home by a caregiver. Typically most individuals feel uneasy about undergoing these procedures; therefore, it is important to get accurate instructions from the physician for providing the care. Follow the directions given by the physician to avoid errors in care. If you are not comfortable completing these tasks, talk to the health care team for support and guidance.

Chapter 18

Common Diseases

SCENARIO

Mr. Martinez has just been told he has diabetes. He is a sales representative in a small store and fears that his employer will not understand that he has to eat frequent meals. His family members are supportive and interested in changing their lifestyle if necessary to treat his disease, but he refuses to discuss it. His children have checked out several library books and have printed a great deal of information from the Internet. They are sure that Mr. Martinez will be able to continue working and that his life will be as full and enjoyable as it was prior to his diagnosis. Mr. Martinez is not as confident.

HYPERTENSION

Hypertension, or high blood pressure, is a treatable chronic disease. People who have hypertension have more stress placed on their circulatory systems than people without high blood pressure. Latest estimates are that more than 50 million Americans suffer from hypertension. Hypertension contributes to death from heart disease and kidney disease. Treatment for hypertension is available, but it must be a permanent part of an individual's daily routine. Bringing blood pressure to an acceptable level does not mean the disease has gone away; it only means that the disease has been brought under control, and this control must be continued.

Symptoms of Hypertension

Hypertension has been called "the silent killer" because it gives no warning. The early stages of this disease often show no symptoms. As the disease develops, people may complain of headaches, vision changes, or problems with their urinary output. If they would consult a physician at this point in their disease, permanent damage to the heart could be avoided. Some people with high blood pressure

343

do not seek help until they have severe problems. By that time, permanent damage to vital organs is common (see Chapter 14 for details of blood pressure readings that can be of concern). Individuals have a higher risk of hypertension if they:

- Have a family history of hypertension, heart disease, or kidney disease
- Smoke cigarettes
- Are overweight
- Use a lot of salt in their diet
- Are African American
- Eat large amounts of saturated fats

Causes and Treatment of Hypertension

Many conditions seem to cause hypertension, and some causes are still unknown. Research scientists are investigating diet, heredity, weight, certain medications, kidney infections, and chemicals as possible causes of this chronic disease. An individualized treatment plan is developed by a physician after a thorough medical examination. Treatment may consist of a combination of diet, medication, and exercise.

YOUR ROLE AS A CAREGIVER

Follow the plan of care for your patient. Support the person you are caring for by complying with her medication plan, diet, and exercise. Report to the appropriate members of the health care team any deviation from the care plan. Assist the patient with incorporating her treatment into her usual daily routine. Because your patient will always be on some treatment for this disease, it is important that the treatment become a regular part of her day.

Listen to your patient. If she has questions about hypertension and/or her treatment, answer her honestly. If you do not know the answer, talk to the appropriate member of the health care team and be sure that the patient receives her answers.

Be observant for possible side effects from any medication that your patient uses. Depending on the drug and the patient, side effects range from a stuffy nose to muscle cramps, weakness, nightmares, and impotence. Careful objective observations and timely reporting of these and other symptoms will result in a treatment plan the patient can live with the rest of her life. If the patient starts taking any medications, including nonprescription drugs, report this to the physician and/or nurse.

HEART ATTACK/MYOCARDIAL INFARCTION

Heart attack is a general term that describes sudden damage to the heart. People have heart attacks for many medical reasons, but they all have the same results; a decrease in the blood supply to the heart eventually leads to heart muscle damage and possibly permanent tissue death.

The word *infarct* means "death of tissue due to lack of blood." The word *myocardial* refers to heart muscle. So a myocardial infarction (MI) is really the death of part of the heart due to a blockage in a blood vessel. If the blood vessel involved is a small one and only a small amount of heart muscle is affected, the patient may suffer only a minor or small heart attack. If the blood vessel involved is a large one and a large portion of the heart is damaged, it is often called a massive heart attack. The ultimate recovery of the injured heart depends on the location of the MI within the heart; the presence of atherosclerosis; and the age, sex, and health history of the individual.

Arteriosclerosis is the hardening of arteries and leads to a decrease in the blood supply to body tissue due to a thickening of vessel walls. Atherosclerosis is a form of arteriosclerosis that takes place in several steps:

- A fatty streak develops in the vessel.
- A fibrous plaque develops on top of the fatty streak. Depending on the size of this plaque, the vessel remains open or becomes completely obstructed.
- Sometimes, a clot develops in the same spot as the fibrous plaque.

If atherosclerosis is discovered and treated after the first stage, the condition is reversible. Once a vessel is completely blocked by plaque, however, it usually remains that way.

Signs of a Heart Attack

The following signs and symptoms may appear in your patient or in a member of the family. Heart disease is the number one cause of death in the United States. Call for emergency help immediately and keep the person quiet and warm until help arrives.

- Chest pain that may or may not radiate to the arm or jaw
- Wet, clammy skin or breaking out into a cold sweat
- Weak and/or rapid pulse rate
- Pale color
- Low blood pressure
- Shortness of breath
- Nausea
- Back pain
- Lightheadedness

The signs and symptoms for men and women are the same; however, women are less likely to believe that they are having a heart attack and thus do not get help as soon as they should. Women are more likely to have the less apparent signs such as nausea, back or jaw pain, and shortness of breath. The single best way to prevent or minimize permanent damage to the heart is to get help at a hospital as soon as possible. Every minute is important!

YOUR ROLE AS A CAREGIVER

After hospitalization, your patient will return with an individualized plan of care based on:

- the type of heart attack she had
- her recovery up to that point
- her home situation
- her prognosis

Allow her as large a part in her care as her activity level permits. The plan of care you receive from the physician will include instructions about:

- activity restrictions
- diet restrictions
- medications
- emotional support

A patient usually receives an exercise regime. If your patient is unable to progress with the exercises or tries to advance too quickly, report this to the appropriate health care team member(s).

While giving care to a person with a cardiac disability, every caregiver balances the desire to allow the individual to be a self-sufficient person and the need to restrict her activity level. Continual discussion with the physician about your patient's condition will assist you in making correct decisions.

After a heart attack, a person may become so fearful of another heart attack that she does not exert herself at all or take any part in her care. She may even remove herself from family relationships. Everything she does is blamed on her heart attack and her fear of another one.

The opposite of this is a total disregard for one's condition. The individual denies any disability. He does not follow any suggestions from his physician, take his medication, or adhere to his diet. This reaction should be reported to the physician.

Some individuals are afraid that a heart attack will affect sexual activities. A person usually will return to a full sexual life after a heart attack; however, a discussion on this topic is best handled by the patient's physician or nurse, who knows what the patient has already been told. Do not give the person any opinions or folktales, but rather say, "I know you are concerned about this, and I will tell the nurse. She will get you the information you want."

A family member may need help in dealing with the stress of lifestyle changes and fear caused by cardiac disease. Suggest that any family member who needs help or expresses these fears seek the assistance of a support group or his or her own physician.

Pacemaker

A pacemaker is an electrical device placed either in the left or right upper chest under the skin. The job of this device is to regulate the heart rhythm. A pacemaker can be temporary or permanent. When a pacemaker is permanent, it requires monitoring that can be done at the medical office or over the telephone. The physician will provide these instructions. There are three types of pacemakers:

1. *Fixed-rate pacemaker:* The stimulation rate is fixed, usually between sixty and seventy beats per minute. This type of pacemaker is used only if the heart is totally dependent on electrical stimulation and is used only temporarily. It is rarely seen in the home.
2. *Synchronous pacemaker:* Stimulation occurs after a predetermined lack of the heart's own activity. This type is not seen often in the home.
3. *Demand pacemaker:* When the heartbeat falls below a predetermined rate, the pacemaker takes over. This is the most common type.

CARE OF A PACEMAKER   It is helpful to know what type of pacemaker your patient has. It is also important to know at what rate it is set. Keep in mind the following guidelines when you have a patient with a pacemaker:

- Electrical appliances may be used around pacemakers.
- Microwave ovens should not be used around pacemakers. Some patients have difficulty being around lawn mowers and cellular telephones.
- If your patient has hiccups, report this immediately to the appropriate health care team member. Hiccups could be an indication that the electrical wires are out of place.
- If your patient's pulse is below the preset level of the pacemaker, report it immediately to the appropriate health care team member.
- Report pain or discoloration near the pacemaker.
- Detecting devices in airports should be avoided.
- Report to the physician any complaints of dizziness, edema (swelling in the arms, hands, legs, or feet), shortness of breath, or irregular heartbeat.
- When moving, lifting, or assisting a patient who has a pacemaker, support her without putting pressure under her arms.
- Batteries have to be replaced from time to time. The physician decides when this is to be done. It varies from patient to patient, but keep to the schedule as determined by your patient's physician.
- Assist your patient with her telephone monitoring procedure. Be sure she understands it so that she can do it when you are not present in the home.

CONGESTIVE HEART FAILURE

Congestive heart failure (CHF) is a condition where the heart has a reduced blood supply, which causes excess fluid to build up around the heart in the chest cavity. This excess fluid continues into the limbs, causing edema. Shows the symptoms of a congestive heart failure episode.

ANGINA

Angina is a brief, temporary pain or heaviness in the chest that results from lack of oxygen to the heart. Usually after resting and medication, the individual no longer experiences discomfort. An episode may be brought on by stress or physical activity. Angina differs from person to person. Changes in your patient's angina signal a change in his cardiac status and should be reported to the physician immediately. Angina is caused by narrowing of the coronary arteries that bring oxygen to the heart. As these vessels narrow, the amount of oxygen decreases, causing pain and discomfort. This is not a heart attack or myocardial infarction because it is a temporary condition. However, if angina is allowed to continue without treatment, the sufferer could have a heart attack and sustain permanent damage to the heart.

Individuals with a higher risk of angina include those who:

- have high blood pressure
- have high blood cholesterol
- smoke cigarettes
- are overweight
- have high stress levels

Treatment for Angina

Angina cannot be cured; however, most people with the disease learn to live productive and meaningful lives. The aim of all treatment is to increase the flow of blood and oxygen to the heart, which is accomplished in several ways:

- *Medication:* The physician will prescribe a regime of medication to help the individual and decrease his pain. The medication will be individualized for the patient's particular condition and should not be altered without consulting her physician.
- *Control of risk factors:* The person may be put on a weight-reducing diet, told to decrease or stop his use of cigarettes, and advised to decrease his stress. These alterations in lifestyle are difficult, and the individual and his family members will need a great deal of encouragement and support to reach the goal.
- *Surgery:* If surgery has been recommended by a physician and your patient or his family members have questions, encourage them to contact the physician to get the answers they need.

YOUR ROLE AS A CAREGIVER

Your role is to help the person you are taking care of, including her family, maintain the regime set up for your patient. Remember, activity levels, diets, and medications are individualized and should not be compared to others or changed without medical consultation.

By providing support to the individual and her family members as she tries to alter her lifestyle and decrease her risk factors, you will be giving the care the person needs. Point out the achievements she has made and the progress she hopes to make in the near future. Do not dwell on her failures. It is usual for a patient who is trying to make changes in her lifestyle to slip back into old patterns from time to time. Do not be judgmental, but rather encourage her to return to the more healthy activities.

Be alert to stress in the family. When there is change in the way the family functions, the other members, not the patient, may exhibit stress. If you notice such family discord, discuss it with the health care team.

DIABETES

When the body cannot change carbohydrates (sugars and starches) into energy because of an imbalance of insulin, the result is the chronic disease known as diabetes mellitus. The pancreas usually produces insulin on a feedback mechanism. When the body needs insulin following a meal or when extra energy is needed, the pancreas is alerted and it pumps extra insulin into the bloodstream. If the body needs insulin and none is produced, however, starches and sugars cannot be converted into energy and absorbed by the cells. Sugar remains in the bloodstream and is eventually excreted in the urine as waste.

Signs of Diabetes

The following are all signs that a patient may be suffering from diabetes:

- Fatigue, tiredness
- Loss of weight
- Sores that heal poorly and slowly
- High blood sugar
- Sugar in the urine (the urine smells sweet)
- Frequent and large amounts of urine
- Excessive thirst that is unsatisfied from drinking fluids
- Poor vision

There are two types of diabetes. Type I is usually diagnosed in children or adolescents and usually results in the person having to take insulin; it is referred to as insulin-dependent diabetes mellitus (IDDM). Type II diabetes, also referred to as non-insulin-dependent diabetes mellitus (NIDDM), usually occurs later in life and can be a result of lifestyle factors or other diseases (i.e., obesity). The pancreas may produce some insulin but not enough for normal body function. In this type of diabetes, the person may be able to control his blood sugar by taking oral medications or just regulating his diet. Because a diabetic has a regulated amount of insulin in his body, his food intake must also be regulated. If the amount of food is greater than the amount of insulin available, there will be too much unmetabolized sugar left in the blood. If the amount of insulin is greater than the amount of food available, there will not be any carbohydrates for the insulin to metabolize, which causes other problems and leads to the need for additional insulin to regulate blood sugar.

Diabetes can be controlled but never cured. A diabetic must maintain a special diet and must sometimes take medication by mouth or insulin by injection forever. A person with diabetes can live a full and productive life if she keeps to a diet and a medication schedule. Diagnosis of this disease can be made only by a physician following laboratory tests.

Diabetic Coma and Insulin Shock

Two conditions may occur if a diabetic does not adhere to a prescribed diet and/or medication regime or has brittle diabetes (meaning that the medications and diet have not been effective and the person's blood sugar spikes up or down without warning). These conditions—diabetic coma and insulin shock—require immediate medical attention.

DIABETIC COMA (HYPERGLYCEMIA/HIGH-BLOOD-SUGAR DIABETIC KETO-ACIDOSIS)   Diabetic coma (ketoacidosis) occurs when the blood has too many carbohydrates and not enough insulin to metabolize it. Symptoms include the following:

- Air hunger; heavy, labored breathing; increased respiration
- Loss of appetite
- Dulled senses
- Nausea and/or vomiting
- Weakness
- Abdominal pains or discomfort
- Increased thirst and a dry tongue
- Sweet or fruity odor of the breath
- Flushed dry skin
- Increased urination

INSULIN SHOCK (HYPOGLYCEMIA/LOW-BLOOD-SUGAR INSULIN REACTION
Insulin shock, or insulin reaction, occurs when a person's blood has more insulin than the amount of carbohydrates available for metabolism. Symptoms include the following:

- Excessive sweating, perspiration
- Faintness, dizziness, weakness
- Hunger
- Irritability, personality change, nervousness
- Numbness of tongue and lips
- Inability to awaken, coma, unconsciousness, stupor
- Headache
- Tremors, trembling
- Blurred or impaired vision

YOUR ROLE AS A CAREGIVER

Your role is to help the patient and her family members learn to live with this disease and the routine of medication and diet. Point out the positive aspects of the individual's situation. Help the family members adapt the prescribed diet to their lifestyle. If the diet seems difficult, obtaining information from the American Diabetics Association may be helpful to the patient and the family. The physician may also prescribe that the patient and the family members work with a nutritionist or dietician, who will try to adapt the diet to the family's needs.

Assist your patient when necessary to ensure that he or she is taking the correct dosage of medication at the correct time of day. Insulin is always taken by injection, not by mouth. Most insulin should be kept in the refrigerator. Notify the physician if the patient does not keep to the prescribed medication schedule or has any reaction to the medication.

The patient's physician or nurse may make it the responsibility of the caregiver to test the individual's urine for sugar and acetone. If you are asked to conduct this test, be sure that you know when and to whom the results should be reported (see Chapter 17 for the procedure on testing blood sugar).

Because a diabetic may have decreased circulation, she may have difficulty with her feet. Observe toenails and toes for signs of infection or pressure areas (redness, peeling skin, blisters, sores, rash, or oozing liquid). Report these signs immediately. Do not cut toenails or fingernails. This procedure should be done by a podiatrist or a family member who has been specially trained. This rule is important because any nick or cut in the foot can turn into a foot wound quickly. The person may have special shoes that will add extra protection to her feet.

As you care for the patient, notice the condition of her skin. Is it dry? Is it flaky? Do you see bruises and any bruises healing? Because a diabetic has a harder time healing than a nondiabetic, it is important to prevent bruises and pressure areas. If the skin is dry, apply lotion. Another risk factor is that dry skin often itches, and an individual who scratches herself could injure the skin, causing bruises or infection.

STROKE

The term *cerebrovascular accident (CVA)*, otherwise known as a stroke, has three important parts:

1. *Cerebro:* having to do with the brain
2. *Vascular:* having to do with the blood vessels
3. *Accident:* something unpredictable and unexpected

CVA (or stroke), the third leading cause of death in the United States, occurs when the blood supply to a part of the brain is stopped by a blocked blood vessel. When blood flow stops, the tissue dies. Because each part of the brain controls a different function, the result of a CVA depends on which blood vessel is blocked and which brain center is destroyed.

It is important to remember that the results of a CVA may be paralysis, loss of speech, or loss of vision, but that the cause of the problem is disruption of nerve impulse transmission from brain tissue damage. In some brains, when a blood vessel is blocked, the surrounding blood vessels take over to supply the injured part of the brain. This is called collateral circulation. In this case, the damage may not be as great as if there were no collateral circulation.

The speech center of the brain is on the left side, so if the CVA occurs on that side, speech may be affected. If the CVA occurs on the right side, varying degrees of muscle weakness may be the result.

Causes of a Stroke

A CVA has four main causes:

1. A blood clot can form elsewhere in the body, travel to the brain, and lodge in a small vessel. This type of blood clot is called an embolus.
2. A blood clot can form in the brain itself and remain there. This is called a thrombus.
3. Plaque can accumulate in the blood vessels and eventually close them.
4. A blood vessel can burst, causing a hemorrhage. This type of CVA is most common in people who have hypertension.

YOUR ROLE AS A CAREGIVER

Caring for a person recovering from a CVA is a team effort. If, at any time, the individual you are caring for shows signs of becoming unstable (change in vital signs, dizziness, weakness, unable to follow usual routine), immediately alert the appropriate team member. You are the team member who will spend the most time with the patient. Your careful, objective observations of the person are important to his eventual recovery.

It is impossible to predict when a body part function will return following a CVA. Encourage the individual to continue with the exercises and use of adaptive equipment prescribed by the health care team. This regimen is the best chance of returning and/or maintaining function.

Follow the principles of good personal care and the instructions of the physical, occupational, and speech therapists. These therapists will plan an individualized program for your patient. You will play an important part in seeing that he and the family follow this routine. The care will be planned with the following in mind:

• Prevention of complications due to decreased mobility
• The need for proper nutrition
• Safety
• Emotional aspects of the chronic condition for both the patient and the family

After you have received the care plans from the therapists, it is your responsibility to make these plans part of the patient's routine throughout the day so that the person does not tire. Having many things to relearn is emotionally painful and at times frustrating. Imagine how you would feel if you had to relearn the alphabet or how to walk, or couldn't clearly communicate. Sadness, anger, and personality changes from the prestroke state are common. Keep the following points in mind:

• Always encourage the patient. Point out the positive aspects of her progress.
• Use simple instructions in words familiar to the person and her family. Speak slowly and clearly while looking at the patient. Do not use baby talk.

CLINICAL ALERT 18.1

After a stroke, medications that thin the blood are often given to prevent further blood clots from forming. Thin blood has dangerous implications, and extra measures to protect the person's skin and avoid cuts and bruises are essential. Read the information that comes from the pharmacy and watch for potential signs that the patient is bleeding internally. Some examples of these signs include dizziness, weakness, unusual bruising, nosebleeds, bleeding of gums, bleeding from cuts that take a long time to stop, menstrual flow or vaginal bleeding that is heavier than normal, pink or brown urine, red or black stools, coughing up blood, or vomiting blood or material that looks like coffee grounds.

- Always demonstrate patience and understanding.
- Have the individual complete only the exercises that are part of the person's care plan. If you have a question, call the appropriate therapist.
- Assist the patient with her medication (see Clinical Alert 18.1). Document which medications were given at what time so that the patient or family members do not give something that has already been given. If visitors tire your patient, tactfully suggest that they leave so the person can rest.
- Listen to the patient and her family members. They may benefit from a mental health clinician or psychiatric nurse to help them cope with the changes in the family system.

ARTHRITIS

Arthritis is inflammation and destruction of joints. At times, there may be other symptoms. The shoulders, ankles, elbows, wrists, fingers, and toes are the most common joints affected by this disease. Arthritis or inflammation can be due to an allergy, injury, or infection. Some causes of arthritis cannot be determined; it just appears. Everyone seems to have a different reaction to this disease.

There are more than 100 types of arthritis, but the following are the four most common types:

Osteoarthritis: Osteoarthritis is the most common type. It is thought that after continual use, the joints and their linings just wear out and become thin. The bony surfaces become thick and develop little spurs that cause pain and inflammation every time the joint moves. Then the bones rub against each other, causing pain and inflammation. This type of arthritis is most common among the elderly.

Rheumatoid arthritis: Rheumatoid arthritis is a crippling, chronic disease. All connective tissue may be affected. If the disease starts in the joints, connective tissue in other organs may eventually be affected. This type of arthritis usually starts in young adulthood or childhood. Three times more women than men have this type of arthritis.

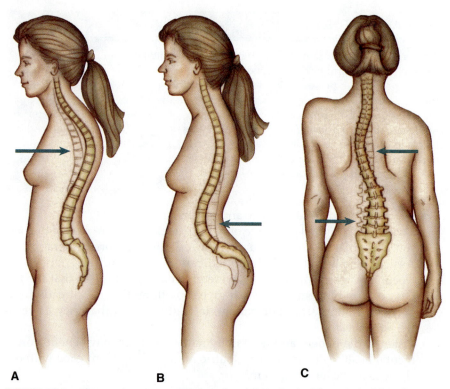

A   **B**   **C**

FIGURE 18.1   Abnormal curvatures of the spine: (A) Kyphosis; (B) Lordosis; (C) Scoliosis.

Gout: This disease is most common among men. Uric acid crystals build up in the blood and lodge in the joints, causing inflammation and pain. This buildup can be sudden and painful. Any joint can be affected.

Kyphosis: This condition is more common in women than in men. It is most often known as humpback and results from an exaggeration of the thoracic curvature. The curvature becomes exaggerated due to a birth defect, disease process (such as tuberculosis, syphilis, or cancer), compression fracture, faulty posture, or hormone changes. Other common curvatures of the spine are depicted in Figure 18.1.

YOUR ROLE AS A CAREGIVER

Remember, arthritis is a chronic disease, which means the individual will have it forever. Help him to establish a safe and efficient routine for daily care that decreases muscle stress and fatigue. Exercise and rest are important parts of the patient's plan of care. Follow the exercise routine. Do not change it unless you have discussed the change with the physician or the appropriate team member. If you notice that your patient's response to the exercises has changed, report it.

Assist the patient with his medication and treatment plan. Each patient is treated differently. Treatment may include diet, weight reduction, rest, and exercise. An occupational therapist and physical therapist may also be involved.

Listen to the patient. He may have many feelings about this disease and may require emotional counseling from a mental health clinician or psychiatric nurse. Ask the patient if he would like counseling and call the appropriate clinician.

CANCER

Cancer, or a malignancy, is a tumor made up of cells that have changed from normal ones to abnormal ones. This change can happen in any organ, at any time, and at any age. As the abnormal cells reproduce and multiply, they destroy the normal tissue and usually form a tumor. The course of the disease depends on many factors:

- Location of the tumor
- Type of tumor
- When the cancer was discovered
- Type of treatment available
- General health of the patient

There is no proven cause of cancer. Although a change in the way your body functions may mean many things (not necessarily cancer), eight changes, usually called early warning signs of cancer, should be reported to a doctor immediately.

The spread of cancer cells from one area of the body to another is called metastasis. Metastasis does not always occur when there is cancer in the body, but it may. The first site of the cancer is called the primary site, and the place it metastasizes to is called the secondary site.

The only way a tumor is known to be malignant (cancerous) or benign (not cancerous) is by taking a small piece of it and examining it under a microscope. This procedure is called a biopsy. It is usually done in the operating room in the hospital.

Cancer Treatment

Treatment varies from patient to patient. The patient may undergo surgery, radiation, chemotherapy, or a combination of the three. The choice of treatment is usually made by the doctor after discussion with the individual and her family.

Sometimes, family members choose not to tell a confused patient that he has cancer. Even though you may not agree with this decision, you must go along with it. It is not your place to give the patient his diagnosis. Discuss this situation with the patient's physician so that you will know what to tell the individual if he asks. Do not lie to the patient; tell her she needs to talk to her family and physician for more information.

YOUR ROLE AS A CAREGIVER

Your role is to give the patient the best care you can, which includes both physical and emotional support. If the patient is terminally ill, you and the health care team will make a plan of care to meet his specific needs. A person is usually said to be terminally ill when there is little or no hope for recovering from the disease and the patient will likely die from the disease. Cancer is not contagious. Encourage the patient's family members to visit and be supportive. Follow the principles of good personal care. Follow the instructions of the therapists within the limits of the patient. Discuss with the therapists your responsibilities for exercises. Encourage the individual to take part in his care. See Chapters 7 and 12 for more information on care of a patient receiving radiation or chemotherapy.

If the patient wishes to talk, let him. If he does not seem to be able to talk to you, ask him if you can call the nurse or someone else. Many people live for many years with cancer. Do not give the person false hope, but do not assume that he will die unless you have been told this. Help family members deal with this diagnosis by letting them take part in the patient's care if they wish. Encourage them to talk to someone who can help them accept this diagnosis.

ALZHEIMER'S DISEASE

Alzheimer's disease is a major cause of mental deterioration in people. It is the diagnosis of more than 50 percent of the nursing home residents in the United States. Most of the victims of this disease, however, receive treatment and care in their homes. This disease is chronic, progressive, and ultimately renders the person totally dependent on others. There is no known cure. Alzheimer's is the sixth leading cause of death in the United States. Those with Alzheimer's live an average of eight years after their symptoms become noticeable to others, but survival can range from three to twenty years, depending on age and other health conditions.

According to the Alzheimer's Association, Alzheimer's is a progressive disease, where symptoms gradually worsen over a number of years. In its early stages, memory loss is mild, but with late-stage Alzheimer's, individuals lose the ability to carry on a conversation and respond to their environment. Alzheimer's disease occurs in seven stages:

Stage 1: No impairment (normal function). The person does not experience any memory problems. An interview with a medical professional does not show any evidence of symptoms.

Stage 2: Very mild cognitive decline (may be normal, age-related changes or earliest signs of Alzheimer's disease). The person may feel as if she is having memory lapses because she is forgetting familiar words or the location of everyday objects. But no symptoms can be detected during a medical examination or by friends, family members, or co-workers.

Stage 3: Mild cognitive decline (early-stage Alzheimer's can be diagnosed in some, but not all, individuals with these symptoms). Friends, family members, or co-workers begin to notice difficulties. During a detailed medical interview, doctors may be able to detect problems in memory or concentration. Common stage 3 difficulties include the following:

- Noticeable problems coming up with the right word or name
- Trouble remembering names when introduced to new people
- Noticeably greater difficulty performing tasks in social or work settings
- Forgetting material that was just read
- Losing or misplacing a valuable object
- Increasing trouble with planning or organizing

Stage 4: Moderate cognitive decline (mild or early-stage Alzheimer's disease). At this point, a careful medical interview should be able to detect clear-cut problems in several areas:

- Forgetfulness of recent events
- Impaired ability to perform challenging mental arithmetic, for example, counting backward from 100 by 7s
- Greater difficulty performing complex tasks, such as planning dinner for guests, paying bills, or managing finances
- Forgetfulness about one's own personal history
- Becoming moody or withdrawn, especially in socially or mentally challenging situations

Stage 5: Moderately severe cognitive decline (moderate or mid-stage Alzheimer's disease). Gaps in memory and thinking are noticeable, and individuals begin to need help with day-to-day activities. At this stage, those with Alzheimer's may:

- Be unable to recall their own address or telephone number or the high school or college from which they graduated
- Become confused about where they are or what day it is
- Have trouble with less challenging mental arithmetic, such as counting backward from 40 by subtracting 4s or from 20 by subtracting 2s
- Need help choosing proper clothing for the season or the occasion
- Still remember significant details about themselves and their family
- Still require no assistance with eating or using the toilet

Stage 6: Severe cognitive decline (moderately severe or mid-stage Alzheimer's disease). Memory continues to worsen, personality changes may take place, and individuals need extensive help with daily activities. At this stage, individuals may:

- Lose awareness of recent experiences as well as of their surroundings
- Remember their own name but have difficulty with their personal history
- Distinguish familiar and unfamiliar faces but have trouble remembering the name of a spouse or caregiver

- Need help dressing properly and may, without supervision, make mistakes such as putting pajamas over daytime clothes or shoes on the wrong feet
- Experience major changes in sleep patterns, for example, sleeping during the day and becoming restless at night
- Need help handling details of toileting, for example, flushing the toilet, wiping, or disposing of tissue properly
- Have increasingly frequent trouble controlling bladder or bowels
- Experience major personality and behavioral changes, including suspiciousness and delusions (such as believing that their caregiver is an impostor) or compulsive, repetitive behavior such as handwringing or tissue shredding
- Wander or become lost

Stage 7: Very severe cognitive decline (severe or late-stage Alzheimer's disease). In the final stage of this disease, individuals lose the ability to respond to their environment, to carry on a conversation, and eventually to control movement. They may still say words or phrases. At this stage, individuals need help with much of their daily personal care, including eating or using the toilet. They may also lose the ability to smile, to sit without support, and to hold their heads up. Reflexes become abnormal. Muscles grow rigid. Swallowing becomes impaired.

Validation of Emotions and Feelings

When an elderly person has Alzheimer's dementia or another type of dementia, it can be difficult to communicate and therefore difficult to care for the individual. Validating your patient's emotions and feelings is important; reminding her that she has dementia or memory loss is not necessary. You can use validating statements such as "That's okay. I'll check and make sure your car is locked" when your patient has just complained to you that she is worried about having left the car unlocked. People with dementia are not likely to remember the reality of the present day; they live in whatever reality their brain remembers and sometimes they live in a reality that never existed. The important thing is to allow the person to keep her respect and dignity while redirecting her if her reality becomes dangerous. For example, your patient may complain daily that she needs to go look for her van. Trying to leave the home to look for the van can be dangerous for your patient. Validating your patient's reality and redirecting her behavior would be prudent. The caregiver might say, "Your van is in the shop getting snow tires put on. Let's go play checkers."

Sometimes, props are necessary to let the individual with dementia live out the reality she is in. For example, if your patient's reality today is that she has young children and is worried about where the children are, you can validate her reality by reassuring her that the children are okay. Other times, a person with dementia will go through the steps of caring for a child, but only with a doll. Parenting the doll by talking to it, putting it to bed, and rocking it to sleep are all comforting to the elder Naomi Feil is an expert on validation therapy and suggests the following for caregivers and family members:

- Try to understand *why* the individual is behaving in a certain way. What's the trigger or underlying concern? Once the trigger is found, figure out a way to address it. For example, if your patient or loved one is hoarding or hiding items, ask what he is fearful of losing. Give him a "safe box" that can be used to store those items.
- Don't get caught up in whether something makes sense. A person with dementia may not be able to piece everything together, but his emotions are still valid. In fact, his distress or anxiety can be amplified when he isn't understood. Accept that your patient's emotions have more validity than the logic that leads to them.
- Ask specific questions about how certain actions or situations make your patient feel. After you receive an explanation of those feelings, validate them with phrases that show your support, such as "I'd be upset too, if that happened to me" or "I understand why you feel that way."
- Allow your patient a graceful exit and be mindful of his ego!

YOUR ROLE AS A CAREGIVER

You are an important part of the care when your patient has Alzheimer's. Follow the care plan carefully. The maintenance of a routine is one way to ease the care of the patient. If you feel the need to change the plan of care, be sure to discuss it with the patient's family members and the health care team. Your continued support is important for the family members of an Alzheimer's victim. Be on time and be conscientious about coming to work. A change of personnel is a disrupting factor in these households.

In addition, keep the following points in mind when caring for a patient who has Alzheimer's:

- Be alert for the safety of the patient. Remember, he is unable to remember your instructions so you must be aware of his activities and movements.
- Provide a quiet, unstressed environment.
- Maintain the personal hygiene of the patient. Careful washing of the perineal area will prevent skin breakdown. Frequent cleaning of the teeth will decrease mouth odor and improve general appearance.
- Maintain a toileting routine. If the patient is incontinent and can no longer participate in his personal hygiene, discuss with the occupational therapist the use of various appliances, for example, toilet riser, commode, urinal, bedpan or adult incontinent briefs.
- Offer small nutritious meals. Frequent sips of water will decrease the chance of dehydration.
- Monitor the patient's sleep habits and report to the appropriate health care team member if they are markedly disturbed or they change.

- Be supportive of family members who care for the patient. Encourage them to leave the house when you are there. Encourage them to seek relief and enjoyment while you are available to care for the patient.
- Be alert to family tension. Report any family tension to the appropriate health care team member, who will discuss with family members the appropriate counseling or support groups.
- Do not be judgmental or compare the care one family gives to the way another family cares for a relative.
- Be alert to your feelings. If you find you cannot continue caring for the patient, discuss your feelings with your health care team so that relief can be arranged.

CHRONIC OBSTRUCTIVE PULMONARY DISEASE

Chronic obstructive pulmonary disease (COPD) refers to all diseases that cause irreversible damage to the lungs over a period of time. This condition is one of the leading causes of death in the United States. People with a diagnosis of asthma and emphysema are often said to have COPD, which means that their lungs cannot expand, remove oxygen from air breathed in, or expel waste products such as carbon dioxide. These individuals also find it difficult to perform activities that require exertion of any kind. Eating and speaking are difficult, and exercise is often impossible. Most of these patients are susceptible to infection due to the pooling of pulmonary secretions in their lungs. When the levels of carbon dioxide and other gases are incorrect, these patients exhibit unusual behavior and cannot make decisions or be left alone. When the blood gases are corrected, this behavior disappears.

Persons with COPD also suffer from a change in body image. They must learn to live with machines as constant companions because they depend on oxygen equipment and sometimes suction equipment to help them breathe. Some patients may have tracheostomy tubes, intravenous (IV) lines, or even feeding tubes.

As the patient demands more and more care, the family function changes. The primary caregiver becomes isolated from friends because the individual's care takes up so much time. Family members become socially isolated and depressed and often suffer from sensory deprivation. Relationships with friends change because the person often is too tired, or even unable, to speak. Visitors may stop coming, and family members often find themselves without any outside activities. While all this is occurring, families must often become accustomed to a change in finances and a change in the work status of the individual.

YOUR ROLE AS A CAREGIVER

Your presence in a home where your patient has COPD is a most important one. You will assist family members by providing a break in their routine. Encourage the other caregivers to go out and tend to personal needs while you are in the house. Assure both patient and family members that you will adhere to the routine they have established and will not make changes without discussing them first. This respite for the caregiver often enables him or her to continue the care for the rest of the day and possibly into the night.

Encourage the patient to adhere to his medication schedule. Report any change in behavior. No change is too small. If you report changes as soon as they occur, the physician or other health care team member can change the plan of care to meet the patient's changing needs. Often, you will be the first person to see a change in behavior, which may mean that the patient's blood gases are incorrect.

Try to interest the patient in eating nutritious, small meals. Because eating is a chore for this individual and his taste buds often are less sensitive, every bit of food should be nutritious and tasty. Fluids may or may not be restricted. Be sure to check. Prepare foods that the person likes.

Expose the patient to activities to occupy his time. If the patient has no hobbies, discuss with him and his family what type of activities he might enjoy. Then keep on trying each one. Do not be discouraged. The patient and the family will appreciate your concern and interest, and you will eventually find an activity that will please the patient. For example, if the person you are caring for likes to play sports but is no longer able to participate in games, be sure to have him listen to the radio when ballgames are on or make him comfortable so he can look at TV. Plan your schedule around these important times in the patient's day.

Many of the patients you care for will be using oxygen therapy. This is not necessarily a problem, except that many of the people who have COPD also smoke. Although the patient and her family members are taught that oxygen cannot run when there is an open flame or someone is smoking in the area, individuals may forget. Be firm, but polite. Tell the patient and the family that oxygen and smoking is a dangerous combination and that you will have to report this situation.

NEUROLOGICAL DISEASES

Three neurological diseases you may see in a home setting are Parkinson's disease, multiple sclerosis (MS), and amyotrophic lateral sclerosis (ALS). Individuals who have these diseases usually remain in the home setting and use adaptive aids. Some remain at home until they die. Although the diseases are different, there are many similarities in the care of these patients. All three diseases result in the need for assistance with care, attention to safety, and support from patients' families. As these diseases progress, patients require a great deal of personal care and protection. Their ability to respond to changes and slight infections becomes progressively worse.

Parkinson's Disease

Parkinson's disease is a progressive disease that affects the part of the brain controlling movement and balance. The first signs are usually tremors of the

CLINICAL ALERT 18.2

Medications used for Parkinson's disease often require a balancing act. One of the side effects of these medications is psychosis (i.e., hallucinations, delusions, or paranoia). If your patient develops this side effect, he may have to take another medication to offset the psychosis. If you notice a change in mood or in the thinking of your patient who is on medication for Parkinson's disease, contact the physician.

hands or legs, difficulty walking, and slowness of movement. Other symptoms may be changes in vision, drooling, difficulty swallowing, and inability to control bowel and bladder function. The cause of the disease is unknown, but patients respond to drug therapy that replaces certain chemicals they seem to be lacking. People with this disease often work many years after the diagnosis. Drugs must be carefully and continuously regulated. Side effects from the drugs often occur many years after the therapy has started. Sometimes, patients may appear to be getting better and conclude that they no longer need the medication or may change their routines. This is a great mistake and should be reported to their physicians immediately (see Clinical Alert 18.2).

Multiple Sclerosis

Multiple sclerosis (MS) is a progressive disease that affects the transmission of impulses through the central nervous system. The first signs are usually fatigue, emotional changes, and difficulty with speech. This disease affects young adults with young families who are in the first stages of their careers. The people who have this disease often work for many years if they are protected from infection and have a safe environment. Medications help some people, but no one medication has been found useful for all patients. The cause is unknown, and the course of the disease varies (see Figure 18.2). For more information and resources on multiple sclerosis, contact your local chapter or the national organization of the Multiple Sclerosis Society.

Amyotrophic Lateral Sclerosis

Amyotrophic lateral sclerosis (ALS), or Lou Gehrig's disease, is a progressive disease that degenerates the neurons that control muscles in the body. The cause is unknown, and most patients die within three years of diagnosis. Many of these patients choose to stay at home. They need assistance with all aspects of personal care and maintenance of a safe environment. Surprisingly, they often maintain cognitive abilities until death.

Huntington's Chorea

Huntington's chorea is a hereditary, progressive, degenerative disorder of the brain. This disease usually begins during the mid- to late thirties. The

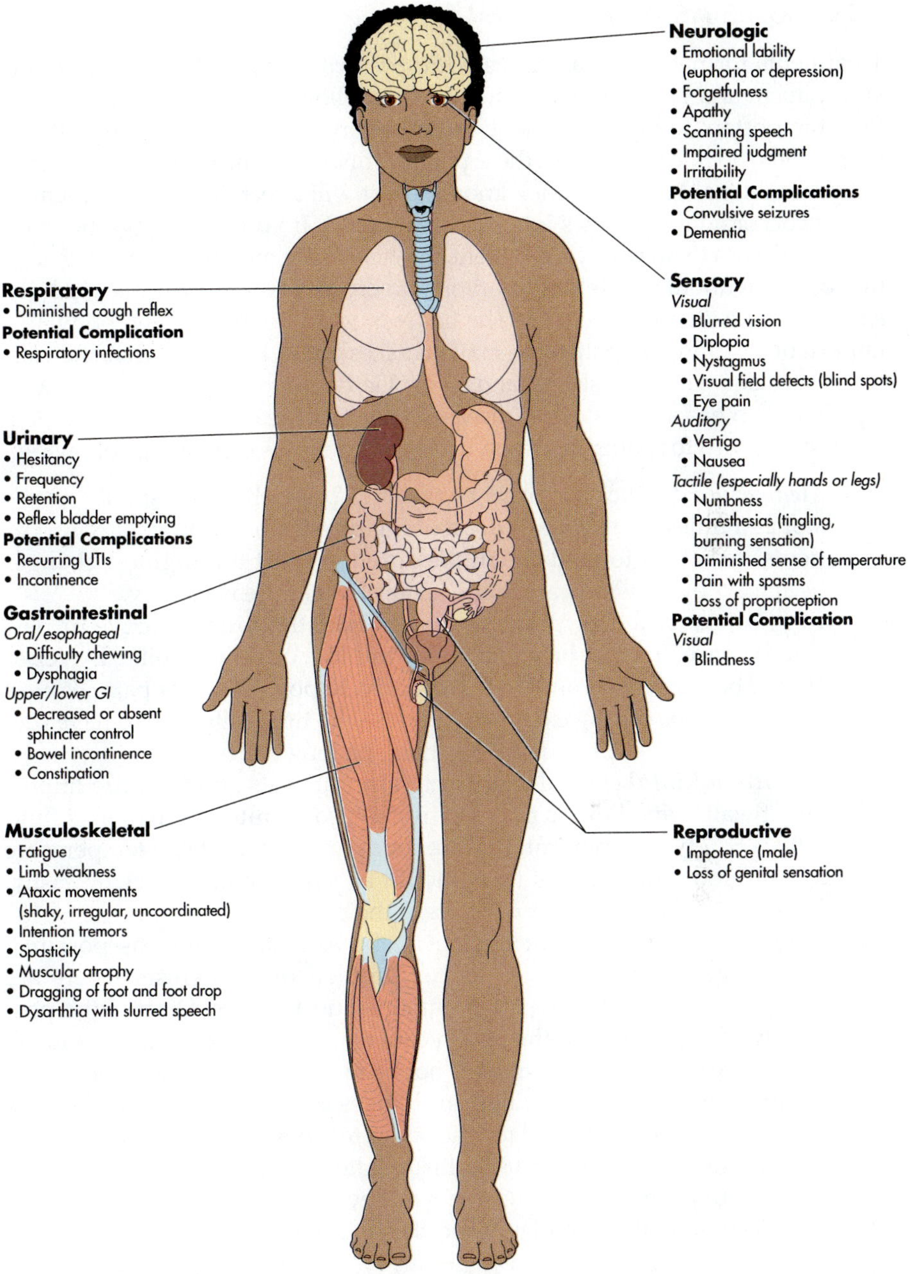

Neurologic
- Emotional lability
  (euphoria or depression)
- Forgetfulness
- Apathy
- Scanning speech
- Impaired judgment
- Irritability

Potential Complications
- Convulsive seizures
- Dementia

Respiratory
- Diminished cough reflex

Potential Complication
- Respiratory infections

Urinary
- Hesitancy
- Frequency
- Retention
- Reflex bladder emptying

Potential Complications
- Recurring UTIs
- Incontinence

Gastrointestinal
Oral/esophageal
- Difficulty chewing
- Dysphagia
Upper/lower GI
- Decreased or absent
  sphincter control
- Bowel incontinence
- Constipation

Musculoskeletal
- Fatigue
- Limb weakness
- Ataxic movements
  (shaky, irregular, uncoordinated)
- Intention tremors
- Spasticity
- Muscular atrophy
- Dragging of foot and foot drop
- Dysarthria with slurred speech

Sensory
Visual
- Blurred vision
- Diplopia
- Nystagmus
- Visual field defects (blind spots)
- Eye pain
Auditory
- Vertigo
- Nausea
Tactile (especially hands or legs)
- Numbness
- Paresthesias (tingling,
  burning sensation)
- Diminished sense of temperature
- Pain with spasms
- Loss of proprioception

Potential Complication
Visual
- Blindness

Reproductive
- Impotence (male)
- Loss of genital sensation

FIGURE 18.2 Multisystem effects of multiple sclerosis.

symptoms include involuntary movements, rigidity, problems with balance, difficulty swallowing, and slurred speech. People with Huntington's disease usually die within fifteen years of being diagnosed. For more information and resources, contact your local chapter or the national organization of the Huntington's Disease Society.

YOUR ROLE AS A CAREGIVER

Treatments for neurological diseases are prescribed by a physician. Support your patient and her family members as they follow the regime. Most patients find it important to follow the same routine every day. This may seem difficult for people who like variety, but these patients find the same routine comforting. They know what to expect. They know how it will affect them. Assist them as they incorporate the regimes into their daily lives. If you have suggestions for change, discuss them with your patient and her family members. Do not change the routine without first telling everyone involved. Having a neurological disease can make the individual feel she has lost control of her life and body. It is important to allow the patient to make choices about her care, what she eats, when she eats, when she sleeps, and so on. Getting into a power struggle with a patient who has a neurological disease is not helpful and should be avoided. Areas of concern for patients with neurological diseases include the following:

- *Medication:* Medication must be taken as prescribed and should not be stopped unless the patient's prescribing physician is notified. Report patients' reactions to medication. Be sure to report the slightest changes because they may indicate that dosage changes are necessary.
- *Regular exercise:* Regular exercise can take the form of active or passive exercise. It could be walking, swimming, or riding a bike. Exercises should be supervised and done regularly. Report fatigue or pain. Be alert to safety needs during exercise. Patients who tire easily should have several short exercise periods rather than one long one.
- *Nutritional intake:* Small meals high in nutrients and fiber are important. Swallowing liquids may be difficult, so monitor the patient's fluid intake. Safety is important. Be sure foods are an acceptable temperature and not too hot. Pieces of food should be small enough to chew easily. Report bowel and bladder changes to the physician.
- *Support:* Encourage your patient to be as independent as possible. Encourage family members to pursue their own interests. There are many local support groups for patients and families. Discuss the possibility of referrals with the health care team. Allow all family members time to express their feelings. Do not be judgmental. Support the family members in their roles. Be alert to changes in roles. Family members, as well as patients, often need to voice their feelings of frustration, fear, and fatigue (see Clinical Alert 18.3). Listen attentively. Offer to put them in touch with professional counselors if they wish. Discussing feelings can be helpful to both the patients and the caregivers.

ACQUIRED IMMUNE DEFICIENCY SYNDROME

Acquired immune deficiency syndrome (AIDS) is a disease that develops from the human immunodeficiency virus (HIV). HIV is spread through contact of blood and body fluids. It cannot be transmitted by holding hands, by giving blood, or by being near someone who has AIDS. There is no evidence that HIV can be spread from sharing the same equipment or bathroom. You

CLINICAL ALERT 18.3

Huntington's disease is hereditary and is often passed on in the males of the family. For example, if a father has the disease, the sons in the family are most likely to have the disease. The sooner the disease is treated, the less the symptoms will interfere with daily living. A blood test is all it takes to find out if one has Huntington's disease. Due to the responsibility parents often feel for conditions their children acquire, parents of children with Huntington's disease may be angry and/or feel guilty, and they may try to overcompensate by doing everything for the individual or never leaving the patient's side. It is important to listen to these parents and to refer them to professional counseling if they present with excessive caregiving and/or guilt. Most physicians will suggest that all immediate family members of someone with Huntington's disease be tested for the gene to provide not only the opportunity for early intervention, but also to give them information related to passing the gene to future generations.

will not get sick if you sit next to someone who has any form of AIDS. The virus is not spread by food or sharing a kitchen. It is transmitted only by contact with blood, seminal fluid, or vaginal fluid in the mouth, rectum, vagina, penis, or open wound on the body.

A person can have a form of AIDS and often not know it. Therefore, it is always important to practice standard precautions (see Chapter 7) with all patients. HIV infection can take one of several forms. Only a physician can diagnose the disease. Anyone who thinks he has been exposed to HIV or AIDS should go to a physician, a hospital, or health department immediately (free confidential testing is available at most health departments). If someone is infected with HIV in any form, he can transmit the infections to others, even though he may not have any symptoms.

Risk Factors of HIV

You are at risk of giving, getting, or having HIV, which leads to AIDS, if:

- you are an IV drug user who shares needles.
- you received a blood transfusion or blood products.
- you have several sexual partners and do not use condoms.
- you do not know your sexual partners well.
- any of your sexual partners have had unprotected sex.
- you have hepatitis B or C.

AIDS Disease Process

AIDS inhibits the immune system from working, and thus any infection or disease that the individual acquires can be very slow to resolve or heal and can take his life. Multiple medication regimes are designed to build the immune system of someone who has AIDS. These regimes can be costly and can have severe side effects. Most of the patients with AIDS will have sores (from slow healing of any cut or bruise), weight loss, and weakness. When taking medication and living a healthy lifestyle (i.e., eating nutritious foods, exercising regularly, and keeping away from people with illness), people with HIV or AIDS can live an average, full life.

YOUR ROLE AS A CAREGIVER

You will be asked to demonstrate standard precautions while caring for the AIDS patients, just as you would when caring for other patients. Use these standard precautions only when necessary so that neither the patients nor their families think you are afraid of catching the disease. AIDS patients are often lonely. At times, due to fear of catching the disease, family and friends do not spend time with them, touch them, or hold their hands. Your demonstration that this activity is without danger will help decrease needless fears and myths.

AIDS patients often take medication and have set routines to conserve strength and maintain their muscle tone. Assist the patients with these medications and maintain routines comfortable for the families and the patients. If family members are unavailable to assist the patient when you are not there, discuss with other members of the health care team the availability of support groups or community volunteers. Make these suggestions carefully so the patients know that you are concerned but not trying to get somebody else to assume the care.

Report all changes in behavior, pain tolerance, activity tolerance, and skin integrity. Protect the patients from friends and neighbors who may have slight colds or infections. If you believe any visitor is not 100 percent healthy, suggest that the guest return at another time or speak to your patient on the telephone.

Should you have any questions about the disease or the safest way to care for the patient, discuss them openly with the health care team to increase your knowledge and decrease your fears. You can also contact the local health department for assistance in gaining knowledge and resources for an AIDS patient.

For additional information on some of the diseases discussed in this chapter and support groups that help with these diseases, see the Resource Page at the end of this book.

Summary

Patients with the diseases covered in this chapter commonly live at home with caregivers assisting with some or all of their daily living needs. The more you understand a disease, the better equipped you are to care for a patient with the disease. Today's technology allows for information to be gathered quickly on the Internet and shared with others. Sharing ideas can be helpful in caregiving and in coping with the deterioration your patient may experience due to the disease. When caring for an individual in her home, be sure to discuss any changes in medication, exercise, or nutrition with the physician and/or other members of the health care team to ensure that you are providing proper care for the patient.

Chapter 19

Emergency Procedures

SCENARIO

Mrs. Soledad has worked all her life as a seamstress. She sews for both her employer and her family and enjoys the creativity and the praise she receives. She is now faced with arthritis in her hands and her hips. Some days she is unable to thread a needle or cut a pattern. Once an outgoing and talkative woman, Mrs. Soledad has become much quieter and has started keeping to herself at lunch. She no longer brings food to share and does not join in any conversations with her co-workers about her family and other aspects of her life. Her employer has mentioned that Mrs. Soledad's work, although still perfect, seems to take longer to complete. Her co-workers notice that, at times, she rubs her hands and finds it difficult to stand up from a sitting position.

EMERGENCY ESSENTIALS

This chapter covers the essentials of emergency procedures in the home. All individuals, especially caregivers, should take an emergency certification course to learn first aid and cardiopulmonary resuscitation (CPR) skills. Contact the local chapter of the American Red Cross or the American Heart Association to obtain more information (also see the Resource Page at the end of this book).

Emergencies are situations that call for immediate action. First aid is the action taken to assist people who suffer injuries or sudden illnesses until medical help arrives. Every home should have an emergency procedure. It should include a plan of whom to call depending on the type of emergency that is occurring, along with the telephone numbers of fire, police, and rescue squads. It is your responsibility to create this plan with the patient and other household members, to be familiar with this plan, and to know the location of the telephone numbers. In many places, the emergency number is 911. In some places, however, the number is different. The communication notebook is a great place to keep emergency information.

As you make a decision about giving first aid, remember that the person is a whole unit and will react physically and emotionally to the emergency situation.

If you are faced with a situation in which nobody can help you or go for help, take care of the person and stay until help arrives. If you face an emergency situation in which more than one person needs help, you will have to review the entire situation to decide whom to help first.

Steps to take in an Emergency

Before you take any action, you must know the following:

- What is the problem or emergency?
- What must be done?
- What are *you* capable of doing?
- Can the person be moved?

Determine the problem or emergency by asking the person, family members, or bystanders what happened or what is wrong. Decide what must be done based on your training. Know what you are capable of doing. For example, if you must lift or move a person, be sure that you can do so without injuring yourself. If the person can be moved, move him to safe, firm ground away from danger of electrical shock, fire, or explosion. Moving an injured person may cause further injury such as increased blood loss, increased pain, and/or paralysis. Do not move the person unless he is in great danger of further injury. Remember, you should do this without causing serious injury to yourself.

Do not leave a person who needs help. Have someone else call for additional help. If the person does not need immediate help to maintain life, your responsibility is to prevent additional injury and to provide comfort and security until medical help arrives. Keep the person warm, comfortable, and safe. If she is on the floor, leave her there until medical help arrives.

A severely injured person is treated according to common first-aid priorities by trained people. If you are not trained to treat severe injuries, wait with the severly injured person until trained medical help arrives.

RESTORE OR MAINTAIN BREATHING FUNCTION

Heart function and breathing function are related. When oxygen to the lungs is cut off, oxygen to the brain also decreases. When this happens, cells that control heart function die and the heart becomes weak. As a caregiver, you will be concerned only with restoring an open airway and restoring or maintaining breathing. You should carry a pocket face shield so that if you perform artificial breathing, you will be protected.

Obstructed Airway

When an object blocks air from getting into a person's lungs, it must be removed or the person will choke to death. A person's airway can be obstructed (blocked) by:

- Foreign matter, such as food, vomitus, blood, or a foreign object, in the mouth, throat, or windpipe
- Unconsciousness leading to relaxed muscles and the tongue falling back into the throat and blocking the airway

A person can have either a partial or a complete airway obstruction. Partial airway obstruction presents with snoring sounds, weak coughs, gurgling, or crowing sounds. These sounds indicate that some air passes to and from the lungs, but that breathing conditions still need to improve. At times a partial airway obstruction will cause the lips, nails, tongue, and skin to have a dark or bluish color. *Do not interfere with the person if he is able to breath, cough, or speak.* Just call for help.

A complete airway obstruction means no air is passing to and from the lungs. The person may be conscious or unconscious. The conscious person will be unable to speak or cough and may clutch his throat. He will become unconscious if the situation is not remedied. The unconscious person has no chest movement.

WHEN CHILDREN ARE HAVING TROUBLE BREATHING   Children and infants less than 50 pounds are treated differently than adults when they have difficulty breathing. *If the child or infant is breathing, speaking, or coughing, do not help, but call for assistance immediately.* If the child or infant has had an infection, has had a high fever, or has taken medication and is having difficulty breathing, call for immediate help.

If the child or infant is unable to speak or cry and is conscious, it is important to act quickly to relieve the obstruction. Use a combination of back blows and chest thrusts on an infant or small child. Back blows are quick, forceful blows between the shoulder blades used to dislodge objects from an infant; chest thrusts are similar to the compressions given in CPR. Do not use back blows on a child if you cannot lift the child in the same manner as you would lift an infant.

For the infant or small child:

- Call out for help.
- Turn the infant face down on your forearm and support her head in your hand. Rest your arm on your thigh for support and keep the infant's head lower than her body (see Figure 19.1).
- Deliver up to five back blows forcefully between the shoulder blades with the heel of one hand.
- Sandwich the infant between your arms and turn the infant over as you continue to support her head in your hands. Again, support her on your thigh.

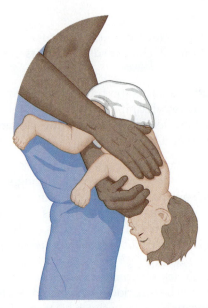

FIGURE 19.1 Hold the infant on your leg while sitting so that head and body are supported.

- Provide up to five quick downward chest thrusts with two fingers in the same location as for chest compressions (the lower third of the sternum, approximately one finger-width below the nipple line). Again, support the infant on your thigh (see Figure 19.2).
- Open the infant's mouth and look for the object. If you see it, turn the infant on her side and allow the object to roll out or turn the infant upside down and allow the object to fall out.
- Open the airway and attempt rescue breathing. If no air enters the infant's lungs, reposition the head and attempt rescue breathing again. If the airway is still obstructed, repeat these steps until the airway is clear (see Figure 19.3).

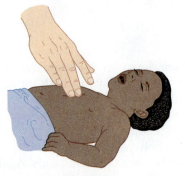

FIGURE 19.2 Provide up to five quick downward chest thrusts with two fingers in the same location as for chest compressions during CPR.

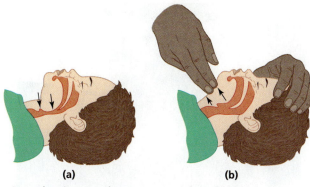

FIGURE 19.3   Open the airway and attempt rescue breathing.

ABDOMINAL THRUST FOR THE CONSCIOUS ADULT   Manual thrusts are a series of quick movements to the upper abdominal area or chest area to force the obstruction to move. An abdominal thrust, also called the Heimlich maneuver, is used when the person cannot breathe, cough, or speak. Talk to the person as you are doing this. Tell her you are going to do the Heimlich maneuver to help her breathe easier. Do not use the Heimlich maneuver on pregnant women, infants, or small children.

When the person is sitting or standing and conscious:

- Stand behind the person and wrap your arms around her waist.
- Put the thumb side of your hand on the abdomen between the navel and the end of the breastbone (sternum).
- Grasp this hand with the other hand and press it into the abdomen with a quick upward movement (see Figure 19.4).
- Repeat and continue the thrusts until the object is expelled. Each thrust should be separate and distinct.

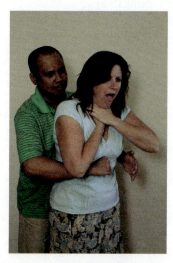

FIGURE 19.4   Abdominal thrusts on a choking adult.

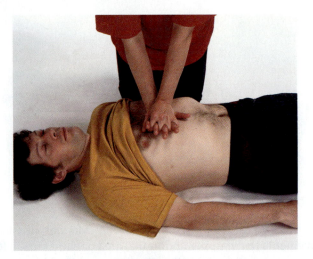

FIGURE 19.5 Chest compressions on a choking unconscious adult.

CHEST COMPRESSIONS FOR THE UNCONSCIOUS ADULT When the person is lying down and unconscious:

- Position the person on his back. Open his airway and attempt to ventilate. If no air enters, reposition his head and attempt to ventilate again. If unsuccessful, perform the following steps:
  - Kneel beside him close to his chest.
  - Place the heel of your hand two fingers above the lower half of the breastbone.
  - Put your other hand on top of this hand, and lean forward. As you do so, compress the chest downward 2 inches. Give five of these chest compressions (see Figure 19.5).
  - Open the person's mouth and look for the object. If you see it, turn the person on his side and allow the object to roll out.
  - Attempt to ventilate. If unsuccessful, reposition his head and attempt to ventilate again.
  - If unsuccessful, repeat the steps until the obstruction is dislodged.

CHEST COMPRESSIONS ON A PREGNANT WOMAN OR LARGE PERSON The chest compression is also a useful procedure when the person with an obstruction is large and your arms do not reach around her abdomen but do reach around her chest. It is also used when the person is pregnant (see Figure 19.6).

When the person is standing or sitting and conscious:

- Put your arms around the person's chest.
- Put the thumb side of your fist on his breastbone (sternum) just above the lower end.
- Grasp this hand with your other one and push quickly directly backward.
- Repeat until the airway is clear.

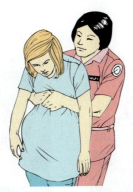

FIGURE 19.6 On a large person or pregnant woman, use the chest compressions to dislodge any obstructions.

When the person is lying down and unconscious, follow the procedure listed above for an unconscious adult.

RESCUE BREATHING Rescue breathing is the exchange of air between you and (1) an unconscious, nonbreathing person; (2) a person who loses consciousness while you are trying to dislodge an obstruction; (3) or the person who cannot breathe on her own but does have a pulse. Remember, you must dislodge the obstruction first or you will not be able to ventilate the person.

To provide rescue breathing, perform the following steps:

- Check for a response. If there is no response, call or send someone for medical assistance.
- Check for a pulse by placing two fingers on the carotid artery in the neck. Feel for a pulse in the artery. If there is a pulse, continue by checking the airway.
- Open the airway by tilting the head back with one hand on the forehead and lifting the chin with the other hand. Do not put your hand under the person's neck to open the airway (see Figure 19.7).
- Open your mouth and take a deep breath. When giving mouth-to-mouth ventilation, use a barrier device or mouth shield if one is available.
- Blow into the one-way valve on the barrier device (or blow into the person's mouth, keeping a seal between your mouth and the victim's mouth) and watch for the chest to rise. Give two initial breaths, about two seconds per breath (see Figure 19.8).
- Remove your mouth and allow the person to exhale passively. You should be able to see the chest fall. If you are using a breathing device, you do not have to remove it because the air will escape through a vent in the one-way valve.
- If the person's chest rises and falls, it means the airway is unobstructed. Continue mouth-to-mask resuscitation until medical help arrives or

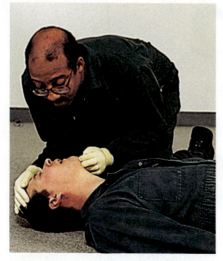

FIGURE 19.7 Open the airway.

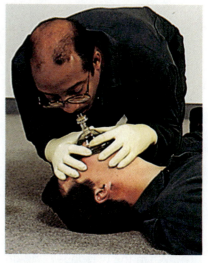

FIGURE 19.8 Give two breaths, 2 seconds long, 2 seconds apart and watch for the chest to rise.

the person starts breathing on his own. Give ten to twelve breaths per minute.

• Once the person is breathing on his own, turn him on his side in case he vomits. This action can prevent choking from occurring.

The only difference with ventilating infants and small children is that you deliver just enough air to make the chest rise.

CARDIOPULMONARY RESUSCITATION GUIDELINES (2010): HANDS ONLY Cardiopulmonary resuscitation (CPR) can save a person's life if her heart has stopped beating. The American Heart Association determined in 2010 that the most important piece of the CPR routine is the chest compressions. Therefore, the guidelines have changed. If a person is unconscious:

• Check for response. If there is no response, call or send someone for medical assistance.
• Check for a pulse by placing two fingers on the carotid artery in the neck. Feel for a pulse in the artery. If there is no pulse, start chest compressions.
• Place the heel of your hand two fingers above the lowest end of the breastbone.
• Put your other hand on top of this hand, and lean forward. As you do so, compress the chest downward two inches. Perform these compressions at 100 beats per minute.
• Continue compressions until medical personnel arrive and take over.

CONTROLLING BLEEDING

Severe blood loss or hemorrhage leads to several serious effects on the body, including shock, which is discussed later in this chapter. Blood loss causes:

- damage to body cells due to lack of circulating oxygen
- a drop in blood pressure, which means that oxygen and nutrients do not reach tissues
- the heart to pump too fast in an attempt to circulate the remaining blood

Emergency Procedures for Controlling Bleeding

External blood loss (bleeding outside the body) can come from an artery, a vein, or a capillary. External blood loss, no matter what its origin, must be controlled in the same way, as follows:

- Don gloves.
- Apply direct pressure over the wound. Use any clean cloth. Keep pressure for ten to thirty minutes while someone else calls for help. If the dressing becomes saturated with blood, put another one on top of it. Do not remove the saturated dressing or ease up on the pressure over the wound.
- If the wound is on an extremity, elevate the limb if possible to decrease the blood supply and cover the cloth with a bandage.
- Remain with the person until help arrives.

POISONING

A poison is any substance to which the body has a bad reaction. What is poisonous to one person may not be to another. Quick action and careful observation are necessary if poisoning or an overdose of medication is suspected. General guidelines for dealing with a possible poisoning include the following:

- Look for a container that might have held the poison. Do not follow antidotes on the bottle. Call the poison control center.
- Check in and around the mouth for chemical burns.
- Check the breath for odors.
- Gather as much information as possible about this incident before you act. A person can be poisoned by:
  a. swallowing a poison
  b. inhaling a poison through his mouth and nose
  c. injecting himself or being injected (drugs, insect bites) with it
  d. absorbing it through his skin

Emergency Procedures for Poisonings

The following subsections list points to keep in mind for specific types of poisonings, but report *all* poisoning incidents to your supervisor.

SWALLOWED POISONS If the person is conscious and does not have convulsions:

- Do not cause the person to vomit until you check with the poison control center. Some poisons burn tissue and would cause more damage as the person vomited.
- Call the poison control center with as much information as you have. Follow the instructions given to you by the poison control center.
- Save any vomitus, if possible, in a bag, bowl, or other available container.

If the person is unconscious:

- Do not give anything by mouth.
- Position the person on her side. If she vomits, it will drain out.
- Maintain a clear airway. If the person stops breathing, give rescue breathing with a barrier device.
- Call for help and remain with the person until someone arrives.

INHALED POISONS Chemicals and gases can poison people and cause various reactions, such as irritation of eyes, throat, and/or skin; difficulty seeing, hearing, and/or speaking; hallucinations; fatigue; and/or collapse. Follow these steps if someone has inhaled a poisonous substance:

- If you can move the person to a safe area away from the poison, do so, but do not expose yourself to a hazardous environment.
- Send someone for help. Ventilate the area, if possible.
- Loosen tight clothing around the person's neck.
- Call the poison control center.
- Keep the person warm and comfortable.

Rescue breathing may be necessary if the person stops breathing.

INJECTED POISONS

- Insect bites can cause allergic reactions. If the person experiences difficulty breathing, tingling, swelling, and/or redness in the area of the bite, call for assistance immediately.
- If you suspect that someone has experienced a drug overdose, call for help. Do not leave the person alone, and be alert for changes in his condition.

ABSORBED POISONS

- Some chemicals react violently with water. Powders should be brushed off the person's body.
- Call the poison control center.
- Poison ivy and related plants can cause irritation and rashes. Wash the area with clear water but not soap.

SHOCK

Shock is the failure of the heart and vascular system to pump enough blood to all parts of the body. Shock may have many causes, such as loss of blood or an experience the person finds traumatice, but the result is the same.

Signs and Symptoms of Shock

- Eyes are dull and pupils are wide.
- The face is pale and may be bluish in color. (Lips and nail beds will be dusky blue.)
- The person may be nauseated.
- Respirations are shallow, irregular, and labored.
- The pulse is rapid and weak.
- The skin is cold and clammy.
- The person is restless.
- The person is weak and may collapse.

Emergency Procedures for Someone in Shock

- Send someone for help. Talk to the person and make her comfortable until help arrives.
- Position the person with her head lower than her legs. Keep her warm. Blood loss makes a person cold, so cover her. If you cannot move the person because of injury, keep her warm until help arrives.

BURNS

A burn is tissue damage caused by excessive heat regardless of the source. The heat may come from fire, electricity, chemicals, the sun, or steam. Any heat source can cause damage to the skin and sometimes to various organs. By acting quickly and correctly, you can stop the burning process and prevent further injury.

A burn is labeled a superficial burn, which is the least severe burn and causes only reddening of the skin; a partial thickness burn, which causes blistering and destruction of underlying tissue; or a full thickness burn, which indicates near-destruction of the body part.

Complications from burns are many and include infection, shock, pain, loss of body heat and fluid, swelling of breathing passages, and death. All treatment for burns is aimed at preventing complications and speeding the healing process.

Emergency Procedures for Burns

SMALL BURN AREAS (SUPERFICIAL—REDDENING OF SKIN)

- Put the body part in cool water, if possible. Let it remain there for two to five minutes. Do not put ice on the burn.
- Cover the area with a sterile or clean cloth.

- Continue to put cool water over the dressing.
- Get medical help. Stay until someone arrives.

LARGER, DEEPER BURN AREAS (PARTIAL THICKNESS—BLISTERING; FULL THICKNESS—CHARRING)

- Stop the burning, if necessary, by dowsing with cool water.
- Check to see if the person is breathing. Resuscitation may be necessary.
- Keep the person's airway open.
- Cover the area with a sterile or clean dry cloth or sheet.
- Do not wet the dressing—it will chill the person and cause shock.
- Call for medical help. Stay until someone arrives.

CHEMICAL BURNS

- Flush with water for at least twenty minutes.
- Wrap the area with a clean cloth or sheet.
- If the person complains of burning, flush the area again.
- For lime burns, first brush away most of the powder, then flush with water.
- Call for medical help.

CHEST PAIN

The heart is a muscle that has its own blood supply. Any damage to the heart's blood supply may lead to damage to the heart muscle, which is a heart attack or myocardial infarction. Therefore, anyone who has any type of chest pain should seek medical attention immediately! Most heart attacks do not necessarily follow unusual physical activity but may occur during sleep or after eating.

Symptoms of a heart attack can include the following:

- Pain like a vise or a belt around the chest that may radiate to the jaw, neck, or inner left arm
- Wet, clammy skin
- Perspiration
- Rapid and weak pulse rate
- Pale skin color
- Generalized weakness
- Low blood pressure
- Shortness of breath
- Nausea
- Shallow and difficult respirations

Emergency Procedure for Chest Pain

- If the person is unconscious, check for a pulse. If there is no pulse, call for help and initiate CPR.

- If there is a pulse, attempt rescue breathing with a barrier device. If the person is conscious and if it is feasible, help the person into a comfortable position. Loosen her clothing if it is tight. If she wants to walk around, tell her it is important to rest and remain quiet.
- Reassure her. Continue to talk to her. Tell her what you are doing. If she asks you if she is having a heart attack, tell her that her chest pain could be caused by many things, but it is safest to treat it as though it were a heart attack.
- Do not give her anything to eat or drink.

CEREBROVASCULAR ACCIDENT

When a blood vessel to the brain is damaged and a part of the brain no longer has its own blood supply, it dies. This occurrence is called a stroke, or cerebrovascular accident (CVA), as discussed in Chapter 18. If you suspect that a person is having a CVA, treat him as though he were, in fact, experiencing a stroke.

Signs and Symptoms of a Stroke

- Headache
- Difficulty with speech or vision
- Change in state of consciousness or orientation
- Paralysis in an extremity or one side of the face
- Seizure
- Difficulty breathing
- Unequal size of pupils
- Weakness on one side of the body or inability to use an arm or leg
- Uncontrolled drooling
- Loss of bowel or bladder control

Emergency Procedure for a Possible Stroke Victim

- Call for help
- Provide CPR or ventilation, if needed
- If the person is conscious, assist him into a comfortable, safe position. Position paralyzed extremities in proper body alignment
- Be sure that the person can control his saliva. If he is lying down, position him on his side for drainage
- Do not give the person anything to eat or drink
- Remain with the person and reassure him that help is coming

TERRORISM AND NATURAL DISASTERS

In recent years, awareness has been increasing regarding the possibility of both terrorism and bioterrorism. Bioterrorism is the use of a biological substance to hurt, cause fear, infect, or kill. Terrorism is the use of random force or weapons to cause hurt, fear, and/or death. Unfortunately both types of incidents may occur at any time or anywhere. Although we do not want to live our lives in a state of fear, we should be aware of such possibilities. Keep the following precautions in mind:

- If you see any package that you do not believe is either appropriate or in the appropriate place, do not touch it. Call the local authorities immediately!
- Do not transport any package for anyone you do not know.
- If someone threatens you, leave the area as soon as possible and call the authorities.

Natural disasters are unstoppable occurrences in nature such as floods, fires, and volcanic eruptions. Sometimes we get warnings that these events will happen and sometimes they happen suddenly and without warning.

- Heed a warning, whether it comes on the radio or television or you receive a telephone call. Act as the warning dictates.
- Call the authorities if you are in doubt about what to do.

Emergency Procedure for Handling a Natural Disaster

- Know the family's emergency plan pertaining to natural disasters.
- Know the telephone numbers for local authorities in case of emergency.
- Know all the exits and entrances to the home in which you are working.
- Always try to leave an area that is under duress. Do not stay to watch what happens.
- Follow the directions of the agency (i.e., police, fire department, Federal Emergency Management Association [FEMA], or other emergency control department) in charge of the disaster.
- It is always a good idea to have a small disaster kit available. The disaster kit should include bottled water, candles, matches, a flashlight, and a portable radio.

Summary

Being prepared for emergencies is essential to caring for someone in the home. Keep in mind prevention of accidents, which is covered throughout this book. As for emergencies that can occur at any time, be prepared by having lifesaving supplies (i.e., first aid supplies, breathing mask, emergency phone numbers, etc.) on hand in an easy-to-find location. Finally, when in the midst of an emergency, stay calm and focused. Do the best you can in each situation and you will succeed in your home health care work.

INDEX

A

Abdominal respiration, 281
Abdominal thrust, 371
Abuse
  child (*see* Child abuse)
  defined, 67, 76
  elderly, 67
  substance (*see* Substance abuse)
Abusive words, 42
Acetone, 335
Acquired immunodeficiency syndrome
      (AIDS), 117
Activities of daily living (ADL), 250
Activity tolerance, patient's, 170, 250
Acute illness, 39
Acute pain, 287
ADL. *see* Activities of daily living (ADL)
Adults
  abdominal thrust for conscious, 371
  chest compressions for unconscious, 372
  vital signs, 263
Advance health care directive, 43,
      102–108
  defined, 102
  DNR order, 103, 108
  sample, 104–107
Affordable Care Act, 2011, 3–5
Aging, 52–53. *see also* Elderly
  caregiver role, 59
  cognitive changes, 57–58
  defined, 52
  physical changes of, 53–57
  process, phases of, 53, 54
  social changes, 58–59
AIDS (acquired immunodeficiency
      syndrome), 117, 364–366. *see also*
      Human immunodeficiency virus (HIV)
  caregiver role in, 366
  disease process, 365–366
Airway obstruction, 369
Alignment, body, 168, 171
Allergies, food, 154
ALS. *see* Amyotrophic lateral sclerosis (ALS)
Alzheimer's disease, 356–360
  caregiver role in, 359–360
  defined, 356
  patient's emotions/feelings and, 358–359
  stages of, 356–358
Ambulation, 235–236
Amyotrophic lateral sclerosis (ALS), 362
Aneroid sphygmomanometer, 285, 286
Angina, 348–349
  caregiver role in, 348–349
  causes of, 348

defined, 347
  treatment for, 348
Aphasia
  defined, 242–244
  expressive, 242–243
  receptive, 243
Apical pulse, 277
  measuring, 280
Apical-radial deficit, 279
  measuring, 280–281
Arteriosclerosis, 345
Arthritis, 353–355
  caregiver role in, 354–355
  defined, 353
  types of, 353–354
Asepsis, 302
Aseptic techniques, 117
Atherosclerosis, 345
Aura, 334
Aural/tympanic thermometers, 274, 275–276
Axillary temperature, measuring, 273

B

Backrub, 205–207
Bacteria
  spores, 117
Balancing, 167–168
Base of support, 167
Bathing
  adaptive equipment, 255
  complete, 199, 200–202
  guideline, 200, 254–255
  infants, 92–93
  occupational therapy, 251, 252, 253
  partial, 202, 203–204
  patients, 199–205
  shower, 203
  sponge baths, 92–93
  tub baths, 93, 94–95, 202, 204
Bathrooms
  cleaning, 132–133
  safety in, 133, 144
  toileting in, 254
Bed making, 135
  guidelines, 136–137
  occupied bed, 135, 137, 138–140
Bedpans
  defined, 213
  offering, 214–215
Bioterrorism, 379
Birth defects, 70, 71–72
Bleeding
  emergency procedures for controlling, 375